Tips to Eat Well When Eating Out

How food is prepared influences whether it's healthy. Look for these phrases on the menu:

Low fat, healthier choices	Higher fat with lots of calories
In its own juice/au jus	Marinated in oil
Roasted	Creamy/cream sauce/creamed
Steamed or simmered	Buttery/butter sauce/buttered
Broiled/charbroiled	Gravy/hollandaise/Béarnaise sauce
Poached	Au gratin/cheese sauce/cheese-filled
Grilled/sautéed	Fried/pan fried/deep fried
Baked	Breaded/crispy/golden

Key Elements Used in Nutrition Words

Element	Meaning
amyl-	starch
an-	without
anti-	against
-ase	an enzyme
di-	two
-emia	found in the blood
gastro-	referring to the stomach
gly-	referring to sugars
hydr-, hydro-	water (*also:* hydrogen)
hyper-	above normal
hypo-	below normal
lact-, lacti-, lacto-	milk
lip-, lipo-	fat
macro-	large
micro-	very small
mono-	one
-ose	sugar
tri-	three

Easy Ways to Cut Calories

- Use low-fat or no-fat dairy products
- Use sugar substitutes instead of sugar
- Eat more whole fruits and vegetables
- Cut the fruit juice and sweetened beverages
- Cook and serve poultry without skin
- Limit high-fat, oily salad dressings
- Make open-face sandwiches with just one slice of bread
- Eliminate high-fat ingredients in any dish
- Read Nutrition Facts tables — choose wisely
- Choose proper portions, and eat Food Guide servings

For Dummies: Bestselling Book Series for Beginners

Nutrition For Canadians For Dummies®

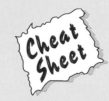

Cheat Sheet

When You May Need Extra Nutrients

- When you're pregnant, you need extra amounts of some vitamins, minerals, and protein to meet the needs of your growing baby.

  Ditto for when you're nursing your baby.

- Some medicines reduce your body's ability to absorb and use certain vitamins and minerals. When your doctor writes a prescription, ask whether you need supplements.

- What? You still smoke? You need more vitamin C than non-smokers.

- Are you a woman approaching menopause? Time for extra calcium and vitamin D to maintain healthy bones.

  Older men also need extra calcium and vitamin D.

- Is your diet strictly vegan — meaning no food of animal origin, not even milk and eggs? You need extra vitamin B12. You may also need extra calcium, zinc, vitamin D, and iron.

How to Keep Food Safe as Well as Nutritious

- Wash your hands before (and after) touching food.

- Wash all fruits and vegetables before you use them.

- Follow the directions on the food package for storing and preparing food safely.

- Handle all raw meat, fish, and poultry as if it's contaminated (sometimes, it is!).

- Cook foods thoroughly.

- Keep hot foods hot, cold foods cold.

- Never eat or drink anything containing raw eggs.

- Use a separate cutting board for raw meat, fish, and poultry.

- Never taste any questionable food "just to be sure it's all right." When in doubt, throw it out.

The 22 Essential Vitamins and Minerals

- Vitamin A
- Vitamin B12
- Vitamin D
- Choline
- Vitamin E
- Calcium
- Vitamin K
- Phosphorous

- Vitamin C
- Magnesium
- Thiamin (vitamin B1)
- Iron
- Riboflavin (vitamin B2)
- Zinc
- Niacin
- Iodine

- Vitamin B6
- Selenium
- Folate
- Potassium
- Copper
- Chromium

For Dummies: Bestselling Book Series for Beginners

Nutrition
For Canadians
FOR
DUMMIES®

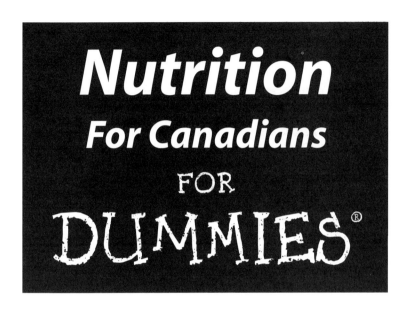

Nutrition
For Canadians
FOR
DUMMIES®

**by Carol Ann Rinzler and
Doug Cook, RD, MHSc, CDE**

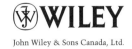

John Wiley & Sons Canada, Ltd.

Nutrition For Canadians For Dummies®

Published by
John Wiley & Sons Canada, Ltd.
6045 Freemont Blvd.
Mississauga, ON L5R 4J3
www.wiley.com

Library and Archives Canada Cataloguing in Publication Data

Rinzler, Carol Ann
     Nutrition for Canadians for dummies / Carol Ann Rinzler, Doug Cook.
Includes index.
ISBN 978-0-470-15307-9
     1. Nutrition. 2. Food. I. Cook, Doug, 1964– II. Title.
TX353.R535 2008   613.2   C2008-907584-3
Printed in Canada

1 2 3 4 5 TRI 12 11 10 09 08

Distributed in Canada by John Wiley & Sons Canada, Ltd.

For general information on John Wiley & Sons Canada, Ltd., including all books published by Wiley Publishing Inc., please call our warehouse, Tel. 1-800-567-4797. For reseller information, including discounts and premium sales, please call our sales department, Tel. 416-646-7992. For press review copies, author interviews, or other publicity information, please contact our marketing department, Tel. 416-646-4584, Fax 416-236-4448.

For authorization to photocopy items for corporate, personal, or educational use, please contact in writing The Canadian Copyright Licensing Agency (Access Copyright). For an Access Copyright license, visit www.accesscopyright.ca or call toll free 1-800-893-5777.

WILEY

About the Authors

Carol Ann Rinzler is a noted authority on health and nutrition and holds an MA from Columbia University. She has written a nutrition column for the *New York Daily News* and is the author of more than 20 health-related books, including *Controlling Cholesterol For Dummies*, *Weight Loss Kit For Dummies*, and the highly acclaimed *Estrogen & Breast Cancer: A Warning to Women*. Rinzler lives in New York with her husband, wine writer Perry Luntz, and their amiable cat, Kat.

Doug Cook, RD, MHSc, CDE, is a Registered Dietitian/Nutritionist and Certified Diabetes Educator. He currently works at St. Michael's Hospital in Toronto, and also has a private practice. He contributes to the "Vice Squad" column in the *Toronto Star*. In addition, he served as a nutrition expert for the Ontario Ministry of Health's Web site www.healthyontario.com.

Dedication

From Carol: This book is dedicated to my husband, Perry Luntz, a fellow writer who, as always, stayed patient as a saint and even-tempered beyond belief while I was racing pell-mell (and not always pleasantly) to deadline.

From Doug: This book is dedicated to my family and friends, who over the years have supported and believed in me, enabling me to fulfill my dreams and to reach new goals that have afforded me the invaluable opportunity to work on a project such as this.

Authors' Acknowledgements

From Carol: This new book has given me the opportunity to work with yet another group of thoroughly pleasant professionals at the Dummies group of Wiley Publishing. Acquisitions Editor Michael Lewis enthusiastically welcomed the new edition and kept the project moving smoothly. Senior Project Editor Natalie Harris was incredibly soothing to the author, not to mention totally in command of the hundreds, maybe even thousands, of details it takes to update a nutrition book. I appreciate Danielle Voirol, maybe more than she knows; medical and science writers understand very well that without skillful, knowledgeable copy editors, we would be walking over factual cliffs every day of our writing lives. Finally, I am grateful to Alfred Bushway, PhD, for once again reading and commenting on the manuscript. Thanks, guys.

From Doug: Editor Robert Hickey successfully guided me thorough the process of adapting an existing manuscript and, as a result, has allowed me the chance to have my name attached to this project. Another goal realized. Thank you.

Publisher's Acknowledgements

We're proud of this book; please send us your comments through our Dummies online registration form located at www.dummies.com/register/.

Some of the people who helped bring this book to market include the following:

Acquisitions, Editorial, and Media Development

Executive Editor: Robert Hickey

Project Editor, U.S. edition: Natalie Faye Harris

Technical Review: Stephanie Demaio, BASc, RD

Copy Editor: Edna Barker

Cover photo: © Masterfile

Cartoons: Rich Tennant
(www.the5thwave.com)

Composition Services

Vice-President Publishing Services: Karen Bryan

Project Manager: Elizabeth McCurdy

Project Coordinator: Lindsay Humphreys

Layout and graphics: Reuben W. Davis, Alissa D. Ellet, Brooke Graczyk, Stephanie D. Jumper, Ronald Terry, Christine Williams

Proofreaders: Laura L. Bowman, Susan Moritz

Indexer: Belle Wong

John Wiley & Sons Canada, Ltd.

  Bill Zerter, Chief Operating Officer

  Jennifer Smith, Vice-President and Publisher, Professional and Trade Division

Publishing and Editorial for Consumer Dummies

  Diane Graves Steele, Vice-President and Publisher, Consumer Dummies

  Joyce Pepple, Acquisitions Director, Consumer Dummies

  Kristin A. Cocks, Product Development Director, Consumer Dummies

  Michael Spring, Vice-President and Publisher, Travel

  Kelly Regan, Editorial Director, Travel

Publishing for Technology Dummies

  Andy Cummings, Vice-President and Publisher, Dummies Technology/General User

Composition Services

  Gerry Fahey, Vice-President of Production Services

  Debbie Stailey, Director of Composition Services

Contents at a Glance

Table of Contents

Introduction

● ●

*O*nce upon a time people simply sat down to dinner, eating to fill up an empty stomach or just for the pleasure of it. Nobody said, "Wow, that cream soup is loaded with calories," or asked whether the bread was a high-fibre loaf, or fretted about the chicken being served with the skin still on. No longer. Today, the dinner table can be a battleground between health and pleasure. You plan your meals with the precision of a major general moving the troops into the front lines, and like most people, the fight to eat what's good for you rather than what tastes good has become a lifelong struggle.

This book is designed to end the war between your need for good nutrition and your equally compelling need for tasty meals. In fact (listen up, here!), what's good for you can also be good to eat — and vice versa.

About This Book

Nutrition For Canadians For Dummies doesn't aim to send you back to the classroom, sit you down, and make you take notes about what to put on the table every day from now until you're 104 years old. You're reading a reference book, so you don't have to memorize anything — when you want more info, just jump in anywhere to look it up.

Instead, this book means to give you the information you need to make wise food choices — which always means choices that please the palate and soul, as well as the body. Some of what you'll read here is really, *really* basic: definitions of vitamins, minerals, proteins, fats, carbohydrates, and — can you believe this? — plain old water. You'll also read tips about how to put together a nutritious shopping list and how to use food to make meals so good you can't wait to eat them.

For those who know absolutely nothing about nutrition except that it deals with food, this book is a starting point. For those who know more than a little about nutrition, this book is a refresher course to bring you up to speed on what has happened since the last time you checked out a calorie chart.

For those who want to know absolutely everything, *Nutrition For Canadians For Dummies* is up to date, with hot new info from the 2007 revision of Canada's Food Guide, new recommended daily allowances for all the nutrients a healthy body needs, plus all the twisty "this is good for you" and "this is really, really rotten" bits and pieces of food info that nutrition scientists have come up with.

Conventions Used in This Book

The following conventions are used throughout the text to make things consistent and easy to understand:

- ✔ All Web addresses appear in `monofont`.
- ✔ New terms appear in *italic* and are closely followed by an easy-to-understand definition.
- ✔ **Bold** is used to highlight the action parts of numbered steps, as well as key words in bulleted lists.
- ✔ Nutrition experts commonly use metric terms such as gram (g), milligram (mg), and microgram (mcg) to describe quantities of protein, fat, carbohydrates, vitamins, minerals, and other nutrients.

What You Don't Have to Read

What? Not read something printed in a book? Well, yeah. Some small parts of this book are fun or informative but not necessarily vital to your understanding of nutrition. For example:

- ✔ **Text in sidebars:** The sidebars are the shaded boxes that appear here and there. They share personal stories and observations but aren't necessary reading.
- ✔ **Anything with a Technical Stuff icon attached:** This information is interesting but not critical to your understanding of nutrition.
- ✔ **The stuff on the copyright page:** No kidding. You'll find nothing here of interest unless you're inexplicably enamoured by legal language.

Foolish Assumptions

Every book is written with a particular reader in mind, and this one is no different. As we wrote this book, we made the following basic assumptions about who you are and why you plunked down your hard-earned cash for an entire volume about nutrition:

- ✔ You didn't study nutrition in high school or university and now you've discovered that you have a better shot a staying healthy if you know how to put together well-balanced, nutritious meals.

✔ You're confused by conflicting advice on vitamins and minerals, protein, fats, and carbs. In other words, you need a reliable road map through the nutrient maze.

✔ You want basic information, but you don't want to become an expert in nutrition or spend hours digging your way through medical textbooks and journals.

How This Book Is Organized

The following is a brief summary of each part in *Nutrition For Canadians For Dummies*. You can use this guide as a fast way to check out what you want to read first. One really nice thing about this book is that you don't have to start with Chapter 1 and read straight through to the end. *Au contraire,* as the French like to say when they mean "on the contrary." You can dive in absolutely anywhere and still come up with tons of tasty information about how food helps your body work.

Part I: The Basic Facts about Nutrition

Chapter 1 defines nutrition and its effects on your body. This chapter also tells you how to read a nutrition study and how to judge the value of nutrition information in newspapers, magazines, and on TV. Chapter 2 is a really clear guide to how your digestive system works to transform food and beverages into the nutrients you need so you can sustain a healthy body. Chapter 3 concentrates on calories, the energy factor in food and beverages. Chapter 4 tells you how much of each nutrient you need to stay in tiptop form. Chapter 5 details some of the rules on dietary supplements — the pills, powders, and potions that add nutritional punch to your regular diet.

Part II: What You Get from Food

Chapter 6 gives you the facts about protein: where you get it and what it does in your body. Chapter 7 does the same job for dietary fat, while Chapter 8 explains carbohydrates: sugars, starches, and that indigestible but totally vital substance in carbohydrate foods — ta-da! — dietary fibre. Chapter 9 outlines the risks and, yes, some newly proven benefits of alcohol beverages.

Chapter 10 is about vitamins, the substances in food that trigger so many vital chemical reactions in your body. Chapter 11 is about minerals, substances that often work in tandem with vitamins. Chapter 12 explains phytochemicals, newly important substances in food. Chapter 13 is about water, the essential liquid that comprises as much as 70 percent of your body weight. This chapter also describes the functions of electrolytes, special minerals that maintain your fluid balance (the correct amount of water inside and outside your body cells).

Part III: Healthy Eating

Chapter 14 is about *hunger* (the need for food) and *appetite* (the desire for food). Balancing these two eating factors makes maintaining a healthful weight possible for you. Chapter 15, on the other hand, is about food preference: why you like some foods and really, really hate others. (Broccoli, anyone?) Chapter 16 tells you how to assemble a healthful diet. It's based on the principles of Health Canada's newly revised Food Guide, so you know it's good for you. Chapter 17 explains how to use nutritional guidelines to plan nutritious, appetizing meals at home. Chapter 18 shows you how to take the guidelines out to dinner so that you can judge the value of foods in all kinds of restaurants, from the posh white-tablecloth ones to fast-food havens.

Part IV: Food Processing

Chapter 19 asks and answers this simple question: What is food processing? Chapter 20 shows you how cooking affects the way food looks and tastes, as well as its nutritional value. Chapter 21 does the same for freezing, canning, drying, and irradiating techniques. Chapter 22 gives you the lowdown on chemicals used to keep food fresh.

Part V: Food and Medicine

Chapter 23 explains why some food gives some people hives, then presents strategies for identifying and avoiding the food to which you may be allergic. Chapter 24 is about how eating or drinking certain foods and beverages may affect your mood — a hot topic these days with nutrition researchers. Chapter 25 tells you how foods may interact with medical drugs — an important subject for anyone who ever has taken, now takes, or ever plans to take medicine. Chapter 26 tells you how some foods may actually act as preventive medicine or relieve the symptoms of certain illnesses ranging from the horrible-but-not-really-serious common cold to the Big Two: heart disease and cancer.

Part VI: The Part of Tens (And Twelves)

Could there even be a *For Dummies* book without The Part of Tens? Not a chance. This part (Chapters 27, 28, and 29) provides 10 great nutritional Web site addresses, lists 12 common foods with near-magical status, and — last but definitely not least — lays out 10 easy ways to cut calories from food.

Icons Used in This Book

Icons are a handy *For Dummies* way to catch your attention as you slide your eyes down the page. The icons come in several varieties, each with its own special meaning:

Nutrition is full of stuff that "everybody knows." This masked marvel clues you in to the *real* facts when (as often happens) everybody's wrong!

This little guy looks smart because he's marking the place where you find definitions of the words used by nutrition experts.

The Official Word icon says, "Look here for scientific studies, statistics, definitions, and recommendations used to create standard nutrition policy."

This time, the same smart fella is pointing to clear, concise explanations of technical terms and processes — details that are interesting but not necessarily critical to your understanding of a topic. In other words, skip them if you want, but try a few first.

Bull's-eye! This is time- and stress-saving information you can use to improve your diet and your health.

This is a watch-out-for-the-curves icon, alerting you to nutrition pitfalls such as (oops!) leaving the skin on the chicken — turning a low-fat food into one that is high in fat and cholesterol. This icon also warns you about possible physical dangers to avoid (for example, supplements) because they may do more damage than good to your health.

Where to Go from Here

Ah, here's the best part. *For Dummies* books are not linear (a fancy way of saying they proceed from A to B to C . . . and so on). In fact, you can dive right in anywhere, say at L, M, or N, and still make sense of what you're reading because each chapter delivers a complete message.

For example, if carbohydrates are your passion, go right to Chapter 8. If you want to know how to pick and choose from a menu when you're eating out, skip to Chapter 18. If you've always been fascinated by food processing, your choice is Chapter 19. You can use the Table of Contents to find broad categories of information or use the Index to look up more specific things.

If you're not sure where you want to go, why not just begin at the beginning? Part I gives you all the basic info you need to understand nutrition, and points to places where you can find more detailed information.

Part I
The Basic Facts about Nutrition

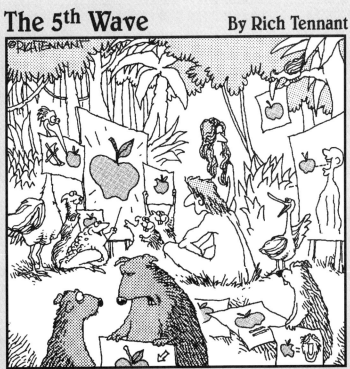

The 5th Wave   By Rich Tennant

"Yes, we told them about the pectin and flavonoids, but they seem a little slow to catch on. Maybe if we just left them alone with the snake a while..."

In this part . . .

To use food wisely, you need a firm grasp of the basics. In this part, we define nutrition and give you a detailed explanation of digestion (how your body turns food into nutrients). We also explain why calories are useful and set forth a no-nonsense starter guide to your daily requirements of vitamins, minerals, and other good stuff.

Chapter 1

What's Nutrition, Anyway?

*W*elcome aboard! You're about to begin your very own *Fantastic Voyage.* (You know. That's the 1966 movie in which Raquel Welch and a couple of guys were shrunk down to the size of a molecule to sail through the body of a politician shot by an assassin who had . . . hey, maybe you should just check out the next showing on your favourite cable movie channel.)

In any event, as you read, chapter by chapter, you can follow a route that carries food (meaning food and beverages) from your plate to your mouth to your digestive tract and into every tissue and cell. Along the way, you'll have the opportunity to see how your organs and systems work. You'll observe firsthand why some foods and beverages are essential to your health. And you'll discover how to manage your diet so you can get the biggest bang (nutrients) for your buck (calories). Bon voyage!

Nutrition Equals Life

Technically speaking, *nutrition* is the science of how the body uses food. In fact, nutrition is life. All living things, including you, need food and water to live. Beyond that, you need good food, meaning food with the proper nutrients, to live well. If you don't eat and drink, you'll die. Period. If you don't eat and drink nutritious food and beverages:

▸ Your bones may bend or break (not enough calcium).

▸ Your gums may bleed (not enough vitamin C).

▸ Your blood may not carry oxygen to every cell (not enough iron).

Essential nutrients for Fido, Fluffy, and your pet petunia

Vitamin C isn't the only nutrient that's essential for one species but not for others. Many organic compounds (substances similar to vitamins) and elements (minerals) are essential for your green or furry friends but not for you, either because you can synthesize them from the food you eat or because they're so widely available in the human diet and you require such small amounts that you can get what you need without hardly trying.

Two good examples are the organic compounds choline and myoinositol. *Choline* is an essential nutrient for several species of animals, including dogs, cats, rats, and guinea pigs. Although choline has now been declared essential for human beings (more about that in Chapter 10), human bodies produce choline on their own, and you can get choline from eggs, liver, soybeans, cauliflower, and lettuce. *Myoinositol* is an essential nutrient for gerbils and rats, but human beings synthesize it naturally and use it in many body processes, such as transmitting signals between cells.

Here's a handy list of nutrients that are essential for animals and/or plants but not for you:

Organic Compounds	*Elements*
Carnitine	Arsenic
Myoinositol	Cadmium
Taurine	Lead
	Nickel
	Silicon
	Tin
	Vanadium

And on, and on, and on. Understanding how good nutrition protects you against these dire consequences requires a familiarity with the language and concepts of nutrition. Knowing some basic chemistry is helpful. (Don't panic: Chemistry can be a cinch when you read about it in plain English.) A smattering of sociology and psychology is also useful, because although nutrition is mostly about how food revs up and sustains your body, it's also about the cultural traditions and individual differences that explain how you choose your favourite foods (see Chapter 15).

To sum it up: The field of nutrition is about why you eat what you eat and how the food you choose affects your body and your health.

First principles: Energy and nutrients

Nutrition's primary task is figuring out which foods and beverages (in what quantities) provide the energy and building material you need for growth and maintenance of every cell, organ, and system (for example, cardiovascular).

To do this, nutrition concentrates on food's two basic attributes: energy (calories) and nutrients (vitamins and minerals).

Energy from food

Energy is the ability to do work. Virtually every bite of food gives you energy, even when it doesn't give you nutrients. The amount of energy in food is measured in *calories,* the amount of heat produced when food is burned (metabolized) in your body cells. You can read all about calories in Chapter 3. But right now, all you need to know is that food is the fuel on which your body runs. Without enough food, you don't have enough energy.

Nutrients in food

Nutrients are chemical substances your body uses to build, maintain, and repair tissues. They allow cells to send messages back and forth to conduct essential chemical reactions, such as the ones that make it possible for you to

- ✔ Breathe
- ✔ Move
- ✔ Eliminate waste
- ✔ Think
- ✔ See
- ✔ Hear
- ✔ Smell
- ✔ Taste

. . . and do everything else natural to a living body.

Food provides two distinct groups of nutrients:

- ✔ **Macronutrients (macro = big):** Protein, fat, carbohydrates, and water
- ✔ **Micronutrients (micro = small):** Vitamins and minerals

What's the difference between these two groups? The amounts you need each day and the amounts that are present in the foods you eat. Your daily requirements for macronutrients generally exceed 1 gram. (There are 28 grams in an ounce.) For example, a man needs about 63 grams of protein a day (slightly more than two ounces), and a woman needs 50 grams (slightly less than two ounces).

Your daily requirements for micronutrients are much smaller. For example, the Recommended Dietary Allowance (RDA) for vitamin C is measured in milligrams ($\frac{1}{1,000}$ of a gram), while the RDAs for vitamin D, vitamin B12, and folate are even smaller and are measured in micrograms ($\frac{1}{1,000,000}$ of a gram). You can find out much more about the RDAs, including how they vary for people of different ages, in Chapter 4.

What's an essential nutrient?

A reasonable person may assume that an essential nutrient is one you need to sustain a healthy body. But who says a reasonable person thinks like a dietitian? In nutritionspeak, an *essential nutrient* is a very special thing:

- ✔ **An essential nutrient cannot be manufactured by the body.** You have to get essential nutrients from food or from a nutritional supplement.

- ✔ **An essential nutrient is linked to a specific deficiency disease.** For example, people who go without protein for extended periods of time develop the protein-deficiency disease *kwashiorkor*. People who don't get enough vitamin C develop the vitamin C–deficiency disease *scurvy*. A diet that supplies an adequate amount of an essential nutrient will prevent a deficiency, but you need the proper nutrient. In other words, you can't cure a protein deficiency with extra amounts of vitamin C.

Not all nutrients are essential for all species of animals. For example, vitamin C is an essential nutrient for human beings but not for dogs. A dog's body makes the vitamin C it needs. Check out the list of nutrients on a can or bag of dog food. See? No C. The dog already has the C it — sorry, he or she — requires.

Essential nutrients for human beings include many well-known vitamins and minerals, several *amino acids* (the so-called building blocks of proteins), and at least two fatty acids. For more about these essential nutrients, see Chapters 6, 7, 10, and 11.

Protecting the nutrients in your food

Identifying nutrients is one thing. Making sure you get them into your body is another. Here, the essential idea is to keep nutritious food nutritious by preserving and protecting its components.

Some people see the term *food processing* as a nutritional dirty word. Or words. They're wrong. Without food processing and preservatives, you and I would still be forced to gather (or kill) our food each morning and down it fast before it spoils. For more about which processing and preservative techniques produce the safest, most nutritious — and yes, delicious — dinners, check out Chapters 19, 20, 21, and 22.

Considering how vital food preservation can be, you may want to think about when you last heard a rousing cheer for the anonymous cook who first noticed that salting or pickling food could extend food's shelf life. Or for the guys who invented the refrigeration and freezing techniques that slow food's natural tendency to degrade (translation: spoil). Or for Louis Pasteur, the man who made it ab-so-lute-ly clear that heating food to boiling kills bugs that might otherwise cause food poisoning. Hardly ever, that's when. So give them a hand, right here. Cool.

Other interesting substances in food

The latest flash in the nutrition sky is caused by phytochemicals. *Phyto* is the Greek word for plants, so *phytochemicals* are simply — yes, you've got it — chemicals from plants. Although the 13-letter name may be new to you, you're already familiar with some phytochemicals. They are *non-nutritive* (meaning you don't require them to stay alive, the way you need vitamins) plant chemicals that have protective or disease-preventive properties. Pigments such as beta carotene, the deep yellow colouring in fruits and vegetables that your body can convert to a form of vitamin A, are phytochemicals.

And then there are *phytoestrogens,* hormonelike chemicals that grabbed the spotlight when someone suggested that a diet high in phytoestrogens, such as the isoflavones found in soybeans, may lower the risk of heart disease and reduce the incidence of reproductive cancers (cancers of the breast, ovary, uterus, and prostate). More recent studies suggest that phytoestrogens may have some problems of their own, so to find out more about phytochemicals, including phytoestrogens, check out Chapter 12.

You are what you eat

Oh boy, I bet you've heard this one before. But it bears repeating, because the human body really is built from the nutrients it gets from food: water, protein, fat, carbohydrates, vitamins, and minerals. On average, when you step on the scale

- About 60 percent of your weight is water.
- About 20 percent of your weight is fat.
- About 20 percent of your weight is a combination of mostly protein (especially in your muscles), plus carbohydrates, minerals, and vitamins.

An easy way to remember your body's percentage of water, fat, and protein and other nutrients is to think of it as the "60-20-20 Rule."

What's a body made of?

Sugar and spice and everything nice . . . oops. What we meant to say was the human body is made of water and fat and protein and carbohydrates and vitamins and minerals.

On average, when you step on the scale, approximately 60 percent of your weight is water, 20 percent is body fat (slightly less for a man), and 20 percent is a combination of mostly protein, plus carbohydrates, minerals, vitamins, and other naturally occurring biochemicals.

Based on these percentages, you can reasonably expect that an average 140-pound person's body weight consists of about

- 38kg (84 pounds) of water

- 13kg (28 pounds) of body fat

- 13kg (28 pounds) of a combination of protein (up to 11kg [25 pounds]), minerals (up to 3kg [7 pounds]), carbohydrates (up to 0.6kg [1.4 pounds]), and vitamins (a trace).

Yep, you're right: Those last figures do total more than 13kg (28 pounds). That's because "up to"

(as in "up to 11kg [25 pounds] of protein") means that the amounts may vary from person to person.

For example, a young person's body has proportionately more muscle and less fat than an older person's, while a woman's body has proportionately less muscle and more fat than a man's. As a result, more of a man's weight comes from protein and calcium, while more of a woman's weight comes from fat. Protein-packed muscles and mineral-packed bones are denser tissue than fat.

Weigh a man and a woman of roughly the same height and size, and he's likely to tip the scale higher every time.

The National Research Council, *Recommended Dietary Allowances* (Washington, D.C.: National Academy Press, 1989); Eleanor Noss Whitney, Corinne Balog Cataldo, and Sharon Rady Rolfes, *Understanding Normal and Clinical Nutrition* (Minneapolis/St. Paul: West Publishing Company, 1994)

Your nutritional status

Nutritional status is a phrase that describes the state of your health as related to your diet. For example, people who are starving do not get the nutrients or calories they need for optimum health. These people are said to be *malnourished* (mal = bad), which means their nutritional status is, to put it gently, definitely not good. Malnutrition may arise from

- **A diet that doesn't provide enough food.** This situation can occur in times of famine or through voluntary starvation because of an eating disorder or because something in your life disturbs your appetite. For example, older people may be at risk of malnutrition because of tooth loss or age-related loss of appetite, or because they live alone and sometimes just forget to eat.

✔ **A diet that, while otherwise adequate, is deficient in a specific nutrient.** This kind of nutritional inadequacy can lead to — surprise! — a deficiency disease, such as beriberi, the disease caused by a lack of vitamin B1 (thiamine).

✔ **A metabolic disorder or medical condition that prevents your body from absorbing specific nutrients, such as carbohydrates or protein.** One common example is diabetes, the inability to produce enough insulin, the hormone your body uses to metabolize (efficiently use) carbohydrates. Another is celiac disease, a condition that makes it impossible for the body to digest gluten, a protein in wheat. Need more info on either diabetes or celiac disease? Check out *Diabetes For Canadians For Dummies* and *Living Gluten-Free For Dummies*. Of course.

Doctors and registered dietitians have many tools with which to rate your nutritional status. For example, they can

✔ Review your medical history to see whether you have any conditions (such as bad teeth) that may make eating certain foods difficult or that interfere with your ability to absorb nutrients.

✔ Perform a physical examination to look for obvious signs of nutritional deficiency, such as dull hair and eyes (a lack of vitamins?), poor posture (not enough calcium to protect the spinal bones?), or extreme thinness (not enough food? An underlying disease?).

✔ Order laboratory blood, urine, and other tests that may identify early signs of malnutrition, such as the lack of red blood cells that characterizes anemia caused by an iron deficiency.

At every stage of life, the aim of a good diet is to maintain a healthy nutritional status.

Fitting food into the medicine chest

Food is medicine for the body and the soul. Good meals make good friends, and modern research validates the virtues of not only Granny's chicken soup but also heart-healthy sulphur compounds in garlic and onions, anti-cholesterol dietary fibre in grains and beans, bone-building calcium in milk and greens, and mood elevators in coffee, tea, and chocolate.

Of course, foods pose some risks as well: food allergies, food intolerances, food and drug interactions, and the occasional harmful substances such as the dreaded *saturated fats* and *trans fats* (quick — Chapter 7!). In other words, constructing a healthful diet can mean tailoring food choices to your own special body. Not to worry: You can do it. Especially after reading through Part V. Would a *For Dummies* book leave you unarmed? Not a chance!

Finding Nutrition Facts

Getting reliable information about nutrition can be a daunting challenge. For the most part, your nutrition information is likely to come from TV and radio talk shows or news, your daily newspaper, your favourite magazine, a variety of nutrition-oriented books, and the Internet. How can you tell whether what you hear or read is really right?

Nutritional people

The people who make nutrition news may be scientists, reporters, or simply people who wandered in with a new theory (Artichokes prevent cancer! Never eat cherries and cheese at the same meal! Vitamin C gives you hives!), the more bizarre the better. But several groups of people are most likely to give you news you can use with confidence. For example:

- **Nutrition scientists:** These are people with graduate degrees (usually in nutritional sciences, chemistry, biology, or biochemistry) engaged in researching the effects of food and nutrients on animals and human beings.

- **Nutrition researchers:** Researchers may be either nutrition scientists or professionals in another field, such as medicine or sociology, whose research (study or studies) concentrates on the effects of food and nutrients on animals and human beings.

- **Registered dietitians:** These people have undergraduate degrees in food and nutritional science from a Dietitians of Canada (DC) accredited university program and often have graduate degrees. The term "dietitian" is protected by law to ensure that national educational and training standards have been met. The letters RD, RDN, P.Dt., Dt.P., and R.Dt. are the legal designations for qualified registered dietitians in Canada.

- **Nutritionists:** Law does not protect the term "nutritionist" in all provinces, so people with different levels of training and knowledge can call themselves nutritionists. Most provinces have a regulatory body for nutrition professionals; contact the regulatory body if you have any questions.

- **Nutrition reporters and writers:** These are people who specialize in giving you information about the medical and/or scientific aspects of food. Like reporters who concentrate on politics or sports, nutrition reporters gain their expertise through years of covering their beat. Most have the science background required to translate technical information into language nonscientists can understand; some have been trained as dietitians, nutritionists, or nutrition scientists; and many interview and liaise with dietitians for their expertise when reporting on a nutrition-related topic.

Consumer alert: Regardless of the source, nutrition news should always pass what you may call *The Reasonableness Test*. In other words, if a story or report or study sounds ridiculous or too good to be true, it probably is.

Want some guidelines for evaluating nutrition studies? Read on.

Can you trust this study?

You open your morning newspaper or turn on the evening news and read or hear that a group of researchers at an impeccably prestigious scientific organization has published a study showing that yet another thing you've always taken for granted is hazardous to your health. For example, the study says drinking coffee stresses your heart, adding salt to food raises blood pressure, or fatty foods increase your risk of cancer or heart disease.

So you throw out the offending food or drink or rearrange your daily routine to avoid the once-acceptable, now-dangerous food, beverage, or additive. And then what happens? Two weeks, two months, or two years down the road, a second, equally prestigious group of scientists publishes a study conclusively proving that the first group got it wrong. In fact, this study shows coffee has no effect on the risk of heart disease — and may even improve athletic performance; salt does not cause hypertension except in certain sensitive individuals; and only *some* fatty foods are risky.

Who's right? Nobody seems to know. That leaves you, a layperson, on your own to come up with the answer. Never fear — you may not be a nutrition expert, but that doesn't mean you can't apply a few commonsense rules to any study you read about, rules that say: "Yes, this may be true," or "No, this may not be true."

Does this study include human beings?

True, animal studies can alert researchers to potential problems, but working with animals alone cannot give you conclusive proof.

Different species react differently to various chemicals and diseases. For example, although cows and horses can digest grass and hay, human beings can't. And while outright poisons such as cyanide clearly traumatize any living body, many foods or drugs that harm a laboratory rat won't harm you. And vice versa. For example, mouse and rat embryos suffer no ill effects when their mothers are given thalidomide, the sedative that's known to cause deformed fetal limbs when given to pregnant monkeys — and human beings — at the point in pregnancy when limbs are developing. (And here's an astounding turn: Modern research shows that thalidomide is beneficial for treating or preventing *human* skin problems related to Hansen's disease [leprosy], cancer, and/or autoimmune conditions, such as rheumatoid arthritis, in which the body mistakenly attacks its own tissues.)

Are enough people in this study?

A study that claims an effect or outcome with a sample size (the number of sub-jects) of 20, 30, or 40, for example, is not considered a strong study. The study must include sufficient numbers and a variety of individuals, too. If you don't have enough people in the study — several hundred to many thousand — to establish a pattern, there's always the possibility that an effect occurred by chance.

If you don't include different types of people, which generally means young and old men and women of different racial and ethnic groups, your results may not apply across the board. For example, the original studies linking high blood cholesterol levels to an increased risk of heart disease and linking small doses of aspirin to a reduced risk of a second heart attack involved only men. It wasn't until follow-up studies were conducted with women that researchers were able to say with any certainty that high cholesterol is dangerous and aspirin is protective for women as well — but not in quite the same way: In January 2006, the *Journal of the American Medical Association* reported that when men take low-dose aspirin, they tend to lower their risk of heart attack. For women, the aspirin reduces the risk of stroke. Vive la difference!

Is there anything in the design or method of this study that may affect the accuracy of its conclusions?

Some testing methods are more likely to lead to biased or inaccurate conclu-sions. For example, a retrospective study (one that asks people to tell what they did in the past) is always considered less accurate than a prospective study (one that follows people while they're actually doing what the researchers are studying), because memory isn't always accurate. People tend to forget details or, without meaning to, alter them to fit the researchers' questions.

Are the study's conclusions reasonable?

When a study comes up with a conclusion that seems illogical to you, chances are the researchers feel the same way. For example, in 1990, the long-running Nurses' Study at the Harvard School of Public Health reported that a high-fat diet raised the risk of colon cancer. But the data showed a link only to diets high in beef. No link was found to diets high in dairy fat. In short, this study was begging for a second study to confirm (or deny) its results.

Chapter 2

Digestion: The 24-Hour Food Factory

*W*hen you see (or smell) something appetizing, your digestive organs leap into action. Your mouth waters. Your stomach contracts. Intestinal glands begin to secrete the chemicals that turn food into the nutrients that build new tissues and provide the energy you need to keep zipping through the days, months, and years.

This chapter introduces you to your digestive system and explains exactly how your body digests the many different kinds of foods you eat, all the while extracting the nutrients you need to keep on truckin'.

Introducing the Digestive System

Your digestive system may never win a Juno, Gemini, or Oscar but it certainly deserves your applause for its ability to turn complex food into basic nutrients. Doing this requires not a cast of thousands but a group of digestive organs, each designed specifically to perform one role in the two-part process. Read on.

The digestive organs

Although exceedingly well organized, your digestive system is basically one long tube that starts at your mouth, continues down through your throat to your stomach, and then goes on to your small and large intestines and past the rectum to end at your anus.

In between, with the help of the liver, pancreas, and gallbladder, the usable (digestible) parts of everything you eat are converted to simple compounds that your body can easily absorb to burn for energy or to build new tissue. The indigestible residue is bundled off and eliminated as waste.

Figure 2-1 shows the body parts and organs that make up your digestive system.

Digestion: A two-part process

Digestion is a two-part process — half mechanical, half chemical:

> ✔ *Mechanical digestion* takes place in your mouth and your stomach. Your teeth break food into small pieces that you can swallow without choking. In your stomach, a churning action continues to break food into smaller particles.

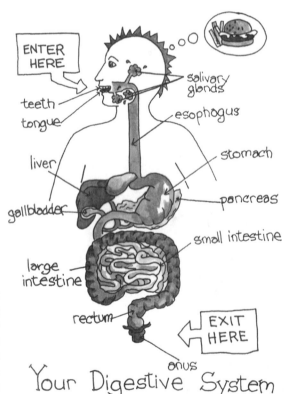

Figure 2-1:
Your digestive system in all its glory.

Your Digestive System

> ✔ *Chemical digestion* occurs at every point in the digestive tract where enzymes and other substances, such as *hydrochloric acid* (from stomach glands) and *bile* (from the liver), dissolve food, releasing the nutrients inside.

Understanding How Your Body Digests Food

Each organ in the digestive system plays a specific role in the digestive drama. But the first act occurs in two places that are never listed as part of the digestive tract: your eyes and nose.

The eyes and nose

When you see appetizing food, you experience a conditioned response. (For the lowdown on how your digestive system can be conditioned to respond to food, see Chapter 14; for information on your food preferences, see Chapter 15.) In other words, your thoughts — "Wow! That looks good!" — stimulate your brain to tell your digestive organs to get ready for action.

What happens in your nose is purely physical. The tantalizing aroma of good food is transmitted by molecules that fly from the surface of the food to settle on the membrane lining of your nostrils; these molecules stimulate the receptor cells on the olfactory nerve fibres that stretch from your nose back to your brain. When the receptor cells communicate with your brain — "Listen up, there's good stuff here!" — your brain sends encouraging messages to your mouth and digestive tract.

In both cases — eyes and nose — the results are the same: "Start the saliva flowing," they say. "Warm up the stomach glands. Alert the small intestine." In other words, the sight and scent of food have made your mouth water and your stomach contract in anticipatory hunger pangs.

But wait! Suppose you hate what you see or smell? For some people, even the thought of liver is enough to make them want to barf — or simply leave the room. At that point, your body takes up arms to protect you: You experience a *rejection reaction* — a reaction similar to that exhibited by babies who taste something bitter or sour. Your mouth purses and your nose wrinkles as if to keep the food (and its odour) as far away as possible. Your throat tightens, and your stomach *turns* — muscles contracting not in anticipatory pangs but in movements preparatory for vomiting up the unwanted food. Not a pleasant moment.

Turning starches into sugars

Salivary enzymes (like amylases) don't lay a finger on proteins and leave fats pretty much alone, but they do begin to digest complex carbohydrates, breaking the long, chainlike molecules of starches into individual units of sugars. Here's a simple experiment that lets you taste first-hand the effects of amylases on carbohydrates:

1. **Put a small piece of plain, unsalted cracker on your tongue.**

   No cheese, no chopped liver — just the cracker, please.

2. **Close your mouth and let the cracker sit on your tongue for a few minutes.**

   Do you taste a sudden, slight sweetness? That's the salivary enzymes breaking a long, complex starch molecule into its component parts (sugars).

3. **Okay, you can swallow now.**

   The rest of the digestion of the starch takes place farther down, in your small intestine.

But assume you like what's on your plate. Go ahead. Take a bite.

The mouth

Lift your fork to your mouth, and your teeth and salivary glands swing into action. Your teeth chew, grinding the food, breaking it into small, manageable pieces. As a result:

- ✔ You can swallow without choking.
- ✔ You break down the indigestible wrapper of fibres surrounding the edible parts of some foods (fruits, vegetables, whole grains) so that your digestive enzymes can get to the nutrients inside.

At the same time, salivary glands under your tongue and in the back of your mouth secrete the watery liquid called *saliva,* which performs two important functions:

- ✔ Moistening and compacting food so that your tongue can push it to the back of your mouth and you can swallow, sending the food down the slide of your *gullet* (esophagus) into your stomach.
- ✔ Providing *amylases,* enzymes that start the digestion of complex carbo- hydrates (starches), breaking the starch molecules into simple sugars. (Check out Chapter 8 for more on carbs.)

No protein digestion occurs in your mouth, though saliva does contain very small amounts of lingual lipases, fat-busting enzymes secreted by cells at the base of the tongue; however, the amount is so small that fat digestion in the mouth is insignificant.

The stomach

If you were to lay your digestive tract out on a table, most of it would look like a simple, rather narrow tube. The exception is your stomach, a pouchy part just below your *gullet* (esophagus).

Like most of the digestive tube, your stomach is circled with strong muscles whose rhythmic contractions — called *peristalsis* — move food smartly along and turn your stomach into a sort of food processor that mechanically breaks pieces of food into ever smaller particles. While this is going on, glands in the stomach wall are secreting *stomach juices* — a potent blend of enzymes, hydrochloric acid, and mucus.

One stomach enzyme — *gastric alcohol dehydrogenase* — digests small amounts of alcohol, an unusual nutrient that can be absorbed directly into your bloodstream even before it's been digested. For more about alcohol digestion, including why men can drink more than women without becoming tipsy, see Chapter 9.

Other enzymes, plus stomach juices, begin the digestion of proteins and fats, separating them into their basic components — amino acids and fatty acids.

Stop! If the words *amino acids* and *fatty acids* are completely new to you and if you are suddenly consumed by the desire to know more about them this instant, stick a pencil in the book to hold your place and flip ahead to Chapters 6 and 7, where you can read about them in detail.

Stop again! For the most part, digestion of carbohydrates comes to a screeching — though temporary — halt in the stomach because the stomach juices are so acidic that they deactivate *amylases,* the enzymes that break complex carbohydrates apart into simple sugars. However, stomach acid can break some carbohydrate bonds, so a bit of carb digestion does take place.

Back to the action. Eventually, your churning stomach blends its contents into a thick soupy mass called *chyme* (from *cheymos,* the Greek word for juice). When a small amount of chyme spills past the stomach into the small intestine, the digestion of carbohydrates resumes in earnest, and your body begins to extract nutrients from food.

The small intestine

Open your hand and put it flat against your belly button, with your thumb pointing up to your waist and your pinkie pointing down.

Your hand is now covering most of the relatively small space into which your 6-metre-long (20-foot) small (6 metres? Who calls that small?) intestine is neatly coiled. When the soupy, partially digested chyme spills from your stomach into this part of the digestive tube, a whole new set of gastric juices is released. These include:

- *Pancreatic amylase and intestinal enzymes* that finish the digestion of carbohydrates into simple sugars

- *Pancreatic trypsin and intestinal enzymes* that finish the digestion of proteins, which started in the stomach, into amino acids

- *Pancreatic lipase and intestinal enzymes* that digest fats into fatty acids

- *Bile,* a greenish liquid (made in the liver and stored in the gallbladder) that enables fats to mix with water

- *Pancreatic bicarbonate* that makes the chyme less acidic so amylases (the enzymes that break down carbohydrates) can go back to work separating complex carbohydrates into simple sugars

- *Intestinal alcohol dehydrogenase,* which digests alcohol not previously absorbed into your bloodstream

While these chemicals are working, contractions of the small intestine continue to move the food mass down through the tube so your body can absorb sugars, amino acids, fatty acids, vitamins, and minerals into cells in the intestinal wall.

The lining of the small intestine is a series of folds covered with projections that have been described as "fingerlike" or "small nipples." The technical name for these small fingers/nipples is *villi.* Each villus is covered with smaller projections called *microvilli,* and every villus and microvillus is programmed to accept a specific nutrient — and no other.

Nutrients are absorbed not in their order of arrival in the intestine but according to how fast they're broken down into their basic parts:

- Carbohydrates — which separate quickly into single sugar units — are absorbed first.

- Proteins (as amino acids) go next.

- Fats — which take longest to break apart into their constituent fatty acids — are last. That's why a high-fat meal keeps you feeling fuller longer than, say, chow mein or plain tossed salad, which are mostly low-fat carbohydrates.

- Vitamins that dissolve in water are absorbed earlier than vitamins that dissolve in fat.

Peephole: The first man to watch a living human gut at work

William Beaumont, M.D., was a surgeon in the United States Army in the early 19th century. His name survives in the annals of medicine because of an excellent adventure that began on June 6, 1822. Alexis St. Martin, an 18-year-old French-Canadian fur trader, was wounded by a musket ball that discharged accidentally and tore through his back and out his stomach, leaving a wound that healed but didn't close.

St. Martin's injury seems not to have affected what must have been a truly sunny disposition: Two years later, when all efforts to close the hole in his gut had failed, he granted Beaumont permission to use the wound as the world's first window on a working human digestive system. (To keep food and liquid from spilling out of the small opening, Beaumont kept it covered with a cotton bandage.)

Beaumont's method was simplicity itself. At noon on August 1, 1825, he tied small pieces of food (cooked meat, raw meat, cabbage, bread) to a silk string, removed the bandage, and inserted the food into the hole in St. Martin's stomach.

An hour later, he pulled the food out. The cabbage and bread were half digested; the meat was untouched. After another hour, he pulled the string out again. This time, only the raw meat remained untouched, and St. Martin, who now had a headache and a queasy stomach, called it quits for the day. But in more than 230 later trials, Beaumont — with the help of his remarkably compliant patient — discovered that although carbohydrates (cabbage and bread) were digested rather quickly, the stomach juices took up to eight hours to break down proteins and fats (the beef). Beaumont attributed this to the fact that the cabbage had been cut into small pieces and the bread was porous. Modern nutritionists know that carbohydrates are simply digested faster than proteins and that digesting fats (including those in beef) takes longest of all.

By withdrawing gastric fluid from St. Martin's stomach, keeping it at 100°F (the temperature recorded on a thermometer stuck into the stomach), and adding a piece of meat, Beaumont was able to clock exactly how long the meat took to fall apart: 10 hours.

Beaumont and St. Martin separated in 1833 when the patient, then a sergeant in the United States Army, was posted elsewhere, leaving the doctor to write "Experiments and Observations on the Gastric Juice and the Physiology of Digestion." The treatise is considered a landmark in the understanding of the human digestive system.

After you've digested your food and absorbed its nutrients through your small intestine the following processes take place:

- The bloodstream carries amino acids, sugars, vitamin C, the B vitamins, iron, calcium, and magnesium to your liver, where they are processed and sent out to the rest of the body.

- Fatty acids, cholesterol, and vitamins A, D, E, and K go into the lymphatic system and then into the blood. They, too, end up in the liver, are processed, and are shipped out to other body cells.

Chew! Chew! All aboard the Nutrient Express!

Think of your small intestine as a busy train station whose apparent chaos of arrivals and departures is actually an efficient, well-ordered system.

The small intestine resembles a three-level, miniature Grand Central Terminal:

✔ Level 1 is the *duodenum* (at the top, right after your stomach).

✔ Level 2 is the *jejunum* (in the middle).

✔ Level 3 is the *ileum* (the last part before the colon).

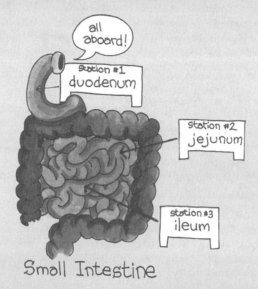

This three-station tube hums away as nutrients arrive and depart, with millions of "trains" (the nutrients) running on millions of "tracks" (the microvilli) designed to accommodate only one kind of train — and no other.

The system absorbs and ships out nutrients that account for more than 90 percent of all the protein, fat, and carbohydrates you consume, plus smaller percentages of vitamins and minerals. The train schedule looks something like this:

Level 1	Duodenum	Vitamin A, B1, the minerals iron and calcium, simple sugars (the end products of carbohydrate digestion), amino acids (the end products of protein metabolism), and fatty acids (the end products of fat digestion)
Level 2	Jejunum	More of the simple sugars, amino acids and fatty acids, the water-soluble vitamins (vitamin C and the B vitamins, other than vitamin B12), the fat-soluble vitamins D, E, and K, the minerals copper, zinc, potassium, iodine, calcium, magnesium, and phosphorus
Level 3	Ileum	Vitamin B12, and the minerals chloride, sodium, and potassium

Inside the cells, nutrients are *metabolized* — burned for heat and energy or used to build new tissues. The metabolic process that gives you energy is called *catabolism* (from *katabole,* the Greek word for casting down). The metabolic process that uses nutrients to build new tissues is called *anabolism* (from *anabole,* the Greek word for raising up).

How the body uses nutrients for energy and new tissues is, alas, a subject for another chapter. In fact, this subject is enough to fill seven different chapters, each devoted to a specific kind of nutrient. For information about metabolizing proteins, turn to Chapter 6. You'll find fats in Chapter 7, carbohydrates in Chapter 8, alcohol in Chapter 9, vitamins in Chapter 10, minerals in Chapter 11, and water in Chapter 13.

The large intestine

After every useful, digestible ingredient other than water has been wrung out of your food, the rest — indigestible waste such as fibre — moves into the top of your large intestine, the area known as your *colon.* The colon's primary job is to absorb water from this mixture and then to squeeze the remaining matter into the compact bundle known as feces.

Feces (whose brown colour comes from leftover bile pigments) are made of indigestible material from food, plus cells that have sloughed off the intestinal lining, plus bacteria — quite a lot of bacteria. In fact, about 30 percent of the entire weight of the feces is bacteria. No, these bacteria aren't a sign you're sick. On the contrary, they prove that you're healthy and well. These bacteria are good guys, micro-organisms that live in permanent colonies in your colon, where they:

- ✓ Manufacture vitamin B12, which is absorbed through the colon wall

- ✓ Produce vitamin K, also absorbed through the colon wall

- ✓ Break down amino acids and produce nitrogen (which gives feces a characteristic odour)

- ✓ Feast on indigestible complex carbohydrates (fibre), excreting the gas that sometimes makes you physically uncomfortable — or a social pariah

When the bacteria have finished, the feces — perhaps the small remains of yesterday's copious feast — pass down through your rectum and out through your anus. But not necessarily right away: Digestion of any one meal may take longer than a day to complete.

After that, digestion's done!

Chapter 3
Calories: The Energizers

. . . .

In This Chapter

▶ Discovering what a calorie is

▶ Understanding why not all calories deliver the same nutrition

▶ Explaining why men generally need more calories than women

▶ Estimating whether you're at a healthful weight

. . . .

Automobiles burn gasoline to get the energy they need to move. Your body burns *(metabolizes)* food to produce energy in the form of heat. This heat warms your body and (as energy) powers every move you make.

 Nutrition scientists measure the amount of heat produced by metabolizing food in units called kilocalories. A *kilocalorie* is the amount of energy it takes to raise the temperature of 1 kilogram of water 1 degree Centigrade (Celsius) at sea level.

In common use, nutritionists substitute the word *calorie* for *kilocalorie*. This common usage isn't scientifically accurate: Strictly speaking, a calorie is really ⅟₁₀₀₀ of a kilocalorie. But the word calorie is easier to say and easier to remember, so that's the term you see whenever you read about the energy in food. And few nutrition-related words have caused as much confusion and concern as the lowly calorie. Read on to find out what calories mean to you and your nutrition.

Counting the Calories in Food

When you read that a serving of food — say, one banana — has 105 calories, that means metabolizing the banana produces 105 calories of heat that your body can use for work.

Measuring the number of calories

Nutrition scientists measure the number of calories in food by actually burning the food in a *bomb calorimeter*, which is a box with two chambers, one inside the other. The researchers weigh a sample of the food, put the sample on a dish, and put the dish into the inner chamber of the calorimeter. They fill the inner chamber with oxygen and then seal it so the oxygen can't escape. The outer chamber is filled with a measured amount of cold water, and the oxygen in the first chamber (inside the chamber with the water) is ignited with an electric spark. When the food burns, an observer records the rise in the temperature of the water in the outer chamber. If the temperature of the water goes up 1 degree per kilogram, the food has 1 calorie; 2 degrees, 2 calories; and 235 degrees, 235 calories — or one 250 mL (8-ounce) chocolate malt!

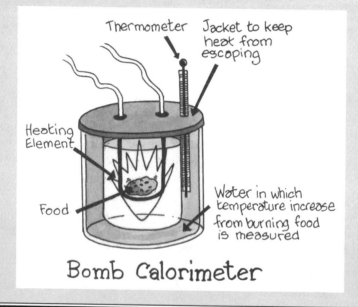

Bomb Calorimeter

You may wonder which kinds of food have the most calories. Here's how the calories measure up in 1 gram of the following nutrients:

- ✔ **Protein:** 4 calories

- ✔ **Carbohydrate:** 4 calories

- ✔ **Alcohol:** 7 calories

- ✔ **Fat:** 9 calories

In other words, ounce for ounce, proteins and carbohydrates give you fewer than half as many calories as fat. That's why — again, ounce for ounce — high-fat foods, such as cheese, are high in calories, while lower-fat foods, such as apples, are not.

Sometimes foods that seem to be equally low in calories really aren't. You have to watch all the angles, paying attention to fat in addition to protein and carbohydrates. Here's a good example: A chicken breast and a hamburger are both high-protein foods. Both should have the same number of calories per gram. But if you serve the chicken without its skin, it contains very little fat, while the hamburger is (sorry about this) full of it. An 85 gram (3-ounce) serving of skinless chicken provides 140 calories, while an 85 gram (3-ounce) burger yields 230 to 245 calories, depending on the cut of the meat.

Empty calories

All food provides calories. All calories provide energy. But not all calories come with a full complement of extra benefits such as amino acids, fatty acids, fibre, vitamins, and minerals. Some foods are said to give you *empty calories*. This term has nothing to do with the calorie's energy potential or with calories having a hole in the middle. It describes a calorie with no extra benefits.

The best-known, empty-calorie foods are table sugar and *ethanol* (the kind of alcohol found in beer, wine, and spirits). On their own, sugar and ethanol give you energy — but no nutrients. (See Chapter 8 for more about sugar and Chapter 9 for more about alcohol.)

People who abuse alcohol aren't always thin, but the fact that they often substitute alcohol for food can lead to nutritional deficiencies, most commonly a deficiency of thiamin (vitamin B1), resulting in loss of appetite, an upset stomach, depression, and an inability to concentrate. (For more on vitamin deficiency problems, check out Chapter 10.)

Of course, it's only fair to point out that sugar and alcohol are ingredients often found in foods that do provide other nutrients. For example, sugar is found in bread, and alcohol is found in beer — two very different foods that both have calcium, phosphorus, iron, potassium, sodium, and B vitamins.

Throughout Canada, some people are malnourished because they can't afford enough food to get the nutrients they need. But many Canadians who can afford enough food nevertheless are malnourished because they simply don't know how to choose a diet that gives them nutrients as well as calories. For these people, eating too many foods with empty calories can cause significant health problems, such as having weak bones; being underweight (yes, being too thin can be a problem); getting bleeding gums, skin rashes, and other nasties; and developing mental disorders, including depression and preventable retardation.

Every calorie counts

People who say that "calories don't count" or that "some calories count less than others" are usually trying to convince you to follow a diet that concentrates on one kind of food to the exclusion of most others. One common example that seems to arise like a phoenix in every generation of dieters is the *high-protein diet.*

The high-protein diet says to cut back or even entirely eliminate carbohydrate foods on the assumption that because your muscle tissue is mostly protein, the protein foods you eat will go straight from your stomach to your muscles, while everything else turns to fat. In other words, this diet says that you can stuff yourself with protein foods until your eyes bug out, because no matter how many calories you get, they'll all be protein calories and they'll all end up in your muscles, not on your hips. Boy, wouldn't it be nice if that were true? The problem is, it isn't. Here's the absolute truth: All calories, regardless of where they come from, give you energy. If you take in more energy (calories) than you spend each day, you'll gain weight. If you take in fewer than you use up, you'll lose weight. This nutrition rule is an equal opportunity, one-size-fits-all proposition that applies to everyone.

How Many Calories Do You Need?

Think of your energy requirements as a bank account. You make deposits when you consume calories. You make withdrawals when your body spends energy on work. Dietitians divide the amount of energy you withdraw each day into two parts:

- The energy you need when your body is at rest
- The energy you need to do your daily "work"

To keep your energy account in balance, you need to take in enough each day to cover your withdrawals. As a general rule, infants and adolescents burn more energy per kilogram than adults do, because they're continually making large amounts of new tissue. Similarly, an average man burns more energy than an average woman because his body is larger and has more muscle, thus leading to the totally unfair but totally true proposition that a man who weighs, say, 68.2 kg (150 pounds) can consume about 10 percent more calories than a woman who weighs 68.2 kg (150 pounds) and still not gain weight. For the numbers, check out the next section and Table 3-1.

Resting energy expenditure (REE)

Even when you're at rest, your body is busy. Your heart beats. Your lungs expand and contract. Your intestines digest food. Your liver processes nutrients. Your glands secrete hormones. Your muscles flex, usually gently. Cells send electrical impulses back and forth among themselves, and your brain continually signals to every part of your body.

The energy that your resting body uses to do all this stuff is called (surprise! surprise!) *resting energy expenditure,* abbreviated REE. The REE, also known as the *basal metabolism,* accounts for a whopping 60 to 70 percent of all the energy you need each day.

To find your resting energy expenditure (REE), you must first figure out your weight in kilograms (kg). One kilogram equals 2.2 pounds. So to get your weight in kilograms, divide the number in pounds by 2.2. For example, if you weigh 150 pounds, that's equal to 68.2 kg (150 ÷ 2.2). Plug that into the appropriate equation in Table 3-1 — and bingo! You have your REE.

Table 3-1 How Many Calories Do You Need When You're Resting?

Sex and Age	Equation to Figure Out Your REE
Males	
18–30 years	(15.3 × weight in kg) + 679
31–60 years	(11.6 × weight in kg) + 879
Older than 60 years	(13.5 × weight in kg) + 487
Females	
18–30 years	(14.7 × weight in kg) + 496
31–60 years	(8.7 × weight in kg) + 829
Older than 60 years	(10.5 × weight in kg) + 596

The National Research Council, Recommended Dietary Allowances (Washington, D.C.: National Academy Press, 1989)

Sex, glands, and chocolate cake

A *gland* is an organ that secretes *hormones,* which are chemical substances that can change the function — and sometimes the structure — of other body parts. For example, your pancreas secretes *insulin,* a hormone that enables you to digest and metabolize carbohydrates. At puberty, your sex glands secrete either the female hormones estrogen and progesterone or the male hormone testosterone; these hormones trigger the development of secondary sex characteristics, such as the body and facial hair that make us look like either men or women.

Hormones can also affect your REE, how much energy you use when your body's at rest. Your pituitary gland, a small structure in the centre of your brain, stimulates your thyroid gland (which sits at the front of your throat) to secrete hormones that influence the rate at which your tissues burn nutrients to produce energy.

When your thyroid gland doesn't secrete enough hormones (a condition known as *hypothyroidism*), you burn food more slowly and your REE drops. When your thyroid secretes excess amounts of hormones (a condition known as *hyperthyroidism*), you burn food faster and your REE is higher.

When you're frightened or excited, your adrenal glands (two small glands, one on top of each kidney) release *adrenalin*, the hormone that serves as your body's call to battle stations. Your heartbeat increases. You breathe faster. Your muscles clench. And you burn food faster, converting it as fast as possible to the energy you need for the reaction commonly known as *fight or flight*. But these effects are temporary. The effects of the sex glands, on the other hand, last as long as you live. Read on.

How your hormones affect your energy needs

If you're a woman, you know that your appetite rises and falls in tune with your menstrual cycle. In fact, this fluctuation parallels what's happening to your REE, which goes up just before or at the time of ovulation. Your appetite is highest when menstrual bleeding starts and then falls sharply. Yes, you really are hungrier (and need more energy) just before you get your period.

Being a man (and making lots of testosterone) makes satisfying your nutritional needs on a normal Canadian diet easier. Your male bones are naturally denser, so you're less dependent on dietary or supplemental calcium to prevent *osteoporosis* (severe loss of bone tissue) late in life. You don't lose blood through menstruation, so you need only two-thirds as much iron. Best of all, you can consume about 10 percent more calories than a woman of the same weight without adding pounds.

Teenage boys developing wide shoulders and biceps while teenage girls get hips is no accident. Testosterone, the male hormone, promotes the growth of muscle and bone. Estrogen gives you fatty tissue. As a result, the average male body has proportionally more muscle; the average female body, proportionally more fat.

Muscle is active tissue. It expands and contracts. It works. And when a muscle works, it uses more energy than fat (which insulates the body and provides a source of stored energy but does not move an inch on its own). What this muscle versus fat battle means is that the average man's REE is about 10 percent higher than the average woman's. In practical terms, that means a 63.5 kg (140-pound) man can hold his weight steady while eating about 10 percent more than a 63.5 kg (140-pound) woman who is the same age and performs the same amount of physical work.

No amount of dieting changes this unfair situation. A woman who exercises strenuously may reduce her body fat so dramatically that she no longer menstruates — an occupational hazard for some professional athletes. But she'll still have proportionately more body fat than an adult man of the same weight. If she eats what he does, and they perform the same amount of physical work, she still requires fewer calories than he to hold her weight steady.

And here's a really rotten possibility. Muscle weighs more than fat. This interesting fact is one that many people who take up exercise to lose weight discover by accident. One month into the barbells and step-up-step-down routine, their clothes fit better, but the scale points slightly higher because they've traded fat for muscle — and you know what that means: Sometimes you can't win for losing.

Energy for work

Your second largest chunk of energy is the energy you withdraw to spend on physical work. That's everything from brushing your teeth in the morning to hoeing a row of petunias in the garden or working out in the gym.

Your total energy requirement (the number of calories you need each day) is your REE plus enough calories to cover the amount of work you do.

Does thinking about this use up energy? Yes, but not as much as you'd like to imagine. To solve a crossword puzzle — or write a chapter of this book — the average brain uses about 1 calorie every four minutes. That's only one-third the amount needed to keep a 60-watt bulb burning for the same length of time.

Table 3-2 defines the energy level of various activities ranging from the least energetic (sleep) to the most (playing football, digging ditches). Table 3-3 shows how many calories you use in an hour's worth of different kinds of work.

Table 3-2	How Active Are You When You're Active?
Activity Level	**Activity**
Resting	Sleeping, reclining
Very light	Seated and standing activities, painting, driving, laboratory work, typing, sewing, ironing, cooking, playing cards, and playing a musical instrument
Light	Walking on a level surface at 4 to 4.8 kph (2.5 to 3 mph), garage work, electrical trades, carpentry, restaurant trades, housecleaning, child care, golfing, sailing, and table tennis
Moderate	Walking 5.6 to 6.4 kph (3.5 to 4 mph), weeding and hoeing, carrying a load, cycling, skiing, tennis, and dancing
Heavy	Walking with a load uphill, tree felling, heavy manual digging, basketball, climbing, football, and soccer
Exceptionally heavy	Professional athletic training

The National Research Council, Recommended Dietary Allowances (Washington, D.C.: National Academy Press, 1989)

Table 3-3	How Many Calories Do You Need to Do the Work You Do?
Activity Level	**Calories Needed for This Work for One Hour**
Very light	80–100
Light	110–160
Moderate	170–240
Heavy	250–350
Exceptionally heavy	350+

"Food and Your Weight," House and Garden Bulletin, No. 74 (Washington, D.C.: U.S. Department of Agriculture)

Enjoying the extras

Can you have your cake and eat it too? It's possible to eat a well-balanced diet and still leave room for extras. If, for example, you need 2,000 calories per day, and you manage to get all the high-quality carbohydrates, lean protein, heart-healthy fats (see Chapter 8 for the story on carbohydrates, Chapter 16 on how to ensure your protein choices are healthy, and Chapters 7 and 16 for the low-down on fats), vitamins, and minerals you require into 1,800 calories, then there's wiggle room to enjoy some treats. Use the "leftover" 200 calories — called *discretionary calories* — for anything that makes your mouth water. Naturally, some expert spoilsports disagree. They say that giving you an inch (those leftover calories) means you'll take a mile (three pieces of chocolate cake). Prove them wrong, and celebrate your smarts. Yum!

How Much Should You Weigh?

How much a person "should" weigh has been the topic of much debate and frustration. Through the years, a number of charts have purported to lay out *standard weights* or *healthy weights* for adults.

The most famous set of weight recommendations is probably the Metropolitan Life Insurance Company's standard height-weight tables for men and women, which were introduced in 1943 and were designed for adults aged 25 to 59 years. Although these reference tables were created in the United States, they were also adopted in Canada as guides to determining what the average person should weigh.

The main criticism of the recommendations from healthy weight charts was that they set the figures for body weight so low that you can hardly get there without severely restricting your diet — or being born again with a different body, preferably with light bones and no curves.

Studying weight charts

Table 3-4 is one moderate, eminently usable set of weight recommendations that originally appeared in the 1990 edition of *Dietary Guidelines for Americans* published by the U.S. Department of Agriculture and the U.S. Department of Health and Human Services. (The Canadian government uses a different means of determining healthy weight, which we examine in the section "Looking at Canada's weight guidelines.") The weights in this chart are listed in ranges for people (men and women) of specific heights. Naturally, height is measured without shoes, and weight is measured without clothes. (For more — much more — on dietary guidelines, see Chapter 16.)

Because most people gain some weight as they grow older, Table 3-4 does a really sensible thing by dividing the ranges into two broad categories, one for men and women ages 19 to 34, the other for men and women age 35 and older.

People with a small frame and proportionately more fat tissue than muscle tissue (muscle is heavier than fat) are likely to weigh in at the low end. People with a large frame and proportionately more muscle than fat are likely to weigh in at the high end. As a general (but by no means invariable) rule, that means that women — who have smaller frames and less muscle — weigh less than men of the same height and age.

Table 3-4	How Much Should You Weigh?	
Height cm (feet)	**Weight kg (pounds) for 19- to 34-Year-Olds**	**Weight kg (pounds) for 35-Year-Olds and Older**
152 (5')	44–58 (97–128)	49–63 (108–138)
155 (5'1")	46–60 (101–132)	50–65 (111–143)
158 (5'2")	47–62 (104–137)	52–67 (115–148)
160 (5'3")	49–64 (107–141)	54–69 (119–152)
163 (5'4")	50–66 (111–146)	55–71 (122–157)
165 (5'5")	52–68 (114–150)	57–74 (126–162)
167 (5'6")	54–70 (118–155)	59–76 (130–167)
170 (5'7")	55–73 (121–160)	61–78 (134–172)
173 (5'8")	57–75 (125–164)	63–81 (138–178)
175 (5'9")	59–77 (129–169)	65–83 (142–183)
178 (5'10")	60–79 (132–174)	66–85 (146–188)
180 (5'11")	62–81 (136–179)	69–88 (151–194)
183 (6')	64–84 (140–184)	70–90 (155–199)
185 (6'1")	65–86 (144–189)	72–93 (159–205)
188 (6'2")	67–89 (148–195)	75–95 (164–210)
191 (6'3")	69–91 (152–200)	76–98 (168–216)
193 (6'4")	71–93 (156–205)	79–101 (173–222)
196 (6'5")	73–96 (160–211)	80–104 (177–228)
198 (6'6")	75–98 (164–216)	83–106 (182–234)

Nutrition and Your Health: Dietary Guidelines for Americans, 3rd ed. (Washington D.C.: U.S. Department of Agriculture, U.S. Department of Health and Human Services, 1990)

What do they mean when they say that you're fat?

Obesity is a specific medical condition in which the body accumulates an overabundance of fatty tissue. One way to determine who's obese is to compare a person's weight with the figures on the weight/height charts (see Table 3-4):

✔ If your weight is 20 to 40 percent higher than the chart recommends, you're mildly obese.

✔ If your weight is 40 to 99 percent higher, you're moderately obese.

✔ If your weight is more than double the weight on the chart, you're severely obese.

Another way to rate your weight: Calculating your BMI

Run your finger down the chart in Table 3-4, but remember that the numbers are guidelines — no more, no less.

Squeezing people into neat little boxes is a reassuring exercise, but in real life, human beings constantly confound the rules. We all know chubby people who live long and happy lives and trim and skinny ones who leave us sooner than they should. However, the fact remains that people who are overweight have a higher risk of developing conditions such as osteoarthritis, some types of cancer (such as breast, colon, prostate, and kidney), Type 2 diabetes, high blood pressure, and cardiovascular disease (such as stroke and coronary heart disease), so you need a way to find out whether your current weight puts you at risk.

One good guide is the *Body Mass Index (BMI),* a number that measures the relationship between your weight and your height and offers some predictive estimates of your risk of weight-related disease.

Canada has used the BMI for its weight guidelines since 1988, with the publication of the *Canadian Guidelines for Healthy Weights.* Researchers deemed the BMI to be precise, reliable, and cheap to use — you just need a scale and a tool to measure height, and probably a calculator if you don't want to calculate by hand. To select appropriate cut-off points for BMIs, researchers reviewed Canadian and international data. They established the cut-off points for BMI categories by analyzing subjects' BMI in relationship to various levels of morbidity (presence of disease) and mortality (death).

To calculate your BMI, divide your weight (in kilograms) by your height (in metres) squared.

For example, if you are 160 cm (or 1.6 metres) tall and weigh 62.7 kg, the equation for your BMI looks like this:

$$BMI = \frac{62.7}{(1.60 \times 1.60)} = 24.5$$

Not yet used to the metric system? Well, to convert your height from inches into centimetres, multiply the number of inches by 2.54. To convert your weight in pounds to kilograms, simply divide the weight by 2.2.

Currently, the healthiest BMI seems to be 21.0. A BMI higher than 28 (76 kg or 168 pounds for a 1.5 metre or 5'5" woman; 88.5 kg or 195 pounds for a 1.75 metre or 5'10" man) appears to double the risk of diabetes, heart disease, and death.

Looking at Canada's weight guidelines

In 2003, Health Canada released its new *Canadian Guidelines for Body Weight Classification in Adults,* an update of the weight classification system from the 1988 guidelines. This was in response to recent research on the role of weight on health, and to address the appropriateness of the international adaptation of the World Health Organization's weight classification released in 2000. The revised guidelines introduced a new definition of both underweight and overweight.

The 2003 guidelines identify an *underweight* individual as having a BMI less than 18.5. Some people are naturally thin and some races such as South East Asian are naturally lighter than others, so the old lowest BMI cut-off of 20, from the 1988 guidelines, would suggest that those individuals are underweight and at an increased risk for disease, too — which isn't necessarily the case.

Although some people naturally weigh less than others, a letter in the November 2004 *Canadian Medical Association Journal* made the point that health professionals need to be aware that by lowering the cut-offs, some individuals who are at risk for malnutrition or eating disorders may be missed.

The revised guidelines define *overweight* individuals as having a BMI between 25 and 30; a BMI of 30–34.9 is Class 1 obese, 35–39.9 is Class 2 obese, and 40+ is Class 3 obese. What do the different classes of obesity mean? In a nutshell, they signify increased health risks. The risk of developing health problems goes from high risk with Class I obesity, to very high risk with Class 2 obesity, to extremely high risk with Class 3 obesity.

Measuring your waist circumference

The Body Mass Index is limited in its ability to predict health risk because it doesn't indicate where a person carries his or her fat (mostly on the hips and butt or around the gut, for example). Waist circumference is important for predicting longer term health: The more fat a person has around his or her midsection, the greater the risk for obesity-related diseases. The *Canadian Clinical Practice Guidelines on the Management and Prevention of Obesity in Adults and Children 2006* (what a catchy title), which was put together by dozens of experts across the country under the auspices of Obesity Canada, advises physicians to measure belly girth as part of a person's regular checkup.

Determining the waist circumference provides measurements of both the fat that lies just below the skin *(subcutaneous fat)* and the fat that surrounds the internal organs *(visceral fat)*. Higher amounts of visceral fat are associated with several risk factors that can lead to heart disease and diabetes.

Measure your waist circumference using a tape measure placed around your body at the level of the uppermost part of your hipbone — usually at the level of your navel. Increased risk of health problems occurs with a waist circumference greater than 102 centimetres (40 inches) for men and greater than 88 centimetres (35 inches) for women.

How reliable are the numbers? Considering confounding variables

Weight charts and tables and numbers and stats are so plentiful that you may think they're totally reliable in predicting who's healthy and who's not. So here's a surprise: They aren't.

The problem is that real people and their differences keep sneaking into the equation. For example, the value of the Body Mass Index in predicting your risk of illness or death appears to be tied to your age. If you're in your 30s, a lower BMI is clearly linked to better health. If you're in your 70s or older, no convincing evidence points to how much you weigh playing a significant role in determining how healthy you are or how much longer you'll live. In between, from age 30 to age 74, the relationship between your BMI and your health is, well, in-between — more important early on, less important later in life.

In other words, the simple evidence of your own eyes is true. Although North Americans sometimes seem totally obsessed with the need to lose weight, the fact is that many larger people, even people who are clearly obese, do live long, happy, and healthy lives. To figure out why, many nutrition scientists now are focusing not only on weight or weight/height (the BMI) but on the importance of *confounding variables,* which is science speak for "something else is going on here."

Here are three potential confounding variables in the obesity/health equation:

- ✔ Maybe people who are overweight are more prone to illness because they exercise less, in which case stepping up the workouts may reduce the perceived risk of being overweight.

- ✔ People who are overweight may be more likely to be sick because they eat lots of foods containing high-calorie ingredients, such as saturated fat, which can trigger adverse health effects; in this case, the remedy may simply be a change in diet.

- ✔ Maybe people who are overweight have a genetic predisposition to a serious disease. If that's true, you'd have to ask whether losing 20 pounds really reduces their risk of disease to the level of a person who is naturally 20 pounds lighter. Perhaps not: In a few studies, people who successfully lost weight actually had a higher rate of death.

Adding to the confusion is the fact that an obsessive attempt to lose weight may itself be hazardous to your health (see Chapter 14). Every year, North Americans spend billions (yes, you read that right) on diet clubs, special foods, and over-the-counter remedies aimed at weight loss. Often the diets, the pills, and the foods don't work, which can leave dieters feeling worse than they did before they started.

The chance that the diet will fail is only half the bad news. Here's the rest: Some foods that effectively lower calorie intake and some drugs that effectively reduce appetite have potentially serious side effects. For example, some individuals are sensitive to sugar substitutes like aspartame and sucralose, and some prescription diet drugs, such as the combination once known as Phen-Fen, are linked to serious, even fatal, diseases.

Facing the numbers when they don't fit your body

Right about here, you probably feel the strong need for a really big chocolate bar (not such a bad idea now that nutritionists have discovered that dark chocolate is rich in disease-fighting antioxidants). But it also makes sense to consider the alternative: realistic rules that enable you to control your weight safely and effectively. Check out the following:

✔ **Rule No. 1: Not everybody starts out with the same set of genes — or fits into the same pair of jeans.** Some people are naturally larger and heavier than others. If that's you, and all your vital stats satisfy your doctor, don't waste time trying to fit someone else's idea of perfection. Relax and enjoy your own body.

✔ **Rule No. 2: If you're overweight and your doctor agrees with your decision to lose weight, you don't have to set world records to improve your health.** Even a moderate drop in weight can be highly beneficial. According to *The New England Journal of Medicine* (www.nejm.org on the Net), losing just 10 to 15 percent of your body weight can lower high blood sugar, high cholesterol, and high blood pressure, reducing your risks of diabetes, heart disease, and stroke.

✔ **Rule No. 3: Moderation is the best path to weight control.** Moderate calorie deprivation on a sensible diet produces healthful, moderate weight loss; this diet includes a wide variety of different foods containing sufficient amounts of essential nutrients. Abusing this rule and cutting calories to the bone can turn you literally into skin and bones, depriving you of the nutrients you need to live a normal healthy life. For more on the potentially devastating effects of starvation, voluntary and otherwise, check out Chapter 14.

✔ **Rule No. 4: Be more active.** Doing exercise allows you to take in more calories and still lose weight. In addition, exercise reduces the risk of many health problems, such as heart disease. Sounds like a recipe for success.

How many calories do you really need?

Figuring out ex-act-ly how many calories to consume each day can be a, well, consuming task. The 1990 Nutrient Recommendations have set daily energy requirements according to age, sex, and activity level. They lay out a list of the average daily calorie allowance using the theoretical estimates of average energy requirements using procedures proposed by the Food and Agriculture Organization, World Health Organization, and the United Nations University Report. The report made recommendations calculated for three levels of occupational activities for healthy adults with a healthy BMI — 21.5 for women and 22.5 for men — based on the amount of activity a person performs each day (Table 3-5).

Note that in this context, *lightly active* means a lifestyle that includes physical activity for daily living and the equivalent of about 20 minutes of exercise daily; *moderately active* means a lifestyle that adds physical activity equal to about 40 minutes per day; and *heavily active* means adding physical activity equal to an hour or more of daily exercise.

Calorie recommendations such as the ones in Table 3-5 are estimates to serve as guidelines; actual requirements will vary from person to person. As a rule, men have proportionately more active tissue (muscle) than women do, so an average man's calorie requirements are about 10 percent higher than an average woman's.

Table 3-5	Matching Daily Calories with Daily Lifestyle		
Gender/Age	Calories If Lightly Active	Calories If Moderately Active	Calories If Heavily Active
Female			
19–24 years	2,100	2,200	2,500
25–49	2,100	2,200	2,400
50–74	1,900	2,000	2,300
75 Years+	1,800	1,900	2,100
Male			
19–24	2,700	3,100	3,600
25–49	2,600	2,900	3,500
50–74	2,300	2,600	3,100
75 Years+	2,100	2,400	2,800

The Report of the Scientific Review Committee: Nutrition Recommendations (Health and Welfare Canada, 1990)

The last word on calories

Calories are not your enemy. On the contrary, they give you the energy you need to live a healthy life.

The trick is managing your calories and not letting them manage you. After you know that fat has twice as many calories as protein or carbohydrate and that ultimately it is how much you eat that determines weight gain or loss and that your body burns food to make energy, you can strategize your energy intake to match your energy expenditure, and vice versa. Here's how: Turn straight to Chapter 16 to find out about a healthful diet and Chapter 17 to find out about planning nutritious meals.

Weighty issues in Canada

The Canadian population is growing in more ways than one. We're a society of increasingly fatter people. The most recent data on the weight of Canadians come from the 2004 Canadian Community Health Survey, which revealed that approximately 6.8 million Canadian adults (58.8 percent) ages 20 to 64 were overweight, and an additional 4.5 million (23.4 percent) were obese. These findings mirror trends worldwide. Globally, the human race is at its fattest ever. More alarming than the fact that the absolute number of overweight adults is greater than it was when similar surveys were first conducted in 1970–1972, a report released by Statistics Canada in 2005 suggests an unhealthy outlook should the trend continue. The study found that approximately one-third of people who were classified as normal weight in 1994–1995 had become overweight by 2002–2003. Nearly one-quarter of those who were initially overweight were now classified as obese.

So are there more obese adults in one part of the country compared to another? Not really. Compared to the national prevalence rate of 23.4 percent, the rates didn't vary greatly from region to region save a couple of exceptions. Prevalence of obesity among men was significantly higher in both Newfoundland and Labrador (33.3 percent) and Manitoba (30.4 percent). For women, the provincial rates again exceeded the national rate in Newfoundland and Labrador (34.5 percent), Saskatchewan (32.9 percent), and Nova Scotia (30.3 percent). Coming in as the leanest province is British Columbia with 18 percent of men and 20 percent of women classified as obese — could the stereotype of everyone in B.C. being outdoorsy and active be true?

Chapter 4

How Much Nutrition Do You Need?

- -

In This Chapter

▶ Unveiling what the Recommended Nutrient Intakes (RNIs) are

▶ Looking at nutrition a new way: The Dietary Reference Intake (DRI)

▶ Discovering how who you are determines the amount of nutrients you need

- -

A healthful diet provides sufficient amounts of all the nutrients that your body needs. The question is, how much is enough?

Today, Canadians can turn to a new set of recommendations called the *Dietary Reference Intake (DRI),* an umbrella term that includes several innovative categories of nutrient recommendations created by a collaboration of Health Canada, the Food and Nutrition Board (FNB) of the Institute of Medicine (IOM), and the National Academy of Sciences in the U.S. The new DRIs replace Canada's earlier nutrient guidelines, which were called the *Recommended Nutrient Intakes* or *RNIs.*

Confused? Not to worry. This chapter spells it all out.

RNIs: Guidelines for Good Nutrition

In 1983, Health Canada developed a set of nutrient intake standards called the *Recommended Nutrient Intakes (RNIs),* which represented the highest recommended intake of a given nutrient for the majority of each age and sex group. The RNIs presented the highest recommended intake because different people need nutrients in different amounts; some people require different amounts based on genetics, and everyone absorbs and utilizes nutrients differently. By setting the RNIs high, but not too high to risk toxicity, Health Canada hoped to meet everyone's different needs.

For example, the estimated average requirement of vitamin C for an adult male is 27 milligrams a day. Some men will need less and some will need more, so to meet the needs of 98 percent of all adult males, the RNI was set higher, at 40 milligrams a day.

The amounts recommended by the RNIs provide a margin of safety for healthy people, but they're not therapeutic. In other words, RNI servings won't cure a nutrient deficiency, but they can prevent one from occurring.

After examining available nutrition and public health research at that time, the report, *Nutrition Recommendations,* was released by the Scientific Review Committee in 1990. The intent of the report was to balance two previous nutrition goals: A healthy diet must provide sufficient amounts of nutrients to prevent deficiencies and, at the same time, to reduce the risk of chronic diseases. *Canada's Guidelines for Healthy Eating* put nutrition theory into practice by giving consumers action-oriented messages which include:

- ✔ Enjoy a variety of foods.
- ✔ Emphasize cereals, breads, other grain products, vegetables, and fruits.
- ✔ Choose lower-fat dairy products, leaner meats, and foods prepared with little or no fat.
- ✔ Achieve and maintain a healthy body weight by enjoying regular physical activity and healthy eating.
- ✔ Limit salt, alcohol, and caffeine.

DRI: A Newer Nutrition Guide

Because science, including nutrition, is a journey of discovery, guidelines change, and in some cases are completely overhauled because of new information. In 1993, the U.S. Food and Nutrition Board's Dietary Reference Intakes committee established several panels of experts to start the process of reviewing the RDAs (the U.S. equivalent of our RNIs) and other recommendations for major nutrients (vitamins, minerals, and other food components) in light of new research and insights.

In 1995, a bunch of nutrition gurus and bureaucrats got together to discuss the pros and cons of harmonizing Canada's dietary standards and RNIs with those of the U.S., and supported harmonization.

The first order of business was to establish a new standard for nutrient recommendations called the *Dietary Reference Intake (DRI)*. DRI is a broad term that includes several categories of nutritional measurements for vitamins, minerals, and other nutrients. It includes:

✔ **Estimated Average Requirement (EAR):** The amount that meets the nutritional needs of half the people in any one group (such as teenage girls or people older than 70). Nutritionists use the EAR to assess whether an entire population's normal diet provides adequate amounts of nutrients, and is not used to assess individuals.

✔ **Recommended Dietary Allowance (RDA):** The RDA, now based on information provided by the EAR, and still a daily average for individuals, is the amount of any one nutrient known to protect against deficiency.

✔ **Adequate Intake (AI):** The AI is a new measurement that provides recommendations for nutrients for which no RDA is set. These include:

- Pantothenic acid
- Biotin
- Choline
- Calcium
- Molybdenum
- Manganese
- Fluoride
- Chromium
- Vitamin K
- Vitamin D

✔ **Tolerable Upper Intake Level (UL):** The UL is the highest amount of a nutrient you can consume each day without risking an adverse effect.

This is the level that you *do not* want to exceed — a real concern with popping too many supplements without appropriate guidance from a nutrition professional.

This chapter is all about the RDAs: those recommended amounts of nutrients that help individuals achieve and maintain health. Although the EAR, AI, and UL are all DRIs, discussing them in detail when they don't apply to you, the reader, directly, might be TMI (too much information).

The DRI panel's first report, listing new recommendations for calcium, phosphorus, magnesium, and fluoride, appeared in 1997. Its most notable change was upping the recommended amount of calcium from 800 mg to 1,000 mg for adults age 31 to 50, as well as post-menopausal women taking estrogen supplements; for post-menopausal women not taking estrogen, the recommendation is 1,500 mg.

The second DRI panel report appeared in 1998. The report included new recommendations for thiamin, riboflavin, niacin, vitamin B6, folate, vitamin B12, pantothenic acid, biotin, and choline. The most important revision was increasing the folate recommendation to 400 mcg a day based on evidence showing that folate reduces a woman's risk of giving birth to a baby with spinal cord defects and lowers the risk of heart disease for men and women. (See the sidebar "Reviewing terms used to describe nutrient recommendations" in this chapter, and the Cheat Sheet at the front of the book, to brush up on your metric abbreviations.)

As a result of the 1998 DRI Panel report, the FDA in the U.S. ordered food manufacturers to add folate to flour, rice, and other grain products. (Many multivitamin products already contain 400 mcg of folate.) To help reduce the incidence of neural tube defects, Canada's food industry began to voluntarily add folate to grain products such as white wheat flour, enriched pasta, and enriched cornmeal in 1996 at the suggestion of Health Canada. Fortification of these food ingredients became mandatory in 1998. Nutrient intake surveys conducted after mandatory fortification reveal improved dietary folate intakes, with 86 percent of women meeting the EAR of 320 mcg per day, compared to only 36 percent prior to fortification. Intakes of folate increased, for example, from 296 to 470 mcg per day in British Columbian women and from 262 to 318 mcg per day in Newfoundland women after fortification. As well, in both men and women, the average blood folate levels and the average red blood cell folate levels (a more accurate measure of folate status) increased after fortification, and the prevalence of folate insufficiency decreased between 59 and 77 percent after fortification.

A DRI report with revised recommendations for vitamin C, vitamin E, the mineral selenium, beta-carotene, and other antioxidant vitamins was published in 2000. In 2001, new DRIs were released for vitamin A, vitamin K, arsenic, boron, chromium, copper, iodine, iron, manganese, molybdenum, nickel, silicon, vanadium, and zinc. And in 2004, the Institute of Medicine (IOM) released a final report on the new recommendations for sodium, potassium, chloride, and water, plus a special report on recommendations for two groups of older adults (ages 50 to 70 and 71 and older). Put these findings all together, and they spell out the recommendations you find in this chapter.

The essentials

RDAs offer recommendations for carbohydrate, protein, and 17 essential vitamins and minerals, which include:

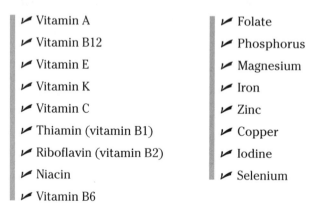

- Vitamin A
- Vitamin B12
- Vitamin E
- Vitamin K
- Vitamin C
- Thiamin (vitamin B1)
- Riboflavin (vitamin B2)
- Niacin
- Vitamin B6

- Folate
- Phosphorus
- Magnesium
- Iron
- Zinc
- Copper
- Iodine
- Selenium

The newest essential nutrient, choline, won its wings in 2002, but no RDAs have yet been established. Calcium has an Adequate Intake (AI) rather than an RDA.

Minimum requirements for carbohydrate and protein

Of the three macronutrients, carbohydrate, protein, and fat (flip to Chapter 1 for more), only carbohydrate and protein have an RDA. This is because the body has a minimum requirement, which it needs to stay healthy. All dietary carbohydrate (sugars and starches) is eventually metabolized into glucose so it can be used by the body's trillions of cells for much-needed fuel. The brain and nervous tissue in particular are known as *glucose obligate* tissues, meaning their preferred fuel is glucose (unlike muscle, which can use both glucose and fat for energy). The brain and nervous tissue are glucose guzzlers and have a minimum amount they need every day. The Recommended Dietary Allowance (RDA) for carbohydrate is set at 130 grams (4.5 ounces) per day for adults and children "based on the average minimum amount of glucose utilized by the brain. This level of intake, however, is typically exceeded to meet energy needs while consuming acceptable intake levels of fat and protein" according to the DRI report. The median intake of carbohydrates is approximately 220 to 330 grams (8 to 11.5 ounces) per day for men and 180 to 230 grams (6.5 to 8 ounces) per day for women.

Protein is the major structural component of all cells in the body — it's your bricks and mortar. Proteins also have a variety of functions. For example, an *enzyme* is a protein molecule that aids in metabolic processes and that also helps transport other nutrients, like minerals and other compounds, throughout the body. Your body is capable of making most of the protein it needs every day from carbohydrate and from recycling other proteins. This isn't 100 percent efficient, however, so some protein must come from your diet each day, to give your body what it needs.

The Recommended Dietary Allowance (RDA) for both men and women is 0.8 grams of good-quality protein for each kilogram of body weight (or 0.04 ounces for every 2.2 pounds). This amount is actually quite small. If a person weighs, for example, 70 kilograms (155 pounds), his or her total protein requirement would be 56 grams (2 ounces). This amount would be met with an average bowl of cereal with milk, a tuna sandwich, 250 mL (1 cup) of rice, and 28 grams (1 ounce) of cheese. This amount of food wouldn't provide enough calories, and because most people would need to eat more, they'd end up eating more protein as well.

Higher-protein foods such as meat, poultry, and fish are relatively inexpensive and abundant in Canada, so most of us get anywhere from two to three times the protein we need for our basic physiological requirements. Not to fret! The body is able to digest and get rid of any extra protein.

Those with liver and/or kidney disease, however, may need to restrict their protein intake — be sure to check with your doctor if you have any concerns.

Recommendations for fats, dietary fibre, and alcohol

What nutrients are missing from the RDA list of essentials? Fibre, fat, and alcohol. When it comes to fat, the reason is simple: If your diet provides enough carbohydrate, protein, vitamins, and minerals, it's probably providing more than enough fat. Fat is a major source of energy for the body and aids in the absorption of fat-soluble vitamins and carotenoids (pigments that give plants their colour and which have health-promoting properties).

There is neither an AI or RDA for total fat because there is insufficient evidence to determine a level of fat intake at which risk of inadequacy or prevention of chronic disease occurs. Nor is there a UL, because there is no defined upper level of total fat intake at which adverse effects (or toxicity) occurs. There is, however, an acceptable range of calories that can come from fat, referred to as the Acceptable Macronutrient Distribution Range (AMDR) — this states that 20 to 35 percent of energy can come from fat (see Chapter 7 for more on dietary fat).

Fibre has an AI of 38 grams per day for young men and 25 grams per day for young women, based on the intake level observed to protect against coronary heart disease.

Alcohol didn't make the RDA list because it isn't essential for life (although some might disagree). However, if you do drink alcohol, Health Canada recommends that no more than 5 percent of your total energy intake should be from alcohol. This works out to roughly one drink per day for women and two for men. This begs the obvious question: What's one drink? Here's the answer:

- 354 mL (12 ounces) of regular beer (150 calories)
- 142 mL (5 ounces) of wine (100 calories)
- 42 mL (1½ ounces) of 80-proof (40 percent alcohol) distilled spirits (100 calories)

Health Canada strongly recommends that pregnant women abstain from drinking alcohol.

Different people, different needs

Because different bodies require different amounts of nutrients, RDAs currently address as many as 22 specific categories of human beings: boys and girls, men and women, from infancy through middle age. The RDAs recently were expanded to include recommendations for groups of people ages 50 to 70 and 70 and older. Eventually, recommendations will be made for people older than 85. These expanded groupings are a really good idea because the Canadian population is living longer than ever before — according to the 2001 census, there were more than 3.8 million Canadians 65 years or older. That's about 13 percent of the total population.

But who you are affects the recommendations. If age is important, so is sex. For example, because women of child-bearing age lose iron when they menstruate, their RDA for iron is higher than the RDA for men. On the other hand, because men who are sexually active lose zinc through their ejaculations, the zinc RDA for men is higher than the zinc RDA for women.

Finally, sex affects body composition, which influences RDAs. Consider protein: The RDA for protein is set in terms of grams of protein per kilogram (2.2 pounds) of body weight. Because the average man weighs more than the average woman, his RDA for protein is higher than hers. The RDA for an adult male, age 19 or older, is 56 grams (2 ounces); for a woman, it's 46 grams (1.6 ounces).

Running through the Recommended Daily Allowances

Table 4-1 shows the most recent RDAs for vitamins for healthy adults; Table 4-2 shows RDAs for minerals for healthy adults. Where no RDA is given, an AI is indicated by an asterisk (*) next to the column heading. The complete reports on which this table is based are available online. Go to www.nap.edu. Prefer hard copy? The print version is available for purchase from the IOM Web site. (If you want an idea of what kinds of foods provide these vitamins, check out Chapter 10.)

Table 4-1	Vitamin RDAs for Healthy Adults				
g = gram	RE = retinol equivalent				
mg = milligram	a-TE = alpha-tocopherol equivalent				
mcg = microgram	NE = niacin equivalent				

Age (Years)	Vitamin A (RE/IU)†	Vitamin D (mcg/IU)‡*	Vitamin E (a-TE)	Vitamin K (mcg)*	Vitamin C (mg)
Males					
19–30	900/2,970	5/200	15	120	90
31–50	900/2,970	5/200	15	120	90
51–70	900/2,970	10/400	15	120	90
Older than 70	900/2,970	15/600	15	120	90
Females					
19–30	700/2,310	5/200	15	90	75
31–50	700/2,310	5/200	15	90	75
51–70	700/2,310	10/400	15	90	75
Older than 70	700/2,310	15/600	15	90	75
Pregnant (age-based)	750–770/ 2,475–2,541	5/200	15	75–90	70
Nursing (age-based)	1,200–1,300/ 3,960–4,290	5/200	19	76–90	95

*Adequate Intake (AI)
† The "official" RDA for vitamin A is still 1,000 RE/5,000 IU for a male, 800 RE/4,000 IU for a female who isn't pregnant or nursing; the lower numbers listed on this chart are the currently recommended levels for adults.
‡ The current recommendations are the amounts required to prevent vitamin D deficiency disease; recent studies suggest that the optimal levels for overall health may actually be higher, in the range of 800–1,000 IU a day.

Age (Years)	Thiamin (Vitamin B1) (mg)	Riboflavin (Vitamin B2) (mg)	Niacin (NE)	Pantothenic acid (mg)*	Vitamin B6 (mg)	Folate (mcg)	Vitamin B12 (mcg)	Biotin (mcg)*
Males								
19–30	1.2	1.3	16	5	1.3	400	2.4	30
31–50	1.2	1.3	16	5	1.3	400	2.4	30
50–70	1.2	1.3	16	5	1.7	400	2.4	30
Older than 70	1.2	1.1	16	5	1.7	400	2.4	30
Females								
19–30	1.1	1.1	14	5	1.3	400	2.4	30
31–50	1.1	1.1	14	5	1.3	400	2.4	30
51–70	1.1	1.1	14	5	1.5	400	2.4	30
Older than 70	1.1	1.1	14	5	1.5	400	2.4	30
Pregnant	1.4	1.1	18	6	1.9	600	2.6	30
Nursing	1.4	1.1	17	7	2.0	500	2.8	35

* Adequate Intake (AI)

Table 4-2		Mineral RDAs for Healthy Adults				
Age (Years)	Calcium (mg)*	Phosphorus (mg)	Magnesium (mg)	Iron (mg)	Zinc (mg)	Copper (mcg)
Males						
19–30	1,000	700	400	8	11	900
31–50	1,000	700	420	8	11	900
51–70	1,200	700	420	8	11	900
Older than 70	1,200	700	420	8	11	900
Females						
19–30	1,000	700	310	18	8	900
31–50	1,000	700	320	18	8	900
51–70	1,000/1,500**	700	320	8	8	900
Older than 70	1,000/1,500**	700	320	8	8	900
Pregnant	1,000–1,300	700–1,250	350–400	27	11–12	1,000
Nursing	1,000–1,300	700–1,250	310–350	9–10	12–13	1,300

* Adequate Intake (AI)
** The lower recommendation is for post-menopausal women taking estrogen supplements; the higher figure is for post-menopausal women not taking estrogen supplements.

Age (Years)	Iodine (mcg)	Selenium (mcg)	Molybdenum (mcg)	Manganese (mg)*	Fluoride (mg)*	Chromium (mcg)*	Choline (mg)*
Males							
19–30	150	55	45	2.3	4	36	550
31–50	150	55	45	2.3	4	36	550
50–70	150	55	45	2.3	4	30	550
Older than 70	150	55	45	2.3	4	30	550
Females							
19–30	150	55	45	1.8	3	25	425
31–50	150	55	45	1.8	3	25	425
51–70	150	55	45	1.8	3	20	425
Older than 70	150	55	45	1.8	3	20	425
Pregnant	220	60	50	2.0	1.5–4.0	29–30	450
Nursing	290	70	50	2.6	1.5–4.0	44–45	550

*Adequate Intake (AI)
Adapted with permission from Recommended Dietary Allowances (Washington D.C.: National Academy Press, 1989), and DRI panel reports, 1997–2004

NUTRITION SPEAK

Reviewing terms used to describe nutrient recommendations

Nutrient listings use the metric system. RDAs for protein are listed in grams. The RDAs and AIs for vitamins and minerals are shown in milligrams (mg) and micrograms (mcg). A milligram is ¹⁄₁₀₀ of a gram; a microgram is ¹⁄₁₀₀ of a milligram.

Vitamin A, vitamin D, and vitamin E are special cases. For instance, one form of vitamin A is *pre-formed vitamin A,* a form of the nutrient that your body can use right away. Preformed vitamin A, known as *retinol,* is found in food from animals — liver, milk, and eggs. Carotenoids (red or yellow pigments in plants) also provide vitamin A. But to get vitamin A from carotenoids, your body has to convert the pigments to chemicals similar to retinol. Because retinol is a ready-made nutrient, the RDA for vitamin A is listed in units called retinol equivalents (RE). One mcg (microgram) RE is approximately equal to 3.33 international units (IU, the former unit of measurement for vitamin A).

Vitamin D consists of three compounds: vitamin D1, vitamin D2, and vitamin D3. Cholecalciferol, the chemical name for vitamin D3, is the most active of the three, so the RDA for vitamin D is measured in equivalents of cholecalciferol.

Your body gets vitamin E from two classes of chemicals in food: tocopherols and tocotrienols. The compound with the greatest vitamin E activity is a tocopherol called *alpha*-tocopherol. The RDA for vitamin E is measured in milligrams of *alpha*-tocopherol equivalents (a-TE).

WARNING!

The slogan "No Sale Ever Is Final," printed on the sales slips of favourite clothing stores, definitely applies to nutritional numbers. RNIs and DRIs should always be regarded as works in progress, subject to revision at the first sign of a new study. In other words, in an ever-changing world, here's one thing of which you can be *absolutely* certain: The numbers in this chapter will change. Sorry about that.

Chapter 5

A Supplemental Story

Seventy-one percent of Canadians report that they regularly take vitamins and minerals, herbal products, homeopathic medicines, and other nutritional supplements — products that, in Canada, are now referred to as natural health products (NHPs). You can stir up a good food fight in any group of nutrition experts simply by asking whether all these supplements are (a) necessary, (b) economical, or (c) safe. But when the argument's over, you still may not have a satisfactory *official* answer, so this brief chapter aims to provide the information you need to make your own sensible choices.

Introducing Natural Health Products

The vitamin pill you may pop each morning is a natural health product (NHP). So are the calcium antacids many Canadian women consider standard nutrition. Echinacea, the herb reputed to short-circuit your winter cold, is, too, and so is the vanilla-flavoured, meal-in-a-can liquid your granny chug-a-lugs every afternoon just before setting off on her daily power walk. Under the Natural Health Products Regulation, which came into effect on January 1, 2004, NHPs include

- Vitamins and minerals
- Herbal medicines
- Homeopathic medicines
- Traditional medicines such as traditional Chinese medicine

> ✔ Probiotics
>
> ✔ Other products, such as amino acids and essential fatty acids

"NHPs must be safe for consideration as over-the-counter products, be available for self-care and self-selection, and not require a prescription to be sold" according to Health Canada.

Examining Why People Use Natural Health Products

In a country where food is plentiful and affordable, you have to wonder why so many people opt to scarf down pills instead of just plain food.

Many people consider vitamin and mineral supplements a quick and easy way to get nutrients without so much shopping and kitchen time and without all the pesky fats and sugars in food. Others take supplements as nutritional insurance (for more on recommended dietary allowances of vitamins and minerals, see Chapter 4). And some even use supplements as substitutes for medical drugs. In general, nutrition experts, including Dietitians of Canada and Health Canada, prefer that you invest your time and money whipping up meals and snacks that supply the nutrients you need in a balanced, tasty diet. Nonetheless, every expert worth his or her vitamin C admits that in certain circumstances, supplements can be a definite plus.

In fact, the majority of Canadians could probably benefit from taking a multivitamin or mineral. An article in the *Canadian Journal of Public Health* in 2000 and the Canadian Community Health Survey 2004 revealed that more than 50 percent of Canadian adults are getting almost one-third of their daily calories from foods low in nutrients (but high in fat and sugar). However, Health Canada offers no official recommendation on supplements to address this nutritional imbalance.

The revised Canada Food Guide does recommend vitamin supplements for two specific groups: women of child-bearing age and adults older than 50. All women who could become pregnant and those who are pregnant or breast-feeding need a multivitamin containing folic acid (a B vitamin that is shown to reduce the risk of neural tube defects), and pregnant women should make sure their multivitamin contains iron. According to Canada's Food Guide, adults older than 50 should take a daily vitamin D supplement of 10 mcg (400 IU). For more on Canada's Food Guide, see Chapter 17.

When food isn't enough

Illness, age, diet preferences, and some sex-related conditions may put you in a spot where you can't get all the nutrients you need from food alone.

Digestive illnesses, unfriendly drugs, injury, and chronic illness

Certain metabolic disorders and diseases of the digestive organs (liver, gallbladder, pancreas, and intestines) interfere with the normal digestion of food and the absorption of nutrients. Some medicines may also interfere with normal digestion, meaning you need supplements to make up the difference. People who suffer from certain chronic diseases, who have suffered a major injury (such as a serious burn), or who have just been through surgery may need more nutrients than they can get from food. In these cases, a doctor may prescribe supplements to provide the hard-to-get vitamins, minerals, and other nutrients.

Checking with your doctor, pharmacist, or dietitian before opting for a supplement you hope will have medical effects (make you stronger, smooth your skin, ease your anxiety) is a smart idea. The bad old days when doctors were total ignoramuses about nutrition may not be gone forever, but they're fading fast. Besides, your doctor is the person most familiar with your health, knows what medications you're taking, and can warn you of potential side effects — assuming that you have an open and honest discussion with him or her. When it comes to your health, being silent and withholding information is not the way to go.

Vegetarianism

Vitamin B12 is found only in food from animals, such as meat, milk, and eggs. (Some seaweed does have B12, but the suspicion is that the vitamin comes from micro-organisms living in the plant.) Without these foods, *vegans* — vegetarians who don't eat any foods of animal origin — almost certainly have to get their vitamin B12 from supplements or fortified foods.

Using supplements as insurance

Healthy people who eat a nutritious diet still may want to use supplements to make sure they're getting adequate nutrition. Plenty of recent research supports their choice.

Protecting against disease

Taking supplements may reduce the likelihood of some types of cancer and other diseases. After analyzing data from a survey of 871 men and women, epidemiologists at Seattle's Fred Hutchinson Cancer Center found that people taking a daily multivitamin for more than ten years were 50 percent less likely to develop colon cancer. In addition, selenium supplements seem to reduce the risk of prostate cancer, and vitamin C seems to lower the risk of cataracts.

Supplementing aging appetites

As you grow older, your appetite may decline, and your senses of taste and smell may falter. If food no longer tastes as good as it once did, if you have to eat alone all the time and don't enjoy cooking for one, or if dentures make chewing difficult, you may not be taking in all the foods you need to get the nutrients you require. Dietary supplements to the rescue!

If you're so rushed that you never get to eat a full, balanced meal, you may benefit from supplements regardless of your age.

Meeting a woman's special needs

And what about women? At various stages of their reproductive lives, they, too, benefit from supplements as insurance:

- ✔ **Before menopause:** Women who lose iron each month through menstrual bleeding rarely get sufficient amounts of iron from a typical North American diet of fewer than 2,000 calories a day. For them, and for women who are often on a diet to lose weight, iron supplements may be the only practical answer.

  Iron is a mineral element, so it may be called "iron" or "elemental iron" on the label. Iron pills contain a compound of elemental iron ("ferrous" or "ferric," from *ferrum,* the Latin word for iron), plus an ingredient such as a sulphur derivative or lactic acid to enable your body to use the iron. On the label, the combination reads "ferrous sulphate" or "ferrous lactate." Different iron compounds dissolve at different rates in your stomach, yielding different amounts of elemental iron, so supplement labels usually list the iron this way: Ferrous sulphate 325 mg / Elemental iron 65 mg. Translation? This pill has 325 milligrams of ferrous sulphate, yielding 65 milligrams of plain old iron. Sometimes the label omits the first part and simply says: Iron 65 mg.

  When doctors say, "Take one 325-milligram pill a day," they mean 325 milligrams iron compound, not plain elemental iron.

- ✔ **During pregnancy and lactation:** Women who are pregnant or nursing often need supplements to provide the nutrients to build new maternal and fetal tissue or to produce nutritious breast milk. In addition, supplements of the B vitamin folate now are known to decrease a woman's risk of giving birth to a child with a neural tube defect (a defect of the spinal cord and column).

  Never self-prescribe supplements while you're pregnant. Large amounts of some nutrients may be hazardous to your baby. For example, taking megadoses of vitamin A while you're pregnant can increase the risk of birth defects.

✔ **Through adulthood:** True, women older than 19 can get the calcium they require (1,000 milligrams a day) from four 250 mL (8-ounce) glasses of non-fat skim milk a day, three 250 mL (8-ounce) containers of yogurt made with non-fat milk, 625 grams (22 ounces) of canned salmon (with the soft edible bones; no, you definitely should not eat the hard bones in fresh salmon!), or any combination of the above. However, expecting women to do this nutritional balancing act every single day may be unrealistic. The simple alternative is calcium supplements.

Supplement Safety: How Natural Health Products Are Regulated in Canada

Health Canada's Natural Health Products Directorate (NHPD) regulates natural health products for sale in Canada. The role of the NHPD is to protect the public by ensuring people have access to NHPs that are safe and effective. Recognizing that people have different cultural and personal beliefs about the use of NHPs, the Directorate aims to support their right to choose for themselves.

The Natural Health Products Regulations set out standards, guidelines, and requirements for the sale of NHPs in Canada. Regulating NHPs brings several advantages to Canadian consumers. Before an NHP can be sold, it's examined by the Bureau of Product Review and Assessment to ensure that, first, what is on the label is what is in the bottle (which isn't always the case), and second, that any health claims made about the product are supported with research.

Regulations also require clear labelling information. NHP labels offer everything you need to know about dosage, treatment, and dangers. They also outline the NHP's premarket review and the NHPD's assessment of the product. Canadians have access to safe, effective NHPs of the highest quality.

Sweet trouble

Nobody wants to choke down a yucky supplement, but pills that look or taste like candy may be hazardous to a child's health. Some nutrients are troublesome — or even deadly — in high doses (see Chapters 10 and 11), especially for kids. For example, Health Canada warns that a lethal dose for young children may be as low as 3 grams (3,000 milligrams) of elemental iron, the amount in 49 tablets with 65 milligrams of iron apiece. If you have youngsters in your house, protect them by buying neutral-tasting supplements, and keep all pills, nutrient and otherwise, in a safe cabinet, preferably high off the floor and locked tight to resist tiny prying fingers.

As with any medication or over-the-counter drug (such as acetaminophen), NHPs are not without potential harm if taken incorrectly. Table 5-1 lists some potentially problematic herbal products you need to approach with caution — or avoid altogether. In many cases, even small amounts are hazardous.

Table 5-1	Some Potentially Hazardous Herbals
Herb	*Known Side Effects and Reactions*
Black cohosh	Nausea, vomiting, dizziness, smooth muscle (such as the uterus) contractions
Chaparral	Liver damage, liver failure
Comfrey	Possible liver damage
Kombuchu tea	Potentially fatal liver damage, intestinal upset
Lobelia (Indian tobacco)	Potentially fatal convulsions, coma
Pennyroyal	Potentially fatal liver damage, convulsions, coma
Senna	Severe gastric irritation, diarrhea
Stephania (also known as magnolia)	Kidney damage (sometimes severe enough to require dialysis or transplant)
Valerian	Severe withdrawal symptoms

"Vitamin and nutritional supplements," Mayo Clinic Health Letter (supplement), June 1997; Nancy Beth Jackson, "Doctors' warning: Beware of herbs' side effects," The New York Times, November 18, 1998; Jane Brody, "Taking a gamble on herbs as medicine," The New York Times, February 9, 1999; Carol Ann Rinzler, The Complete Book of Herbs, Spices, and Condiments, New York: Facts on File, 1990

Choosing the Most Effective Supplements

Okay, you've read about the virtues and drawbacks of supplements. You've decided which supplements you think may do you some good. Now it's crunch time, and all you really want to know is how to choose the safest, most effective products. The guidelines in this section can help.

Read the label

Check the supplement label. Thanks to the NPHD, NHP labels must include a wealth of information. Some of the most important things to note include

✔ The brand name

✔ The dosage form (is the supplement in a capsule, a powder, or a gel?)

Coming soon: Natural Product Numbers

Soon, every natural health product that has been reviewed and approved by the Natural Health Products Directorate will carry either a Natural Product Number (NPN) or a Drug Identification Number-Homeopathic Medicine (DIN-HM). Both the NPN and the DIN-HM will let the consumer know that the product has passed a review of its formulation, labelling, and instructions for use. Many manufacturers are already including NPN on their products, and by January 1, 2010, all NPHs sold in Canada are required to have NPN or DIN-HM on their labels. A list of the currently licensed and approved NHPs can be found on Health Canada's Web site: www.hc-sc.gc.ca.

✔ The name and address of the product licence holder (the manufacturer must have a product licence, which is certification that the NHPD has reviewed information about the product — for example, ingredients, source of ingredients, and product use)

✔ The common and the proper name of each medicinal ingredient (for example, vitamin C is the common name for ascorbic acid)

✔ The amount of medicinal ingredient per dose

✔ The amount of all non-medicinal ingredients

✔ Any cautions, warnings, or potential adverse reactions

✔ The lot number and expiry date

Figure 5-1 shows an example of the new supplement labels.

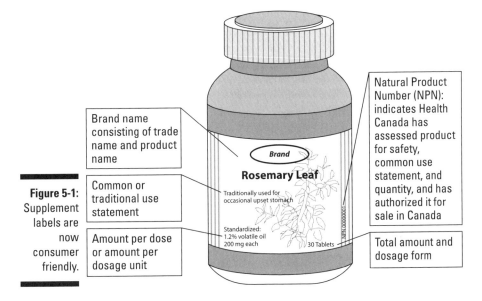

Figure 5-1: Supplement labels are now consumer friendly.

Brand name consisting of trade name and product name

Common or traditional use statement

Amount per dose or amount per dosage unit

Natural Product Number (NPN): indicates Health Canada has assessed product for safety, common use statement, and quantity, and has authorized it for sale in Canada

Total amount and dosage form

Brand

Rosemary Leaf

Traditionally used for occasional upset stomach

Standardized: 1.2% volatile oil 200 mg each

30 Tablets

NPN 00000001

Looking for the expiration date

Over time, all dietary supplements become less potent. Always choose the product with the longest useful shelf life. Don't buy the ones that will expire before you can use all the pills, such as the 100-pill bottle with an expiration date 30 days from now.

Checking the storage requirements

Even when you buy a product with the correct expiration date, it may be less effective if you don't keep it in the right place. Some supplements must be refrigerated; the rest you need to store, like any food product, in a cool, dry place. Avoid putting dietary supplements in a cabinet above the stove or refrigerator — true, the fridge is cold inside, but the motor pulsing away outside emits heat.

Choosing a sensible dose

Unless your doctor prescribes a dietary supplement as medicine, you don't need products marked "therapeutic," "extra-strength," or any variation thereof. Pick one that gives you no more than the RDA for any ingredient.

Avoiding hype

When the label promises something that's too good to be true — "Buy me! You'll live forever" — you know it's too good to be true. The NHPD doesn't permit supplement marketers to claim that their products cure or prevent disease (that would make them medicines that require premarket testing). But the office does allow claims that affect function, such as "maintains your cholesterol" (the no-no medical claim would be "lowers your cholesterol").

Another potential hype zone is the one labelled "natural," as in "natural vitamins are better." If you took Chem 101 in college, you know that the ascorbic acid (vitamin C) in oranges has exactly the same chemical composition as the ascorbic acid some nutritional chemist cooks up in her lab. But the ascorbic acid in a "natural" vitamin pill may come without additives such as colouring agents or fillers used in "regular" vitamin pills. In other words, if you aren't sensitive to the colouring agents or fillers in plain old pills, don't spend the extra dollars for "natural." If you are sensitive, do. What could be simpler? (For more on "natural" versus "synthetic" food ingredients, see Chapter 22.)

Nutrients for the 21st-century body

Hate taking pills? Bored with trying to get all the foods required to meet your nutritional needs? A vitamin company in New South Wales, Australia, has your back. Or should this be, your bottom? AussieBum "Essence" underwear is made with material impregnated with "micro-encapsulated organic substances" that stay functional for up to 15 washings, releasing antioxidant "dermo-protective oils" onto your skin. And they're on, yes, eBay! You can't make this stuff up.

Good Reasons for Getting Nutrients from Food Rather Than Supplements

This chapter focuses on the wonders of supplements, but here are the arguments in favour of healthy people getting all or most of their nutrients from food rather than supplements.

Cost

If you're willing to plan and prepare nutritious meals, you can almost always get your nutrients less expensively from fresh fruits, vegetables, whole grains, lower-fat dairy products, and lean meat, fish, and poultry. Besides, food usually tastes better than supplements.

Unexpected bonuses

Food is a package deal containing vitamins, minerals, protein, fat, carbohydrates, and fibre, plus a cornucopia of as-yet-unidentified substances called phytochemicals (phyto = plant, chemicals = well, chemicals) that may be vital to your continuing good health. Think of lycopene, the red pigment in tomatoes, which scientists recently showed reduces the risk of prostate cancer. Think of genistein and daidzein, the estrogen-like substances in soybeans, which appear to reduce your risk of heart disease. Who knows what else is hiding in your apples, peaches, pears, and plums? Do you want to be the only one on your block who misses out on these goodies? Of course not. For more about the benefits of phytochemicals, see Chapter 12.

Safety

Several common nutrients may be toxic when you scarf them down in *mega-dose servings* (amounts several times larger than the RDAs). Not only are large doses of vitamin A linked to birth defects, but they may also cause symptoms similar to a brain tumour. Niacin megadoses may cause liver damage. Megadoses of vitamin B6 may cause (temporary) damage to nerves in your arms, legs, fingers, and toes. All these effects are more likely to occur with supplements. Pills slip down easily, but regardless of how hungry you are, you probably won't eat enough food to reach toxic levels of nutrients. (To read more about the hazards of megadoses, see Chapters 10 and 11.)

The best statement about the role of supplements in good nutrition may be a paraphrase of Abraham Lincoln's famous remark about politicians and voters: "You can fool all the people some of the time, and some of the people all the time, but you cannot fool all the people all of the time." If Honest Abe were with us now and were a sensible nutritionist rather than president, he might amend his words: "Supplements are valuable for all people some of the time and for some people all the time, but they're probably not necessary for all people all the time."

Part II
What You Get from Food

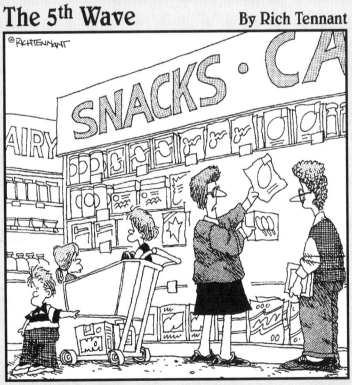

"I'm not actually buying this stuff, I'm just using it to hide the fruit, legumes and greens until we get checked out."

In this part . . .

Here's the lowdown on things you've heard about practically forever: protein, fat, carbohydrates, alcohol, vitamins, minerals, and water, with the absolutely newest numbers available on how much of what nutrients you need to keep your body humming happily.

This is a *For Dummies* book, so you don't have to read straight through from protein to water to see how things work. You can skip from chapter to chapter, back and forth, side to side. Any way you take it, this part is bound to clue you in to the value of the nutrients in food.

Chapter 6

Powerful Protein

· ·

· ·

*P*rotein is an essential nutrient whose name comes from the Greek word *protos,* which means "first." To visualize a molecule of protein, close your eyes and see a very long chain, rather like a strand of pearls. The individual pearls in the strand are *amino acids,* commonly known as the building blocks of protein. In addition to carbon, hydrogen, and oxygen atoms, amino acids contain a nitrogen (amino) group. The *amino group* is essential for synthesizing (assembling) specialized proteins in your body.

In this chapter, you can find out more — maybe even more than you ever wanted to know — about this molecule, how your body uses the proteins you take in as food, and how the body makes some special proteins you need for a healthy life.

Looking Inside and Out: Where Your Body Puts Protein

The human body is chock-full of proteins. Proteins are present in the outer and inner membranes of every living cell. Here's where else protein makes an appearance:

✔ Your hair, your nails, and the outer layers of your skin are made of a protein called keratin. Keratin is a *scleroprotein,* or a protein resistant to digestive enzymes. So if you bite your nails, you can't digest them.

✔ Muscle tissue contains myosin, actin, myoglobin, and a number of other proteins.

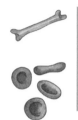

✔ Bone has plenty of protein. The outer part of bone is hardened with minerals such as calcium, but the basic, rubbery inner structure is protein; and bone marrow, the soft material inside the bone, also contains protein.

✔ Red blood cells contain *hemoglobin,* a protein compound that carries oxygen throughout the body. *Plasma,* the clear fluid in blood, contains fat and protein particles known as *lipoproteins,* which ferry cholesterol around and out of the body.

Putting Protein to Work: How Your Body Uses Protein

Your body uses proteins to build new cells, maintain tissues, and synthesize new proteins that make it possible for you to perform basic bodily functions.

About half the dietary protein you consume each day goes into making *enzymes,* the specialized worker proteins that do specific jobs such as digesting food and assembling or dividing molecules to make new cells and chemical substances. To perform these functions, enzymes often need specific vitamins and minerals.

Your ability to see, think, hear, and move — in fact, to do just about everything that you consider part of a healthy life — requires your nerve cells to send messages back and forth to each other and to other specialized kinds of cells, such as muscle cells. To send these messages, your body needs chemicals called *neurotransmitters.* To make neurotransmitters, your body needs — guess what — proteins.

Finally, proteins play an important part in the creation of every new cell and every new individual. Your chromosomes consist of *nucleoproteins,* which are substances made of amino acids and nucleic acids. See the "DNA/RNA" sidebar in this chapter for more information about nucleoproteins.

Packing Back the Protein: What Happens to the Proteins You Eat

The cells in your digestive tract can absorb only single amino acids or very small chains of two or three amino acids called *peptides.* So proteins from food are broken into their component amino acids by digestive enzymes —

which are, of course, specialized proteins. Then other enzymes in your body cells build new proteins by reassembling the amino acids into specific compounds that your body needs so it can function. This process is called *protein synthesis.* Most newly synthesized proteins your body uses come from the recycling of old proteins. During protein synthesis:

- Amino acids hook up with fats to form *lipoproteins,* the molecules that ferry cholesterol around and out of the body. Or amino acids may join up with carbohydrates to form the *glycoproteins* found in the mucus secreted by the digestive tract.

- Proteins combine with phosphoric acid to produce *phosphoproteins,* such as casein, a protein in milk.

- Nucleic acids combine with proteins to create *nucleoproteins,* which are essential components of the cell nucleus and of cytoplasm, the living material inside each cell.

After protein synthesis is complete, the leftover carbon, hydrogen, and oxygen are converted to glucose and used for energy (see Chapter 7). The nitrogen residue (ammonia) isn't used for energy. It's processed by the liver, which converts the ammonia to urea. Most of the urea produced in the liver is excreted through the kidneys in urine; very small amounts are sloughed off in skin, hair, and nails.

DNA/RNA

Nucleoproteins are chemicals in the nucleus of every living cell. They're made of proteins linked to *nucleic acids*— complex compounds that contain phosphoric acid, a sugar molecule, and nitrogen-containing molecules made from amino acids.

Nucleic acids (molecules found in the chromosomes and other structures in the centre of your cells) carry the genetic codes — genes that help determine what you look like, your general intelligence, and who you are. They contain one of two sugars, either *ribose* or *deoxyribose.* The nucleic acid containing ribose is called *ribonucleic acid* (RNA). The nucleic acid containing deoxyribose is called *deoxyribonucleic acid* (DNA).

DNA, a long molecule with two strands twisting about each other (the *double helix*), carries and transmits the genetic inheritance in your chromosomes. In other words, DNA supplies instructions that determine how your body cells are formed and how they behave. RNA, a single-strand molecule, is created in the cell nucleus according to the pattern determined by the DNA. Then RNA carries the DNA's instructions to the rest of the cell.

Knowing about DNA is important because it's the most distinctly "you" thing about your body. Chances that another person on Earth has exactly the same DNA as you are really small. That's why DNA analysis is used increasingly to identify criminals or exonerate the innocent. Some people are even proposing that parents store a sample of their children's DNA so that they'll have a conclusive way of identifying a missing child, even years later.

Your liver can produce only about 80 percent of the protein your body needs, so you have to include enough proteins in your diet to maintain your protein status. If you don't, your body starts digesting the proteins in your muscles — and in extreme cases in your heart muscle.

Examining Protein Types: Not All Proteins Are Created Equal

All proteins are made of building blocks called amino acids, but not all proteins contain all the amino acids you require. This section helps you figure out how you can get the most useful proteins from your varied diet.

Essential and nonessential proteins

To make all the proteins your body needs, you require 20 different amino acids. Ten are considered *essential,* which means you can't synthesize them in your body and must obtain them from food (two of these, arginine and histidine, are essential only for children). Several more are *nonessential:* If you don't get them in food, you can manufacture them yourself from fats, carbohydrates, and other amino acids. Two — glutamine and taurine — are somewhere in between essential and nonessential for human beings and are referred to as *semi-essential:* They're essential only under certain conditions, such as injury or disease.

Essential Amino Acids	*Nonessential Amino Acids*
Arginine*	Alanine
Histidine*	Asparagine
Isoleucine	Aspartate
Leucine	Cysteine
Lysine	Glutamate
Methionine	Glutamine
Phenlyalanine	Glycine
Threonine	Proline
Tryptophan	Serine
Valine	Tyrosine

*Essential for children; nonessential for adults

Super soy: The special protein food

Nutrition fact No. 1: Food from animals has complete proteins. **Nutrition fact No. 2:** Vegetables, fruits, and grains have incomplete proteins. **Nutrition fact No. 3:** Nobody told the soybean.

Unlike other vegetables, including other beans, soybeans have complete proteins with sufficient amounts of all the amino acids essential to human health. In fact, food experts rank soy proteins on par with egg whites and casein (the protein in milk), the two proteins easiest for your body to absorb and use (see Table 6-1).

Some nutritionists think soy proteins are even better than the proteins in eggs and milk, because the proteins in soy come with no cholesterol and very little of the saturated fat known to clog your arteries and raise the risk of heart attack. Better yet, more than 20 recent studies suggest that adding soy foods to your diet can actually lower your cholesterol levels.

There are 14 grams of protein in 125 mL (1/2 cup) of cooked soybeans; 112 grams (4 ounces) of tofu has 13 grams of protein. Either serving gives you approximately twice the protein you get from one large egg or one 250 mL (8-ounce) glass of skim milk, or two-thirds the protein in 84 grams (3 ounces) of lean ground beef. In 250 mL (8 ounces) of fat-free soy milk there are 7 grams of protein — a mere 1 gram less than a similar serving of skim milk — and no cholesterol. Soybeans are also jam-packed with dietary fibre, which helps move food through your digestive tract.

In fact, soybeans are such a good source of food fibre that caution is advised. Take it slow — a little today, a little more tomorrow, and a little bit more the day after that.

High-quality and low-quality proteins

Because an animal's body is similar to yours, its proteins contain similar combinations of amino acids. That's why nutritionists call proteins from foods of animal origin — meat, fish, poultry, eggs, and dairy products — *high-quality proteins* or *complete proteins.* Your body absorbs these proteins more efficiently; they can be used to synthesize other proteins without making much waste. The proteins from plants — grains, fruit, vegetables, legumes (beans), nuts, and seeds — often have limited amounts of some amino acids, which means their nutritional content is not as high as that of animal proteins. These often are referred to as *incomplete proteins.*

The basic standard against which you measure the value of proteins in food is the egg. Nutrition scientists have arbitrarily given the egg a *biological value* of 100 percent, meaning that, gram for gram, it's the food with the best supply of complete proteins. Other foods that have proportionately more protein may not be as valuable as the egg because they lack sufficient amounts of one or more essential amino acids.

Hemp protein: The new kid on the block

Although hemp foods come from the same plant species as marijuana *(Cannabis sativa l.)*, the amount of THC (tetrahydrocannabinol), the psychoactive component, present in hemp is so insignificant that it is considered to be free of it.

Hemp has been around as a food for awhile as hemp seed nut (hemp seeds that resemble tiny nuts), hemp seed nut butter (ground hemp seeds), and hemp seed oil. Now you can get hemp in the form of a protein powder. Hemp protein powder has been getting a lot of attention lately as a very competitive protein source because it contains all the essential amino acids, making it a complete protein (see "High-quality and low-quality proteins" for more about complete proteins). Hemp protein powder is made by pressing hemp seeds to expel the oil, leaving behind a dry "cake." This cake is then sifted and milled at low temperatures. This process helps to remove some of the coarser plant fibre and produces a concentrated form of protein.

Not only is hemp protein complete (making it a vegetarian source of essential amino acids), unlike other plant proteins (except for soy), hemp protein can also supply a significant amount of naturally occurring antioxidants, vitamins, minerals, fibre, and chlorophyll. Hemp is also gluten free, making it suitable for anyone with celiac disease or wheat sensitivities. Hemp also has the unique advantage of an ideal three-to-one balance of omega-6 to omega-3 essential fatty acids (see Chapter 7 for more about fatty acids). This ratio is thought to promote long-term well-being by decreasing the risk of many chronic diseases. Hemp is also a good source of the fatty acid known as gamma-linolenic acid (GLA), an omega-6 fat with anti-inflammatory properties.

For example, eggs are 11 percent protein, and dry beans are 22 percent protein. However, the proteins in beans don't provide sufficient amounts of *all* the essential amino acids, so the proteins in the beans are not as nutritionally complete as the proteins from animal foods. The prime exception is the soybean, a legume that's packed with abundant amounts of all the amino acids essential for adults. Soybeans are an excellent source of proteins for vegetarians, especially *vegans* — vegetarians who avoid all products of animal origin, including milk and eggs.

The term used to describe the value of the proteins in any one food is *amino acid score*. Because the egg contains all the essential amino acids, it scores 100. Table 6-1 shows the protein quality of representative foods relative to the egg.

Table 6-1	Scoring the Amino Acids in Food	
Food	*Protein Content (Grams)*	*Amino Acid Score (Compared to the Egg)*
Egg	33	100
Fish	61	100
Beef	29	100

Food	Protein Content (Grams)	Amino Acid Score (Compared to the Egg)
Milk (cow's whole)	23	100
Soybeans	29	100
Dry beans	22	75
Rice	7	62–66
Corn	7	47
Wheat	13	50
Wheat (white flour)	12	36

Nutritive Value of Foods (Washington, D.C.: U.S. Department of Agriculture, 1991); George M. Briggs and Doris Howes Calloway, Nutrition and Physical Fitness, 11th ed. (New York: Holt, Rinehart and Winston, 1984)

Complete proteins and incomplete proteins

Another way to describe the quality of proteins is to say that they're either complete or incomplete. A *complete protein* contains ample amounts of all essential amino acids; an *incomplete protein* does not. A protein low in one specific amino acid is called a *limiting protein* because it can build only as much tissue as the smallest amount of the necessary amino acid. You can improve the protein quality in a food containing incomplete/limiting proteins by eating a variety of proteins throughout the day.

Homocysteine and your heart

Homocysteine is an *intermediate,* a chemical released when you metabolize (digest) protein. Unlike other amino acids, which are vital to your health, homocysteine can be hazardous to your heart, raising your risk of heart disease: It attacks cells in the lining of your arteries by making them reproduce more quickly (the extra cells may block your coronary arteries) or by causing your blood to clot (ditto).

Years and years ago, before cholesterol moved to centre stage, some smart heart researchers labelled homocysteine the major nutritional culprit in heart disease. Today, they've been vindicated. The American Heart Association cites high homocysteine levels as an independent probable (but not major) risk factor for heart disease, perhaps explaining why some people with low cholesterol have heart attacks.

But wait! The good news is that information from several studies, including the Harvard/Brigham and Women's Hospital Nurses' Health Study in Boston, suggests that a diet rich in the B vitamin folate lowers blood levels of homocysteine. Most fruits, vegetables, and whole grains have plentiful amounts of folate. Stock up on them — they could protect your heart.

The lowdown on gelatin and your fingernails

Everyone knows gelatin is protein that strengthens fingernails. Too bad everyone's wrong. Gelatin is produced by treating animal bones with acid, a process that destroys the essential amino acid tryptophan. Surprise: Bananas are high in tryptophan. Slicing bananas onto your gelatin increases the quality of the protein. Adding milk makes it even better, but that still may not heal your splitting nails. The fastest way to a cure is a visit to the dermatologist, who can tell you whether the problem is an allergy to nail polish, too much time spent washing dishes, a medical problem such as a fungal infection, or just plain peeling nails. Then the dermatologist may prescribe a different nail polish (or none at all), protective gloves, a fungicide (a drug that wipes out fungi), or a lotion product to strengthen the natural glue that holds the layers of your nails together.

Until recently, nutrition experts thought you had to eat the two incomplete proteins in the same meal — for example, beans with rice. Rice has adequate amounts of methionine but lacks lysine. Beans have plenty of lysine but are low in methionine. When you eat any protein, its amino acids enter a reservoir called the *amino acid pool,* and your body can draw on the pool to build new proteins. As long as you eat a variety of foods throughout the day, the amino acids go into this pool, and your body can get what it needs when it needs it.

Here are some foods with incomplete proteins:

- **Grain foods:** Barley, bread, bulgur wheat, cornmeal, kasha, and pancakes
- **Legumes:** Black beans, black-eyed peas, fava beans, kidney beans, lima beans, lentils, peanut butter, peanuts, peas, split peas, and white beans
- **Nuts and seeds:** Almonds, Brazil nuts, cashews, pecans, walnuts, pumpkin seeds, sesame seeds (tahini), and sunflower seeds

In order for the foods to complement each other, they must be consumed throughout the day, and eaten consistently, day after day.

Deciding How Much Protein You Need

The National Academy of Sciences Food and Nutrition Board, which sets the requirements (for example, RDAs) for vitamins and minerals, also sets goals for daily protein consumption. As it does with other nutrients, the board has different recommendations for different groups of people: young or old, men or women.

Calculating the correct amount

As a general rule, the National Academy of Sciences says healthy people need to get 10 to 35 percent of their daily calories from protein. More specifically, the Academy has set a Dietary Reference Intake (DRI) of 45 grams of protein per day for a healthy woman, and 52 grams per day for a healthy man. (Check out Chapter 4 for a complete explanation of the DRI.)

You can get these amounts easily from two 21-gram servings of lean meat, fish, or poultry (3 ounces each). Vegetarians can get their protein from two eggs (12–16 grams), two slices of prepacked fat-free cheese (10 grams), four slices of bread (3 grams each), and one cup of yogurt (10 grams).

As you grow older, you synthesize new proteins less efficiently, so your muscle mass (protein tissue) diminishes while your fat content stays the same or rises. This change is why some folks erroneously believe that muscle "turns to fat" in old age. Of course, you still use protein to build new tissue, including hair, skin, and nails, which continue to grow until you cross over into The Great Beyond. By the way, the idea that nails continue to grow after death — a staple of shock movies and horror comics — arises from the fact that after death, tissue around the nails shrinks, making a corpse's nails simply look longer. Who else would let you in on these secrets?

Dodging protein deficiency

The first sign of protein deficiency is likely to be weak muscles — the body tissue most reliant on protein. For example, children who do not get enough protein have shrunken, weak muscles. They may also have thin hair, their skin may be covered with sores, and tests may show that the level of albumin in their blood is below normal. *Albumin* is a protein that helps the body maintain its fluid balance, keeping a proper amount of liquid in and around body cells.

A protein deficiency may also show up in your blood. Red blood cells live for only 120 days. Protein is needed to produce new ones. People who do not get enough protein may become *anemic,* having fewer red blood cells than they need. Protein deficiency may also show up as fluid retention (the big belly on a starving child), hair loss, and muscle wasting, all caused by the body's attempt to protect itself by digesting the proteins in its own muscle tissue. That's why victims of starvation are, literally, skin and bones.

Given the high protein content of a normal Canadian diet (which generally provides far more protein than you require), protein deficiency is rare in Canada except as a consequence of eating disorders such as *anorexia nervosa* (refusal to eat) and *bulimia* (regurgitation after meals). Protein deficiency also sometimes occurs in elderly people who have lost their appetite for a variety of reasons, or who do not have enough money to buy adequate amounts of food.

Boosting your protein intake: Special considerations

Anyone who's building new tissue quickly needs extra protein. For example, the Dietary Reference Intake for protein for women who are pregnant or nursing is 71 grams per day. Injuries also raise your protein requirements. An injured body releases above-normal amounts of protein-destroying hormones from the pituitary and adrenal glands. You need extra protein to protect existing tissues, and after severe blood loss, you need extra protein to make new hemoglobin for red blood cells. Cuts, burns, and surgical procedures mean you need extra protein to make new skin and muscle cells. Fractures mean extra protein is needed to make new bone. The need for protein is so important when you've been badly injured that if you can't take protein by mouth, you'll be given an intravenous solution of amino acids with glucose (sugar) or emulsified fat.

Do athletes need more proteins than the rest of us? Recent research suggests that the answer may be yes, but athletes easily meet their requirements eating more.

Avoiding protein overload

Yes, you can get too much protein. Several medical conditions make it difficult for people to digest and process proteins properly. As a result, waste products build up in different parts of the body.

People with liver disease or kidney disease either don't process protein efficiently into urea or don't excrete it efficiently through urine. The result may be uric acid kidney stones or *uremic poisoning* (an excess amount of uric acid in the blood). The pain associated with *gout* (a form of arthritis that affects nine men for every one woman) is caused by uric acid crystals collecting in the spaces around joints. Doctors may recommend a low-protein diet as part of the treatment in these situations.

Chapter 7

The Lowdown on Fat and Cholesterol

*T*he chemical family name for fats and related compounds such as choles-terol is *lipids* (from *lipos,* the Greek word for fat). Liquid fats are called *oils;* solid fats are called, well, *fat.* With the exception of *cholesterol* (a fatty substance that has no calories and provides no energy), fats are high-energy nutrients. Gram for gram, fats have more than twice as much energy potential (calories) as protein and carbohydrates (affectionately referred to as *carbs*): 9 calories per gram for fat versus 4 calories per gram for proteins and carbs. (For more calorie facts, see Chapter 3.)

In this chapter, we cut the fat away from the subject of fats and zero in on the essential facts you need to put together a diet with just enough fat (yes, you do need fat) to provide the bounce that every diet requires. And then we deal with that ultimate baddie — cholesterol. Surprise! You need some of that, too. Onward.

Finding the Facts about Fat Stuff

Fats are sources of energy that add flavour to food — the sizzle on the steak, you could say. However, as anyone who's spent the past 30 years on planet Earth knows, fats may also be hazardous to your health. The trick is to sepa-rate the good from the bad. Trust us. It can be done. And this section explains how.

Understanding how your body uses fat

Here's a sentence you probably never thought you'd read: A healthy body needs fat. Your body uses *dietary fat* (the fat you get from food) to make tissue and manufacture biochemicals, such as hormones. Some of the body fat made from food fat is *visible*. Even though your skin covers it, you can *see* the fat in the *adipose* (fatty) *tissue* in female breasts, hips, thighs, buttocks, and belly, or male abdomen and shoulders.

This visible body fat

- ✔ Provides a source of stored energy
- ✔ Gives shape to your body
- ✔ Cushions your skin (imagine sitting in a chair for a while to read this book without your buttocks to pillow your bones)
- ✔ Acts as an insulation blanket that reduces heat loss

Other body fat is invisible. You can't see it because it's tucked away in and around your internal organs. This hidden fat is

- ✔ Part of every cell membrane (the outer skin that holds each cell together)
- ✔ A component of *myelin,* the fatty material that sheathes nerve cells and lets them fire the electrical messages so you can think, see, speak, move, and perform the multitude of tasks natural to a living body; a component of brain tissue
- ✔ A shock absorber that protects your organs (as much as possible) if you fall or are injured
- ✔ A constituent of hormones and other biochemicals, such as vitamin D and bile

Pulling energy from fat

Although fat has more energy (calories) per gram than proteins and carbohydrates, your body has a more difficult time pulling the energy out of fatty foods. Imagine a chain of long balloons — the kind people twist into shapes that resemble dachshunds, flowers, and other amusing things. When you drop one of these balloons into water, it floats. That's exactly what happens when you swallow fat-rich foods. The fat floats on top of the watery food-and-liquid mixture in your stomach, which limits the effect that *lipases* — fat-busting digestive enzymes in the mix below — can have on it. Because fat is digested more slowly than proteins and carbohydrates, you feel fuller (a condition called *satiety*) longer after eating high-fat food.

Into the intestines

When the fat moves down your digestive tract into your small intestine, an intestinal hormone called *cholestokinin* beeps your gallbladder, signalling for the release of bile. *Bile* is an emulsifier, a substance that enables fat to mix with water so that lipases can start breaking the fat into glycerol and fatty acids. These smaller fragments may be stored in special cells (fat cells) in adipose tissue, or they may be absorbed into cells in the intestinal wall, where one of the following happens:

- ✔ They're combined with oxygen (or burned) to produce heat/energy, water, and the waste product carbon dioxide.
- ✔ They're used to make lipoproteins that haul fats, including cholesterol, through your bloodstream.

Into the body

Glucose, the molecule you get by digesting carbohydrates, and fat are the body's basic sources of energy. To get energy, your body burns glucose and fat at the same time, but uses one or the other more as a source of fuel depending on the activity level. When you're sleeping, sitting, or walking, your body is using more fat as fuel. As the intensity of the activity increases, like when you go for a jog or run, your body uses more glucose as fuel. This is because you can get energy faster and more easily by burning glucose.

The first step in burning body fat is for an enzyme in your fat cells to break up stored triglycerides (the form of fat in adipose tissue). The enzyme action releases glycerol and fatty acids, which travel through your blood to body cells, where they combine with oxygen to produce heat/energy, plus water — lots of water — and the waste product carbon dioxide.

As anyone who has used a high-protein/high-fat/low-carb weight-loss diet such as the Atkins regimen can tell you, in addition to all that water, burning fat without glucose produces a second waste product called ketones. In extreme cases, high concentrations of ketones (a condition known as *ketosis*) alter the acid/alkaline balance (or pH) of your blood and may trip you into a coma. Left untreated, ketosis can lead to death. Medically, this condition is most common among people with diabetes. For people on a low-carb diet, the more likely sign of ketosis is stinky urine or breath that smells like acetone (nail polish remover).

Focusing on the fats in food

Food contains three kinds of fats: triglycerides, phospholipids, and sterols. Here's how they differ:

- **Triglycerides:** You use these fats to make adipose tissue, and you burn them for energy.

- **Phospholipids:** These are hybrids — part lipid, part phosphate (a molecule made with the mineral phosphorus) — that act as tiny rowboats, ferrying hormones and fat-soluble vitamins A, D, E, and K through your blood and back and forth in the watery fluid that flows across cell membranes. (By the way, the official name for fluid around cells is *extracellular fluid.* Thus the description "watery fluid.")

- **Sterols (steroid alcohols):** These are fat and alcohol compounds with no calories. Vitamin D is a sterol. So is the sex hormone testosterone. And so is cholesterol, the base on which your body builds hormones and vitamins.

Getting the right amount of fat

Getting the right amount of fat in your diet is a delicate balancing act. Too much, and you increase your risk of obesity, diabetes, heart disease, and some forms of cancer. (The risk of colon cancer seems to be related to fat from meat rather than fat from dairy products.) Too little fat, and infants don't thrive, children don't grow, and everyone, regardless of age, is unable to absorb and use fat-soluble vitamins that smooth the skin, protect vision, bolster the immune system, and keep reproductive organs functioning.

In the fall of 2002, the Institute of Medicine (IOM) recommended that no more than 20 to 35 percent of daily calories should come from fat. On a 2,000-calories-a-day diet, that's 400 to 900 calories from fats.

Because your body doesn't need to get saturated fats, cholesterol, or trans fats from food, the IOM and Health Canada say, "Keep them as low as possible, please."

This advice about fat intake is primarily for adults. Infants and toddlers require fatty acids for proper physical growth and mental development, and they need the extra energy for growth — that's why Mother Nature made human breast milk (see Chapter 28) so high in fatty acids. Never limit the fat in your baby's diet without checking first with your pediatrician.

Essential fatty acids

An *essential fatty acid* is one that your body needs but cannot assemble from other fats. You have to get it whole, from food. Linoleic acid, found in vegetable oils, is an essential fatty acid. Two others — linolenic acid and arachidonic acid — occupy a somewhat ambiguous position. You can't make them from scratch, but you can make them if you have enough linoleic acid on hand, so food scientists can work up a good fight about whether linolenic and arachidonic acids are "essential." In practical terms, who cares? Linoleic acid is so widely available in food, you're unlikely to experience a deficiency (unless you restrict your fat intake too much) of any of the three — linoleic, linolenic, or arachidonic acids — as long as 2 percent of the calories you get each day come from fat.

In 2002, the IOM published the first daily recommendations for two essential fatty acids, alpha-linolenic acid and linoleic acid. The first is an omega-3 fatty acid (more about that later on in this chapter) that's abundant in rapeseed (canola), soybean, flaxseed, perilla, white chia (salba), and hemp, as well as walnuts. The second is an omega-6 fatty acid (ditto) that's abundant in safflower, sunflower, peanut oil, and corn oil. The IOM recommends that

- ✔ Women get 12 grams of linoleic acid and 1.1 grams of alpha-linolenic acid per day
- ✔ Men get 17 grams of linoleic acid and 1.6 grams of alpha-linolenic acid per day

Finding fat in all kinds of foods

As a general rule:

- ✔ Fruits and vegetables have only traces of fat, primarily unsaturated fatty acids.
- ✔ Grains have small amounts of fat, up to 3 percent of their total weight.
- ✔ Dairy products vary. Cream is a high-fat food. Regular milks and cheeses are moderately high in fat. Skim milk and skim milk products are low-fat foods. Most of the fats in dairy products are saturated fatty acids.
- ✔ Meat is moderately high in fat, and most of its fats are saturated fatty acids.
- ✔ Poultry (chicken and turkey), without the skin, is relatively low in fat.
- ✔ Fish may be high or low in fat, primarily unsaturated fatty acids that — lucky for the fish — remain liquid even when the fish is swimming in cold water. (Unsaturated fats don't harden when cooled.)
- ✔ Vegetable oils, butter, and lard are high-fat foods. Most of the fatty acids in vegetable oils are unsaturated; most of the fatty acids in lard and butter are saturated.
- ✔ Processed foods, such as cakes, breads, canned or frozen meats, and vegetable dishes, are generally higher in fat than plain grains, meats, fruits, and vegetables.

A nutritional fish story

When Sir William Gilbert, lyricist to songsmith Sir Arthur Sullivan, wrote, "Here's a pretty kettle of fish!" he may well have been talking about the latest skinny on seafood.

The good news from a 2002 Harvard survey of more than 43,000 male health professionals shows that the ones who eat 85 grams to 140 grams (3 to 5 ounces) of fish just once a month have a 40 percent lower risk of *ischemic stroke,* a stroke caused by a blood clot in a cranial artery. The Harvard study did not include women, but a report on women and stroke published in the *Journal of the American Medical Association* in 2000 says that women who eat about 115 grams (4 ounces) of fish — think one small can of tuna — two to four times a week appear to cut their risk of stroke by a similar 40 percent.

These benefits are, in large part, because of the presence of unique forms of omega-3 fatty acids, *eicosapentaenoic acid (EPA)* and *docosahexaenoic acid (DHA),* which are unsaturated fatty acids found most commonly in fatty fish such as salmon and sardines. EPA and DHA, which nutritionists know as *eicosanoids,* have been associated with many health-promoting benefits such as reduced inflammation, decreased rates of depression, protection from blood clots, better overall blood vessel health, and lower rates of age-related dementia. One 85 gram (3 ounce) serving of Alaskan Red salmon has about 280 mg of EPA and 1,420 mg DHA.

Fish aren't the only sources for eicosanoids, but they're the best ones. Your body is capable of producing EPA and DHA through the conversion of alpha-linolenic acid (ALA), another omega-3 fatty acid. ALA is found in plant oils such as flaxseed oil. Unfortunately, the human body isn't able to wring much EPA and DHA out of ALA; scientists estimate that the conversion of ALA to EPA and DHA is as low as 3 to 10 percent. We need ALA for our health, but we don't require very much — 1.1 grams per day for women and 1.6 grams per day for men. That's not enough ALA to produce EPA or DHA in any beneficial quantities.

Because of the many benefits of EPA and DHA and because of the biological requirement for ALA, it's best to eat a variety of foods that will provide these fats in appropriate amounts so you can get the most benefits from these healthy fats. See the list below for the best food sources.

You can find respectable amounts of omega-3s in

- Anchovies
- Haddock
- Herring
- Mackerel
- Salmon
- Sardines
- Scallops
- Tuna (albacore)
- Broccoli
- Kale
- Spinach
- Soybeans
- Soybean oil
- Canola oil
- Walnuts
- Walnut oil
- Flaxseed, ground
- Flaxseed oil
- Perilla oil
- White chia (salba) seed
- Hemp seed
- Hemp seed oil

Consumer Alert No. 1

Before you shout, "Waiter! Bring me the salmon, mackerel, herring, or whatever," here's the other side of the coin. Earlier research suggests that frequent servings of fish may increase the risk of a stroke caused by bleeding in the brain. This situation is common among Inuit who eat plenty of fish and have a higher than normal incidence of hemorrhagic, or bleeding, strokes. True, the Harvard study found no significant link between fish consumption and bleeding strokes, but researchers say more studies are needed to nail down the relationship — or lack thereof.

Consumer Alert No. 2

Not all omegas are equally beneficial. Omega-6 fatty acids — polyunsaturated fats found in beef, pork, and several vegetable oils, including corn, sunflower, cottonseed, soybean, peanut, and sesame — are chemical cousins of omega-3s, but the omega-6s lack the benefits of the omega-3s.

Consumer Alert No. 3

Wait! Don't go just yet. Despite all the benefits fish bring to a healthful diet, there have been some concerns lately about the amount of mercury in fish, and whether the levels of mercury in certain fish are dangerous to human health. The research doesn't show if the amount of mercury found in our food supply is a problem. Nevertheless, Health Canada has established a guideline level of 0.5 parts per million (ppm) for mercury in most commercial fish. Health Canada advises pregnant women, women of child-bearing age, and young children to limit their intake of certain fish. You can find information on Health Canada's Web site (www.hc-sc.gc.ca). As well, you can download a pocket guide from Sustainable Seafood Canada (www.seachoice.org). This handy guide helps you make ethically and environmentally sound choices when it comes to getting more fish in your diet.

Now it's really a pretty kettle of fish!

Here's a simple guide to finding which foods are high (or low) in fat. Oils are virtually 100 percent fat. Butter and lard are close behind. After that, the fat level drops, from 70 percent for some nuts down to 2 percent for most bread. The rule to take away from these numbers? A diet high in grains and plants always is lower in fat than a diet high in meat and oils.

Fatty acids and dietary fat

Fatty acids are the building blocks of fats. Chemically speaking, a *fatty acid* is a chain of carbon atoms with hydrogen atoms attached and a *carbon-oxygen-oxygen-hydrogen group* (the unit that makes it an acid) at one end.

All the fats in food are combinations of fatty acids. Nutritionists characterize fatty acids as saturated, monounsaturated, or polyunsaturated, depending on how many hydrogen atoms are attached to the carbon atoms in the chain. The more hydrogen atoms, the more saturated the fatty acid. Depending on which fatty acids predominate, a food fat is likewise characterized as saturated, monounsaturated, or polyunsaturated.

- ✔ A *saturated fat,* such as butter, has mostly saturated fatty acids. Saturated fats are solid at room temperature and get harder when chilled.

- ✔ A *monounsaturated fat,* such as olive oil, has mostly monounsaturated fatty acids. Monounsaturated fats are liquid at room temperature; they get thicker when chilled.

- ✔ A *polyunsaturated fat,* such as corn oil, has mostly polyunsaturated fatty acids. Polyunsaturated fats are liquid at room temperature; they stay liquid when chilled.

Exploring the chemical structure of fatty acids

If you don't have a clue about the chemical structure of fatty acids, reading this explanation may be worth your while. The concepts are simple, and the information you find here applies to all kinds of molecules, not just fatty acids.

Molecules are groups of atoms hooked together by chemical bonds. Different atoms form different numbers of bonds with other atoms. For example, a hydrogen atom can form one bond with one other atom; an oxygen atom can form two bonds with other atoms; and a carbon atom can form four bonds with other atoms.

To see how this works, visualize a carbon atom as one of those round pieces in a child's Erector set or Tinkertoy kit. Your carbon atom (C) has — figuratively speaking, of course — four holes: one on top, one on the bottom, and one on each side. If you stick a peg into each hole and attach a small piece of wood representing a hydrogen atom (H) to the pegs on the top, the bottom, and the left, you have a structure that looks like this:

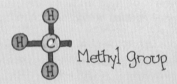

This unit, called a *methyl group,* is the first piece in any fatty acid. To build the rest of the fatty acid, you add carbon atoms and hydrogen atoms to form a chain. At the end, you tack on a group with one carbon atom, two oxygen atoms, and a hydrogen atom. This group is called an *acid group,* and it's the part that makes the chain of carbon and hydrogen atoms a fatty acid.

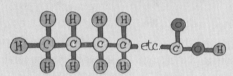

Saturated Fatty Acid

The preceding molecule is a *saturated fatty acid* because it has a hydrogen atom at every available carbon link in the chain. A *monounsaturated fatty acid* drops two hydrogen atoms and forms one double bond (two lines instead of one) between two carbon atoms. A *polyunsaturated fatty acid* drops more hydrogen atoms and forms several (poly) double bonds between several carbon atoms. Every hydrogen atom still forms one bond, and every carbon atom still forms four bonds, but they do so in a slightly different way. These sketches are not pictures of real fatty acids, which have many more carbons in the chain and have their double bonds in different places, but they can give you an idea of what fatty acids look like up close.

Instead of this: You get this:

(a saturated fatty acid)   (a monounsaturated fatty acid)

or

(a polyunsaturated fatty acid)

And that's the whole deal!

So why is margarine, which is made from unsaturated fats such as corn and soybean oil, a solid? First-generation margarines (and some poorer quality ones today) were artificially saturated by food chemists who added hydrogen atoms to unsaturated fatty acids. This process, known as *hydrogenation,* turns an oil, such as corn oil, into a solid fat, which can be used in products such as margarines without leaking out all over the table. The once-liquid oils were turned into shortening, chemically very similar to beef lard or pork suet. A fatty acid with extra hydrogen atoms is called a *hydrogenated fatty acid.* Vegetable oils that have been partially hydrogenated produce trans fatty acids. *Trans fatty acids* are not healthy for your heart. Because of those darned extra hydrogen atoms, they are, well, more saturated. Although not all saturated fats are bad for your heart, some are known for clogging arteries and raising the levels of cholesterol in your blood, mostly by raising the LDL cholesterol. Trans fats are a double threat because they raise the LDL cholesterol (the so-called "bad" cholesterol) *and* they lower the HDL (or "good") cholesterol. Because it would be too time-consuming to worry about which saturated fats raise cholesterol the most, it just makes sense to try to limit your overall intake of all saturated fats. To make it easier for you to control your saturated and trans fat intake, Health Canada has added a new line on the Nutritional Facts label that tells you exactly how many grams of trans fats are in any product you buy.

Margarine fans needn't despair, however. The same smart food chemists who invented hydrogenation have come up with trans fat–free margarines and spreads. These softer margarines are formulated to be spreadable and are very low in saturated fat, so they're appropriate for your heart-healthy diet.

Table 7-1 shows the kinds of fatty acids found in some common dietary fats and oils. Fats are characterized according to their predominant fatty acids. For example, as you can plainly see in the table, nearly 25 percent of the fatty acids in corn oil are monounsaturated fatty acids. Nevertheless, because corn oil has more polyunsaturated fatty acid, it's considered a polyunsaturated fatty acid. Note for math majors: Some of the totals in Table 7-1 don't add up to 100 percent because these fats and oils also contain other kinds of fatty acids in amounts so small that they don't affect the basic character of the fat.

Table 7-1	What Fatty Acids Are in That Fat or Oil?			
Fat or Oil	*Saturated Fatty Acid (%)*	*Monounsaturated Fatty Acid (%)*	*Polyunsaturated Fatty Acid (%)*	*Kind of Fat or Oil*
Canola oil	7	53	22	Monounsaturated
Corn oil	13	24	59	Polyunsaturated
Olive oil	14	74	9	Monounsaturated

(continued)

Table 7-1 *(continued)*

Fat or Oil	Saturated Fatty Acid (%)	Monounsatu-rated Fatty Acid (%)	Polyunsatu-rated Fatty Acid (%)	Kind of Fat or Oil
Palm oil	52	38	10	Saturated
Peanut oil	17	46	32	Monounsaturated
Safflower oil	9	12	74	Polyunsaturated
Soybean oil	15	23	51	Polyunsaturated
Soybean-cottonseed oil	18	29	48	Polyunsaturated
Butter	62	30	5	Saturated
Lard	39	45	11	Saturated*

Because more than one-third of its fats are saturated, nutritionists label lard a saturated fat. Nutritive Value of Foods (Washington, D.C.: U.S. Department of Agriculture); Food and Life (New York: American Council on Science and Health)

Considering Cholesterol and You

We mention earlier in this chapter that your body actually *needs* fat, and here's another sentence that may blow your (nutritional) mind: Every healthy body *needs* cholesterol. Look carefully and you find cholesterol in and around your cells, in your fatty tissue, in your organs, and in your glands. What's it doing there? Plenty of useful things. For example, cholesterol

✔ Protects the integrity of cell membranes

✔ Helps enable nerve cells to send messages back and forth

✔ Is a building block for vitamin D (a sterol), made when sunlight hits the fat just under your skin (for more about vitamin D, see Chapter 10)

✔ Enables your gallbladder to make *bile acids,* digestive chemicals that, in turn, enable you to absorb fats and fat-soluble nutrients such as vitamin A, vitamin D, vitamin E, and vitamin K

✔ Is a base on which you build steroid hormones such as estrogen and testosterone

Cholesterol season

Even if you allow yourself to indulge in (a few) high–saturated fat foods like ice cream cones, doughnuts, and burgers every day of the year, your cholesterol level may still be naturally lower in the summer than in the winter.

The basis for this intriguing culinary conclusion is the 2004 University of Massachusetts SEASONS (Seasonal Variation in Blood Lipids) Study of 517 healthy men and women ages 20 to 70. The volunteers started out with an average cholesterol level of 5.5 mmol/L (women) and 5.77 mmol/L (men). A series of five blood tests during the one-year study showed an average drop of 2 percent in the summer for men and 2.6 percent for women. People with high cholesterol (more than 6.2 mmol/L) did better, dropping as much as 7.5 percent in the summer.

U. Mass cardiologists say one explanation for the summer downswing may be the normal increase in human blood volume in hot weather. Cholesterol levels reflect the total amount of cholesterol in your bloodstream. With more blood in the stream, the amount of cholesterol per litre declines, producing a lower total cholesterol reading. A second possibility is that people tend to eat less and be more active in summer. They lose weight, and weight loss equals lower cholesterol.

The first bit of wisdom from this study is obvious: Being physically active reduces your cholesterol level. The second is that environment matters. In other words, if you're planning to start a new cholesterol-buster diet, you may just do better to start during the cool weather, when your efforts may lower your total cholesterol as much as 5 percent over a reasonable period of time, say, six months. Then, when your doctor runs a follow-up test the following summer, you'll get the added benefit of the seasonal slip to make you feel really, really good about how well you're doing. And there's this: For more on controlling your cholesterol, zip out and get yourself a copy of (what else?) *Controlling Cholesterol For Dummies* (Wiley, 2002).

Cholesterol and heart disease

Doctors measure your cholesterol level by taking a sample of blood and counting the millimoles of cholesterol in one litre of blood. When you get your annual report from the doctor, your total cholesterol level looks something like this: 4.9 mmol/L. Translation: You have 4.9 millimoles of cholesterol in every one litre of blood. Why does this matter? Because cholesterol makes its way into blood vessels, sticks to the walls, and forms deposits that eventually block the flow of blood. The more cholesterol you have floating in your blood, the more cholesterol is likely to cross into your arteries, where it may increase your risk of heart attack or stroke.

As a general rule, the Canadian Guidelines for the management of and treatment of cholesterol say that for adults, a cholesterol level higher than 5.2 mmol/L is a risk factor for cardiovascular disease. However, cholesterol is only one risk factor, and you need to know your total risk assessment profile before you focus on just one number, so read on.

Cholesterol levels alone are not the entire story. Some people with high cholesterol levels live to a ripe old age, and those with low cholesterol levels can develop heart disease. Worse yet, recent research indicates that low cholesterol levels may increase the risk of stroke. In other words, cholesterol is only one of several risk factors for heart disease. Here are some more:

- ✔ An unfavourable ratio of lipoproteins (see the following section)
- ✔ Smoking
- ✔ Obesity
- ✔ Diabetes
- ✔ Hypertension (high blood pressure)
- ✔ Age (being older is riskier)
- ✔ Sex (being male is riskier)
- ✔ A family history of heart disease

To estimate your risk of heart disease or heart attack, check out the Heart and Stroke Foundation's heart attack and stroke assessment at `ww2.heartand stroke.ca/hs_risk.asp`.

Living with lipoproteins

A *lipoprotein* is a fat (lipo = fat, remember?) and protein particle that carries cholesterol through your blood. Your body makes four types of lipoproteins: chylomicrons, very low density lipoproteins (VLDLs), low-density lipoproteins (LDLs), and high-density lipoproteins (HDLs). As a general rule, LDLs take cholesterol into blood vessels; HDLs carry it out of the body.

A lipoprotein is born as a *chylomicron,* made in your intestinal cells from protein and triglycerides (fats). After 12 hours of travelling through your blood and around your body, a chylomicron has lost virtually all of its fats. By the time the chylomicron makes its way to your liver, the only thing left is protein.

The liver, a veritable fat and cholesterol factory, collects fatty acid fragments from your blood and uses them to make cholesterol and new fatty acids. Time out! How much cholesterol you get from food may affect your liver's daily output: Eat more cholesterol, and your liver may make less. If you eat less cholesterol, your liver may make more. And so it goes.

Churning out harmful lipoproteins

Okay, after your liver has made cholesterol and fatty acids, it packages them with protein as very low density lipoproteins (VLDLs), which have more protein and are denser than their precursors, the chylomicrons. As VLDLs travel through your bloodstream, they lose triglycerides, pick up cholesterol, and turn into low-density lipoproteins (LDLs). LDLs supply cholesterol to your body cells, which use it to make new cell membranes and manufacture sterol compounds such as hormones. That's the good news.

The bad news is that both VLDLs and LDLs are soft and squishy enough to pass through blood vessel walls. The larger and squishier they are, the more likely they are to slide into your arteries, which means that VLDLs are more hazardous to your health than plain old LDLs. These fluffy, fatty lipoproteins carry cholesterol into blood vessels, where it can cling to the inside wall, forming deposits, or *plaques*. These plaques may eventually block an artery, prevent blood from flowing through, and trigger a heart attack or stroke. Whew! Got all that?

VLDLs and LDLs are sometimes called "bad cholesterol," but this characterization is a misnomer. They aren't cholesterol; they're just the rafts on which cholesterol sails into your arteries. As they travel through the body, LDLs continue to lose cholesterol. In the end, they lose so much fat that they become mostly protein — turning them into high-density lipoproteins, the particles sometimes called "good cholesterol." Once again, this label is inaccurate. HDLs aren't cholesterol: They're simply protein and fat particles too dense and compact to pass through blood vessel walls, so they carry cholesterol out of the body rather than into arteries.

That's why a high level of HDLs may reduce your risk of heart attack regardless of your total cholesterol levels. Conversely, a high level of LDLs may raise your risk of heart attack, even if your overall cholesterol level is low. Hey, on second thought, maybe that does qualify them as "good" and "bad" cholesterol.

Setting limits on the bad guys

In 2003, the Canadian guidelines for the treatment and management of *dyslipidemia* (a fancy way of saying high blood fats like cholesterol or triglycerides) were updated with new LDL limits. These limits are based on an individual's risk for developing coronary artery disease (CAD).

These guidelines are based on the Framingham Heart Study model, which estimates personal risk based on things like cholesterol levels, family history, and blood pressure. (Your doctor will be familiar with this tool and no doubt uses it when assessing your blood work at your annual physical — you do go for your yearly checkup, don't you?)

There are three main risk categories:

- ✔ High risk: For people whose risk of developing CAD within ten years is greater than 20 percent, the LDL should be less than 2.5 mmol/L. Generally, people in this group have many risk factors including diabetes, family history of heart problems, and high blood pressure.

✔ Moderate risk: People with an 11 to 19 percent chance of developing CAD within ten years should limit their LDL intake to less than 3.5 mmol/L.

✔ Low risk: People with a likelihood of developing CAD of 10 percent or less should have an LDL limit of less than 4.5 mmol/L.

Even newer lipid guidelines from 2006 are calling to rein in the LDL limit for the high risk group to less than 2.0 mmol/L. Several studies have shown that a lower LDL limit results in the reduction of cardiovascular complications amongst the high-risk group. To achieve this lower LDL level, most everyone — if not all — will need cholesterol-busting "statin" drugs such as atorvastatin (Lipitor), rosuvastatin (Crestor), or simvastatin (Zocor). Your physician will determine if there's an added benefit to pushing for such a low LDL limit.

Diet and cholesterol

Most of the cholesterol that you need is made right in your own liver, which churns out about 1 gram (1,000 milligrams) a day from the raw materials in the proteins, fats, and carbohydrates you consume. But you also get cholesterol from food of animal origin: meat, poultry, fish, eggs, and dairy products. Although some plant foods, such as coconuts and cocoa beans, are high in saturated fats, no plants actually have cholesterol. Table 7-2 lists the amount of cholesterol in normal servings of some representative foods.

Because plants don't contain cholesterol, no plant foods are on this list. No grains. No fruits. No veggies. No nuts and seeds. Of course, you can juice plant food up with cholesterol if you really try: butter in the bread dough, cheese on the macaroni, cream sauce on the peas and onions, whipped cream on poached peaches, and so on.

Table 7-2	How Much Cholesterol Is on That Plate?	
Food	*Serving Size*	*Cholesterol (mg)*
Meat		
Beef (stewed), lean and fat	85 g (3 ounces)	87
Beef (stewed), lean	60 g (2.2 ounces)	66
Beef (ground), lean	85 g (3 ounces)	74
Beef (ground), regular	85 g (3 ounces)	76
Beef steak (sirloin)	85 g (3 ounces)	77
Bacon	3 strips	16
Pork chop, lean	70 g (2.5 ounces)	71

Food	Serving Size	Cholesterol (mg)
Poultry		
Chicken (roast), breast	85 g (3 ounces)	73
Chicken (roast), leg	85 g (3 ounces)	78
Turkey (roast), breast	85 g (3 ounces)	59
Fish		
Clams	85 g (3 ounces)	43
Flounder	85 g (3 ounces)	59
Oysters (raw)	250 mL (1 cup)	120
Salmon (canned)	85 g (3 ounces)	34
Salmon (baked)	85 g (3 ounces)	60
Tuna (water canned)	85 g (3 ounces)	48
Tuna (oil canned)	85 g (3 ounces)	55
Cheese		
American	28 g (1 ounce)	27
Cheddar	28 g (1 ounce)	30
Cream	28 g (1 ounce)	31
Mozzarella (whole milk)	28 g (1 ounce)	22
Mozzarella (part skim)	28 g (1 ounce)	15
Swiss	28 g (1 ounce)	26
Milk		
Whole	28 g (1 ounce)	33
2%	28 g (1 ounce)	18
1%	28 g (1 ounce)	18
Skim	28 g (1 ounce)	10
Other dairy products		
Butter	Pat	11

(continued)

Table 7-2 *(continued)*

Food	Serving Size	Cholesterol (mg)
Other		
Eggs, large	1	213
Lard	15 mL (1 tbsp)	12

Nutritive Value of Foods (Washington, D.C.: U.S. Department of Agriculture)

Chapter 8

Carbohydrates: A Complex Story

Carbohydrates — the name means carbon plus water — are sugar compounds that plants make when they're exposed to light. This process of making sugar compounds is called *photosynthesis,* from the Latin words for "light" and "putting together."

This chapter shines a bright light on the different kinds of carbohydrates, illuminating all the nutritional nooks and crannies to explain how each contributes to your vim and vigour — not to mention a yummy daily menu.

Checking Out Carbohydrates

Carbohydrates come in three varieties: simple carbohydrates, complex carbohydrates, and dietary fibre. All are composed of units of sugar. What makes one carbohydrate different from another is the number of sugar units it contains and how the units are linked together.

✔ **Simple carbohydrates:** These carbohydrates have only one or two units of sugar.

• A carbohydrate with one unit of sugar is called a *simple sugar* or a *monosaccharide* (mono = one; saccharide = sugar). Fructose (fruit sugar) is a monosaccharide, and so are glucose, the sugar produced when you digest carbohydrates (blood sugar), and galactose, the sugar derived from digesting lactose (milk sugar).

- A carbohydrate with two units of sugar is called a *double sugar* or a *disaccharide* (di = two). Sucrose (table sugar), which is made of one unit of fructose and one unit of glucose, is a disaccharide. So is *lactose* (milk sugar), which is made of one unit of galactose and one unit of glucose.

✔ **Complex carbohydrates:** Also known as *polysaccharides* (poly = many), these carbs have more than two units of sugar linked together. Carbs with three to ten units of sugar are sometimes called *oligosaccharides* (oligo = few).

  - Raffinose is a *trisaccharide* (tri = three) that's found in potatoes, beans, and beets. It has one unit each of galactose, glucose, and fructose.

  - Stachyose is a *tetrasaccharide* (tetra = four) found in the same vegetables mentioned in the previous item. It has one fructose unit, one glucose unit, and two galactose units.

  - Starch, a complex carbohydrate in potatoes, pasta, and rice, is a definite polysaccharide, made of many units of glucose.

Once upon a time it was believed that because complex carbohydrates are, well, *complex,* with anywhere from three to a zillion units of sugars, your body would take longer to digest them than it took to digest simple carbohydrates. It was thought that because of these structural differences, digesting complex carbohydrates releases glucose into your bloodstream more slowly and evenly than digesting simple carbs. We know now, of course, that this intuitive assumption is false. It turns out that simple structure does not influence how your body digests carbohydrates — enter the glycemic index (the famous GI, discussed later in this chapter).

✔ **Dietary fibre:** This term is used to distinguish the fibre in food from the natural and synthetic fibres (silk, cotton, wool, nylon) used in fabrics. Dietary fibre is a third kind of carbohydrate.

  - Like the complex carbohydrates, dietary fibre (cellulose, hemicellulose, pectin, beta-glucans, gum) is a polysaccharide. Lignin, a different kind of chemical, is also called a dietary fibre.

  - Some kinds of dietary fibre also contain units of soluble or insoluble uronic acids, compounds derived from the sugars fructose, glucose, and galactose. For example, pectin — a soluble fibre in apples — contains soluble galacturonic acid.

Dietary fibre is not like other carbohydrates. The bonds that hold its sugar units together cannot be broken by human digestive enzymes. Although the bacteria living naturally in your intestines convert very small amounts of dietary fibre to fatty acids, dietary fibre is not considered a source of energy. (For more about fatty acids, see Chapter 7.)

Charting the sweetness of carbs

The information in the following table has absolutely no practical value. It's strictly trivia for your own personal nutrition data bank. Of course, you can call it up for use in social situations. For example, suppose you're standing in line at the hot dog stand on a local street corner looking for a way to start up a conversation with the attractive person in front of you. "Wow," you may say. "Did you notice the cola over there is sweetened with both fructose and sucrose — a monosaccharide and a disaccharide, both in the same drink? And given how nutrition-savvy they are here, I bet the hot dog rolls are loaded with polysaccharides." Who could resist such a high-minded, intellectual approach?

Naming the Sugar Units in Carbohydrates

Carbohydrate	Composition
Monosaccharides (1 sugar unit)	
Fructose (fruit sugar)	1 unit fructose
Glucose (sugar unit used for fuel)	1 unit glucose
Galactose (made from lactose [milk sugar])	1 unit galactose
Disaccharides (2 sugar units linked together)	
Sucrose (table sugar)	Glucose + fructose
Lactose (milk sugar)	Glucose + galactose
Maltose (malt sugar)	Glucose + glucose
Polysaccharides (many sugar units linked together)	
Raffinose	Galactose + glucose + fructose
Stachyose	Glucose + fructose + galactose + galactose
Starch	Many glucose units
Cellulose	Many glucose units
Hemicellulose	Arabinose* + galactose + mannose* + xylose** plus uronic acids

(continued)

(continued)

| **(continued)** | |
Carbohydrate	Composition
Pectin	Galactose + arabinose + galacturonic acid
Gums	Mainly galacturonic acid

* This sugar is found in many plants.
** This sugar is found in plants and wood.

The next section is about how your body gets energy from carbohydrates. Because dietary fibre does not provide energy, let's put it aside for the moment and get back to it in the "Dietary Fibre: The Non-Nutrient in Carbohydrate Foods" section, later in this chapter.

Carbohydrates and energy: A biochemical love story

Your body runs on glucose, the molecules your cells burn for energy. (For more information on how you get energy from food, check out Chapter 3.)

Proteins, fats, and alcohol (as in beer, wine, and spirits) also provide energy in the form of calories. And protein does give you glucose, but it takes a long time, relatively speaking, for your body to get it.

When you eat carbohydrates, your pancreas secretes insulin, the hormone that enables you to digest starches and sugars. This release of insulin is sometimes called an *insulin spike,* which means the same thing as "insulin secretion" but sounds a whole lot more sinister.

If you have a metabolic disorder such as diabetes that keeps you from producing enough insulin, you must be careful not to take in more carbs than you can digest. Unmetabolized sugars circulating through your blood can make you dizzy and maybe even trip you into a diabetic coma.

Most people who don't have a metabolic disorder (such as diabetes) that interferes with the ability to digest carbs can metabolize even very large amounts of carbohydrate foods easily. Their insulin secretion rises to meet the demand and then quickly settles back to normal. In other words, although some popular weight-loss programs, such as the South Beach Diet, rely on the glycemic index as a weight-loss tool, the fact remains that for most people, a carb is a carb is a carb, regardless of how quickly the sugar enters the bloodstream. There is more about the GI (and its partner, the glycemic load) later in this chapter.

For info on why the difference between simple and complex carbs can matter for athletes, check out the section called "Who needs extra carbohydrates?"

How glucose becomes energy

Inside your cells, the glucose is burned to produce heat and *adenosine triphosphate,* a molecule that stores and releases energy as required by the cell. By the way, nutrition scientists, who have as much trouble pronouncing polysyllabic words as you probably do, usually refer to adenosine triphosphate by its initials: ATP. Smart cookies!

The transformation of glucose into energy occurs in one of two ways: with oxygen or without it. Glucose is converted to energy with oxygen in the *mitochondria* — tiny bodies in the jellylike substance inside every cell. This conversion yields energy (ATP, heat) plus water and carbon dioxide — a waste product.

Red blood cells do not have mitochondria, so they change glucose into energy without oxygen. This yields energy (ATP, heat) and lactic acid.

Glucose is also converted to energy in muscle cells. When it comes to producing energy from glucose, muscle cells are, well, double-jointed. They have mitochondria, so they can process glucose with oxygen. But if the level of oxygen in the muscle cell falls very low, the cells can just go ahead and change glucose into energy without the oxygen. This is most likely to happen when you've been exercising so strenuously that you (and your muscles) are, literally, out of breath.

Being able to turn glucose into energy without oxygen is a handy trick, but here's the downside: One by-product is lactic acid. Why is that a big deal? Too much lactic acid makes your muscles ache.

How pasta ends up on your hips when too many carbs pass your lips

Your cells budget energy very carefully. They do not store more than they need right now. Any glucose the cell does not need for its daily work is converted to glycogen (animal starch) and tucked away as stored energy in your liver and muscles.

Your body can pack about 400 grams (14 ounces) of glycogen into liver and muscle cells. A gram of carbohydrates — including glucose — has four calories. If you add up all the glucose stored in glycogen to the small amount of glucose in your cells and blood, it equals about 1,800 calories of energy.

If your diet provides more carbohydrates than you need to produce this amount of stored calories in the form of glucose and glycogen in your cells, blood, muscles, and liver, the excess will be converted to fat. And that's how your pasta ends up on your hips.

Other ways your body uses carbohydrates

Providing energy is an important job, but it isn't the only thing carbohydrates do for you. Carbohydrates also protect your muscles. When you need energy, your body looks for glucose from carbohydrates first. If none is available, because you're on a carbohydrate-restricted diet or have a medical condition that prevents you from using the carbohydrate foods you consume, your body begins to pull energy out of fatty tissue and then moves on to burning its own protein tissue (muscles). If this use of proteins for energy continues long enough, you run out of fuel and die.

A diet that provides sufficient amounts of carbohydrates keeps your body from eating its own muscles. That's why a carbohydrate-rich diet is sometimes described as *protein sparing*.

What else do carbohydrates do? They

- Regulate the amount of sugar circulating in your blood so that all your cells get the energy they need

- Provide nutrients for the friendly bacteria in your intestinal tract that help digest food

- Assist in your body's absorption of calcium

- May help lower cholesterol levels and regulate blood pressure (these effects are special benefits of dietary fibre; see "Dietary Fibre: The Non-Nutrient in Carbohydrate Foods" later in this chapter)

Finding the carbohydrates you need

The most important sources of carbohydrates are plant foods — fruits, vegetables, and grains. Milk and milk products contain the carbohydrate lactose (milk sugar), but meat, fish, and poultry have no carbohydrates at all.

In the fall of 2002, the National Academy of Sciences Institute of Medicine (IOM) released a report recommending that 45 to 65 percent of your daily calories come from carbohydrate foods. Canada's Food Guide (see more about that in Chapter 17) makes it easy for you to build a nutritious carb-based diet with portion allowances based on how many calories you consume each day in

> ✔ Six to eight servings of grain products (bread, cereals, pasta, rice)
>
> ✔ Seven to ten servings of vegetables and fruit
>
> ✔ Two to three servings of milk or alternatives

These foods provide simple carbohydrates, complex carbohydrates, and the natural bonus of dietary fibre (with the grains, vegetables, and fruit groups). Table sugar, honey, and sweets — which provide simple carbohydrates — are recommended only on a once-in-a-while basis.

One gram of carbohydrates has four calories. To find the number of calories from the carbohydrates in a serving, multiply the number of grams of carbohydrates by four. For example, one whole bagel has about 38 grams of carbohydrates, equal to about 152 calories (38 × 4). (You have to say "about" because the dietary fibre in the bagel provides no calories, because the body can't metabolize it.) *Wait:* That number does not account for all the calories in the serving. Remember, the foods listed here may also contain at least some protein and fat, and these two nutrients add calories.

Some problems with carbohydrates

Some people have a hard time handling carbohydrates. For example, people with Type 1 ("insulin dependent") diabetes do not produce sufficient amounts of insulin, the hormones needed to carry all the glucose produced from carbohydrates into body cells. As a result, the glucose continues to circulate in the blood until it's excreted through the kidneys. That's why one way to tell whether someone has diabetes is to test the level of sugar in that person's urine.

Other people can't digest carbohydrates because their bodies lack the specific enzymes needed to break the bonds that hold a carbohydrate's sugar units together. For example, many (some say most) Asians, Africans, Middle Easterners, South Americans, and Eastern, Central, or Southern Europeans are deficient in lactase, the enzyme that splits lactose (milk sugar) into glucose and galactose. If they drink milk or eat milk products, they end up with a lot of undigested lactose in their intestinal tracts. This undigested lactose makes the bacteria living there happy as clams — but not the person who owns the intestines: As bacteria feast on the undigested sugar, they excrete waste products that give their host gas and cramps.

Time out for the name game!

Here's an interesting bit of nutritional information. The names of all enzymes end in the letters *ase*. An enzyme that digests a specific substance in food often has a name similar to the substance but with the letters *ase* at the end. For example, *proteases* are enzymes that digest protein; *lipases* are enzymes that digest fats (lipids); and *galactase* is the enzyme that digests galactose.

To avoid this anomaly, many national cuisines purposely are void of milk as an ingredient. (Quick! Name one native Asian dish that's made with milk. No, coconut milk doesn't count.) Does that mean people living in these countries don't get enough calcium? No. They simply substitute high-calcium foods such as greens or soy products for milk.

A second solution for people who don't make enough lactase is to use a *predigested milk product* such as yogourt or buttermilk or sour cream, all made by adding friendly bacteria that digest the milk (that is, break the lactose apart) without spoiling it. Other solutions include lactose-free cheeses and enzyme-treated (lactose-free) milk, but because the lactose is broken down into two single sugars — glucose and galactose — this type of milk tastes sweeter than regular milk. The single sugars are sweeter tasting than the dissacharide lactose.

Who needs extra carbohydrates?

The small amount of glucose in your blood and cells provides the energy you need for your body's daily activities. The 400 grams of glycogen stored in your liver and muscles provide enough energy for ordinary bursts of extra activity.

But what happens when you have to work harder or longer than that? For example, what if you're a long-distance athlete, which means that you use up your available supply of glucose before you finish your competition? (That's why marathoners often run out of gas — a phenomenon called *hitting the wall* — at 32 km or 20 miles, which is 9.6 km or 6 miles short of the finish line.)

If you were stuck on an ice floe or lost in the woods for a month or so, after your body exhausts its supply of glucose, including the glucose stored as glycogen, it starts pulling energy first out of fat and then out of muscle. But extracting energy from body fat requires large amounts of oxygen — which is likely to be in short supply when your body has run, swum, or cycled 32 km (20 miles). So athletes have to find another way to leap the wall. Here it is: They load up on carbohydrates in advance.

Carbohydrate loading is a dietary regimen designed to temporarily increase the amount of glycogen stored in your muscles in anticipation of an upcoming event.

Once upon a time it was believed that the best way to saturate muscle with glycogen was to first "starve" the muscles by exercising to exhaustion starting about one week prior to the event so that your body pulls as much glycogen as possible out of your muscles. Then, for three days, you eat foods high in fat and protein and low in carbohydrates, to keep your glycogen level from rising again. Three days before the big day, reverse the pattern and eat a very high carbohydrate diet, up to 70 percent carbohydrate. This approach was devised during the 1960s. It was phased out after research in the 1980s demonstrated that it was unnecessary to use this approach to achieve maximum muscle glycogen levels.

Nowadays we know differently. The latest from the sport nutrition research has demonstrated that as long as an athlete consistently eats a higher carbohydrate diet (65 to 70 percent of their total calories) every day, muscle glycogen levels will return to normal levels within 24 hours of rest after strenuous training. To ensure that muscles have the maximum amount of glycogen before the big race, an athlete ideally should rest as much as possible while continuing to eat a high-carb diet for the 48-hour period before their event.

This carb-loading diet is not for everyday use, nor will it help people competing in events of short duration. It's strictly for events lasting longer than 90 minutes.

What about while you're running, swimming, or cycling? Will consuming simple sugars during the race give you extra short-term bursts of energy? Yes. Sugar is rapidly digested and used by exercising muscles.

But you don't want *straight sugar* (candy, honey) because it's *hydrophilic* (hydro = water; philic = loving), which means that it pulls water from body tissues into your intestinal tract. Using straight sugar can increase dehydration and make you nauseated. Thus, getting the sugar you want from sweetened sport drinks, which provide fluids along with the energy, is best. The label on the sport drink also tells you the liquid contains salt (sodium chloride). Why? To replace the salt that you lose when perspiring heavily. Turn to Chapter 13 to find out why this is important.

Glycemic index

The concept of the *glycemic index* (GI) was invented by Dr. David J. Jenkins and colleagues in 1981 at the University of Toronto. The GI is a ranking system for carbohydrates based on their ability to raise blood glucose (sugar) — also called the *glycemic response.* Foods are ranked as having either a low GI (55 or less), a medium GI (56 to 69), or a high GI (70 or more).

Why should you be concerned about the GI of foods? A lot of research has shown that when you eat lower GI foods more often than higher GI foods, you'll tend to be more successful at controlling your blood sugar levels (good for those with diabetes), your cholesterol, and your appetite, and you'll be less likely to develop heart disease and type 2 diabetes. See Table 8-1 for examples of foods and their glycemic index.

Table 8-1		Glycemic Index of Some Foods
Classification	*GI Range*	*Examples*
Low GI	55 or less	Most fruit and vegetables (but not potato), basmati rice, oats, All-bran cereal, some ice creams, chickpeas, sweet potato, plain yogourt
Medium GI	56–69	Sucrose (table sugar), Mars bar, some ice creams, beets, banana, oatmeal, brown rice, popcorn
High GI	70 or more	Corn flakes, baked potato, jasmine rice, white bread, popcorn, watermelon, French fries, parsnips, dried dates

One of the first things you might be saying to yourself is, "If foods with a lower GI are better for me, then according to this table, ice cream (GI about 50) or a Mars bar (GI about 69) are healthier than parsnips!" That would be nice, wouldn't it? The reality is that many factors can affect the GI of a food, such as how it is prepared. Pasta cooked *al dente* (slightly firm) has a lower GI than pasta that's overcooked and mushy. The GI of a food can also be affected by the foods with which it's eaten, if those other foods have fibre, protein, or fat. If broccoli (which has fibre) and steak (protein and fat) are eaten at the same time as a baked potato, then the higher GI ranking of the potato is lowered because the potato will be digested more slowly.

Because of the GI, many healthy foods such as carrots have been seen as "off limits" — people think that eating these foods will cause a rapid rise in blood sugar. Conversely, looking at the GI of a chocolate bar might lead someone to believe that it's a better choice than a baked potato. This misconception can be addressed and the GI made more complete with the concept of the glycemic load.

Glycemic load

The *glycemic load* (GL) is a ranking system for carbohydrate content in food portions based on their GI and the portion size. This is much more useful than the GI alone; it's based on the idea that both a high-GI food eaten in small amounts and a low-GI food eaten in large amounts will have a similar effect on blood sugar.

The GL is a relatively new way to assess the impact of carbohydrate consumption that takes the GI into account, but gives a fuller picture than does the GI alone. The GI tells you only how rapidly a particular carbohydrate turns into glucose (blood sugar); however, it doesn't tell you the carbohydrate content of that food. You need to know both things to understand a food's effect on blood sugar. That is where the GL comes in. A GL of 20 or more is high, a GL of 11 to 19 is medium, and a GL of 10 or less is low.

The GL load of a food can be calculated as the amount of carbohydrate content (g), multiplied by its GI, and divided by 100. For example, 100 g of plain baked beans have a GI of 52 and about 21 g of carbohydrate. The equation for the baked beans GL looks like this:

$$21 \times \frac{52}{100} = 11$$

Table 8-2 provides the GL for some common foods.

Table 8-2		Glycemic Load of Some Foods	
Food (serving g)	GI*	Carbohydrate Content (g)*	GL*
Baguette, white, plain (30g)	95	15.9	15.1
Mango, (120g) (Phillipines)	41	15.1	6.2
Carrots, boiled (80g) (Canada)	92	4.2	3.9
Baked beans, canned (150g) (Canada)	40	16.8	6.7
Mashed potatoes (150g) (Canada)	67	18.5	12.4
Rice, boiled white, long grain (150g)	64	42	26.9
Kiwi (76g) (Australia)	58	11	6.4

*All amounts are approximate.
Glycemic Index and GI database (www.glycemicindex.com)
Nutrition Data (www.nutritiondata.com)

So what's the bottom line? Highly processed foods, starchy high-GI foods such as white bread and white rice, and foods and beverages that contain a lot of sugar — cakes, cookies, candy, and soft drinks — generally have high GL values. These foods lack nutrients and fibre, which are crucial to your body's handling of carbs. The foods that are ultimately better choices are those that are closest to nature, in other words, minimally processed whole foods. You got it, whole-grain products, whole vegetables, and fruits, eaten in amounts that support both your activity level and a healthy weight.

Dietary Fibre: The Non-Nutrient in Carbohydrate Foods

Dietary fibre is a group of complex carbohydrates that are not a source of energy for human beings. Because human digestive enzymes cannot break the bonds that hold fibre's sugar units together, fibre adds no calories to your diet and cannot be converted to glucose.

Ruminants (animals, such as cows, that chew the cud) have a combination of digestive enzymes and digestive microbes that enables them to extract the nutrients from insoluble dietary fibre (cellulose and some hemicelluloses). But not even these creatures can pull nutrients out of lignin, an insoluble fibre in plant stems and leaves and the predominant fibre in wood.

But just because you can't digest dietary fibre doesn't mean it isn't a valuable part of your diet. The opposite is true. Dietary fibre is valuable *because* you can't digest it!

The two kinds of dietary fibre

Nutritionists classify dietary fibre as either insoluble or soluble, depending on whether it dissolves in water. Both types of fibre are present in all plant foods, with varying degrees of each according to a plant's characteristics. (Both kinds of fibre resist human digestive enzymes.)

- **Insoluble fibre:** This type of fibre includes cellulose, some hemicelluloses, and lignin found in whole grains and other plants. This kind of dietary fibre is a natural laxative. It absorbs water, helps you feel full after eating, and stimulates your intestinal walls to contract and relax. These natural contractions, called *peristalsis,* move solid materials through your digestive tract.

  By moving food quickly through your intestines, insoluble fibre may help relieve or prevent digestive disorders such as constipation or diverticulitis (infection that occurs when food gets stuck in small pouches in the wall of the colon). Insoluble fibre also bulks up stool and makes it softer, reducing your risk of developing hemorrhoids and lessening the discomfort if you already have them.

- **Soluble fibre:** This fibre, found in pectins in apples and beta-glucans in oats and barley, seems to lower the amount of cholesterol circulating in your blood (your *cholesterol level*). This tendency may be why a diet rich in fibre appears to offer some protection against heart disease.

Here's a benefit for dieters: Soluble fibre forms a gel in the presence of water, which is what happens when apples and oat bran reach your digestive tract. Like insoluble fibre, soluble fibre can make you feel full without adding calories.

Ordinary soluble dietary fibre can't be digested, so your body doesn't absorb it. But in 2002, researchers at Detroit's Barbara Ann Karamonos Cancer Institute fed laboratory mice a form of soluble dietary fibre called *modified citrus pectin*. The fibre, which is made from citrus fruit peel, can be digested. When fed to laboratory rats, it appeared to reduce the size of tumours caused by implanted human breast and colon cancer cells. The researchers believe that the fibre prevents cancer cells from linking together to form tumours. Now, two pharmaceutical companies in the U.S. — one on the east coast and one on the west coast — are investigating the effects of modified citrus pectin in human beings. But the product isn't yet ready for prime time. Although it's being sold as a dietary supplement (not as a medicine), experts warn that its effects on human bodies (and human cancers) remain unproven.

Getting fibre from food

You find fibre in all plant foods — fruits, vegetables, and grains. But you find absolutely no fibre in foods from animals: meat, fish, poultry, milk, milk products, and eggs.

A balanced diet with lots of foods from plants gives you both insoluble and soluble fibre. Most foods that contain fibre have both kinds, although the balance usually tilts toward one or the other. For example, the predominant fibre in an apple is pectin (a soluble fibre), but an apple peel also has some cellulose, hemicellulose, and lignin.

Table 8-3 shows you which foods are particularly good sources of specific kinds of fibre. A diet rich in plant foods (fruits, vegetables, grains) gives you adequate amounts of dietary fibre.

Table 8-3	Sources of Different Kinds of Fibre
Fibre	*Where Found*
Soluble fibre	
Pectin	Fruits (apples, strawberries, citrus fruits)
Beta-glucans	Oats, barley
Gums	Beans, cereals (oats, rice, barley), seeds, seaweed

(continued)

Table 8-3 *(continued)*

Fibre	Where Found
Insoluble fibre	
Cellulose	Leaves (cabbage), roots (carrots, beets), bran, whole wheat, beans
Hemicellulose	Seed coverings (bran, whole grains)
Lignin	Plant stems, leaves, skin

How much fibre do you need?

Health Canada uses recommendations made by the Institute of Medicine to suggest daily fibre intake. But Canadian men and women aren't getting enough fibre. Here's what the IOM suggests:

- ✔ 25 grams (0.8 ounces) a day for women younger than 50
- ✔ 38 grams (1.3 ounces) a day for men younger than 50
- ✔ 21 grams (0.7 ounces) a day for women older than 50
- ✔ 30 grams (1 ounce) a day for men older than 50

The amounts of dietary fibre recommended by the IOM are believed to give you the benefits you want without causing fibre-related — um — unpleasantries.

Fibre factoid

The amount of fibre in a serving of food may depend on whether the food is raw or cooked. For example, as you can see from Table 8-4, a 3½-ounce serving of plain dried prunes has 7.2 grams of fibre, while a 3½-ounce serving of stewed prunes has 6.6 grams of fibre.

Why? When you stew prunes, they plump up — which means they absorb water. The water adds weight but (obviously) no fibre. So a serving of prunes-plus-water has slightly less fibre per ounce than a same-weight serving of plain dried prunes.

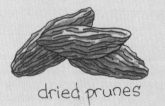

dried prunes

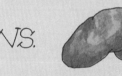

stewed prunes

Unpleasantries? Like what? And how will you know if you've got them?

Trust me: If you eat more than enough fibre, your body will tell you right away. All that roughage may irritate your intestinal tract, which will issue an unmistakable protest in the form of intestinal gas or diarrhea. In extreme cases, if you don't drink enough liquids to moisten and soften the fibre you eat so that it easily slides through your digestive tract, the dietary fibre may form a mass that can end up as an intestinal obstruction (for more about water, see Chapter 13).

If you decide to up the amount of fibre in your diet, follow this advice:

✔ Do so *very* gradually, a little bit more every day. That way you're less likely to experience intestinal distress. In other words, if your current diet is heavy on no-fibre foods such as meat, fish, poultry, eggs, milk, and cheese, and low-fibre foods such as white bread and white rice, don't load up on bran cereal (35 grams of dietary fibre in 3½ ounces) or dried figs (9.3 grams in 3½ ounces) all at once. Start by adding a serving of cornflakes (2.0 grams dietary fibre in 3½ ounces) at breakfast, maybe an apple (2.8 grams in 3½ ounces) at lunch, a pear (2.6 grams in 3½ ounces) at midafternoon, and a half cup of baked beans (7.7 grams in 3½ ounces) at dinner. Four simple additions, and already you're up to 15 grams of dietary fibre.

✔ Always check the nutrition label whenever you shop (for more about these wonderfully informative guides, see Chapter 17). When choosing between similar products, just take the one with the higher fibre content per serving. For example, white pita bread generally has about 1.6 grams dietary fibre per serving. Whole-wheat pita bread has 7.4 grams. From a fibre standpoint, you know which works better for your body. Go for it!

✔ Get enough liquids. Dietary fibre is like a sponge. It sops up liquid, so increasing your fibre intake may deprive your cells of the water they need to perform their daily work (for more about how your body uses the water you drink, see Chapter 13). That's why health professionals recommend you get plenty of fluids when you consume more fibre. How much is enough? Back to Chapter 13.

Table 8-4 shows the amounts of all types of dietary fibre — insoluble plus soluble — in a 100-gram (3½-ounce) serving of specific foods. By the way, nutritionists like to measure things in terms of 100-gram portions so you can compare foods at a glance.

To find the amount of dietary fibre in your own serving, divide the gram total for the food shown in Table 8-4 by 3.5 to get the grams per ounce, and then multiply the result by the number of ounces in your portion. For example, if you're having 1 ounce of cereal, the customary serving of ready-to-eat breakfast cereals, divide the gram total of dietary fibre by 3.5; then multiply by 1. If your slice of bread weighs ½ ounce, divide the gram total by 3.5; then multiply the result by 0.5 (½).

Or — let's get real! — you can look at the nutrition label on the side of the package — it gives you the nutrients per portion.

Finally, the amounts in this table are averages. Different brands of processed products (breads, some cereals, cooked fruits, and vegetables) may have more (or less) fibre per serving.

Table 8-4	Fibre Content in Common Foods
Food	*Grams of Fibre in a 100-Gram (3½-Ounce) Serving*
Bread	2.1
Bran bread	8.5
Pita bread (white)	1.6
Pita bread (whole wheat)	7.4
White bread	1.9
Cereals	
Bran cereal	35.3
Bran flakes	18.8
Cornflakes	2.0
Oatmeal	10.6
Wheat flakes	9.0
Grains	
Barley, pearled (minus its outer covering), raw	15.6
Cornmeal, whole grain	11.0
De-germed	5.2
Oat bran, raw	6.6
Rice, uncooked (brown)	3.5
Rice, uncooked (white)	1.0–2.8
Rice, uncooked (wild)	5.2
Wheat bran	15.0
Fruits	
Apple, with skin	2.8
Apricots, dried	7.8

Food	Grams of Fibre in a 100-Gram (3½-Ounce) Serving
Figs, dried	9.3
Kiwi fruit	3.4
Pear, raw	2.6
Prunes, dried	7.2
Prunes, stewed	6.6
Raisins	5.3
Vegetables	
Baked beans (vegetarian)	7.7
Chickpeas (canned)	5.4
Lima beans, cooked	7.2
Broccoli, raw	2.8
Brussels sprouts, cooked	2.6
Cabbage, white, raw	2.4
Cauliflower, raw	2.4
Corn, sweet, cooked	3.7
Peas with edible pods, raw	2.6
Potatoes, white, baked, w/ skin	5.5
Sweet potato, cooked	3.0
Tomatoes, raw	1.3
Nuts	
Almonds, oil-roasted	11.2
Coconut, raw	9.0
Hazelnuts, oil-roasted	6.4
Peanuts, dry-roasted	8.0
Pistachios	10.8
Other	
Corn chips, toasted	4.4
Tahini (sesame-seed paste)	9.3
Tofu	1.2

Provisional Table on the Dietary Fiber Content of Selected Foods (Washington, D.C.: U.S. Department of Agriculture, 1988)

Fibre and your heart: The continuing saga of oat bran

Oat bran is the second chapter in the fibre fad, which began with wheat bran in about 1980. Wheat bran, the fibre in wheat, is rich in the insoluble fibres cellulose and lignin. Oat bran's gee-whiz factor is the soluble fibre called *beta-glucans*. For more than 30 years, scientists have known that eating foods high in soluble fibre can lower your cholesterol, although nobody knows exactly why. Fruits and vegetables (especially dried beans) are high in soluble fibre, but ounce for ounce, oats have more. In addition, beta-glucans are a more effective cholesterol-buster than pectin and gum, which are the soluble fibres in most fruits and vegetables.

By 1990, researchers at the University of Kentucky reported that people who add ½ cup of dry oat bran (*not* oatmeal) to their regular daily diets could lower their levels of low-density lipoproteins (LDLs), the particles that carry cholesterol into your arteries, by as much as 25 percent (see Chapter 7 for more on cholesterol).

Recently, scientists, funded by Quaker Oats, at the Medical School of Northwestern University enlisted 208 healthy volunteers whose normal cholesterol readings averaged about 5.2 mmol/L (mmol/L is unit of measure for different things in your blood, in this case it stands for "millimoles of cholesterol in one litre of blood") for a study involving oat bran. The volunteers' total cholesterol levels decreased an average of 9.3 percent with a low-fat, low-cholesterol diet supplemented by 2 ounces of oats or oat bran every day. About one-third of the cholesterol reduction was credited to the oats.

Oat cereal makers rounded the total loss to 10 percent, and the National Research Council said that a 10 percent drop in cholesterol could produce a 20 percent drop in the risk of a heart attack.

What happened next? Books on oat bran hit the best-seller list. Cheerios elbowed Frosted Flakes aside to become the number one cereal in the U.S. And people added oat bran to everything from bagels to orange juice.

Today scientists know that although a little oat bran can't hurt, the link between oats and cholesterol levels is no cure-all.

If your cholesterol level is higher than 6.5 mmol/L, lowering it by 10 percent through a diet that contains oat bran may reduce your risk of heart attack without the use of medication. If your cholesterol level is lower than that to begin with, the effects of oat bran are less dramatic. For example:

- If your cholesterol level is below 6.5 mmol/L, a low-saturated, low-trans-fat, low-cholesterol diet alone may push it down 6 percent. Adding oats reduces it another 3½ percent but doesn't take you to the ideal, which is less than 5.2 mmol/L.

- If your cholesterol is already low, say 5.2 mmol/L or less, a low-saturated, low-trans-fat, low-cholesterol diet plus oats may drop it to 4.7 mmol/L, but the oats account for only 3 percent of your loss.

By the way, the soluble pectin in apples and the soluble beta-glucans (gums) in beans and peas also lower cholesterol levels. The insoluble fibre in wheat bran does not.

Chapter 9

Alcohol: Another Form of Grape and Grain

· ·

In This Chapter

▶ Finding out how alcohol is made

▶ Categorizing different kinds of alcohol beverages

▶ Digesting alcohol

▶ Revealing alcohol's effect on your health

· ·

*A*lcohol beverages are among mankind's oldest home remedies and simple pleasures, so highly regarded that the ancient Greeks and Romans called wine a "gift from the gods," and when the Gaels — early inhabitants of Scotland and Ireland — first produced whiskey, they named it *uisge beatha* (whis-key-ba), a combination of the words for "water" and "life." Today, although you may share their appreciation for the product, you know that alcohol beverages may have risks as well as benefits.

By the way, throughout this chapter we refer to beverages made from alcohol as "alcohol beverages." Yes, we know most people probably think the correct term is "alcoholic beverages," but whenever we write or say those words, we get an immediate image of tipsy beer bottles. Besides, you've heard of "milk beverages" but not "milky" ones, or "cola beverages" but not "cola-y" ones. So do please indulge us.

Revealing the Many Faces of Alcohol

When micro-organisms (yeasts) digest (ferment) the sugars in carbohydrate foods, they make two by-products: a liquid and a gas. The gas is carbon dioxide. The liquid is *ethyl alcohol,* also known as *ethanol,* the intoxicating ingredient in alcohol beverages.

This biochemical process is not an esoteric one. In fact, it happens in your own kitchen every time you make yeast bread. Remember the faint, beerlike odour in the air while the dough is rising? That odour is from the alcohol the yeasts make as they chomp their way through the sugars in the flour. (Don't worry; the alcohol evaporates when you bake the bread.) As the yeasts digest the sugars, they also produce carbon dioxide, which makes the bread rise.

From now on, whenever you see the word *alcohol* alone in this book, unless otherwise noted, it means *ethanol,* the only alcohol used in alcohol beverages. (Yes, yes, yes. That definition applies backward, too. If you find the word *alcohol* in a previous chapter, it, too, means ethanol. Gee. Some people are so picky.)

Examining How Alcohol Beverages Are Made

Alcohol beverages are produced either through fermentation or through a combination of fermentation plus distillation.

Fermented alcohol products

Fermentation is a simple process in which yeasts or bacteria are added to carbohydrate foods such as corn, potatoes, rice, or wheat, which are used as starting material, or food. The yeasts digest the sugars in the food, leaving liquid (alcohol); the liquid is filtered to remove the solids, and water is usually added to dilute the alcohol, producing — voilà — an alcohol beverage.

Beer is made this way. So is wine. *Kumiss,* a fermented milk product, is slightly different because it's made by adding yeasts and friendly bacteria called *lactobacilli* (lacto = milk) to mare's milk. The micro-organisms make alcohol, but it isn't separated from the milk, which turns into a fizzy fermented beverage with no water added.

What other alcohols do you have in your home?

Ethanol is the only kind of alcohol used in food and alcohol beverages, but it isn't the only kind of alcohol used in consumer products. Other alcohols may be sitting on the shelf in your bathroom or workshop (though you definitely don't want to drink them):

Methyl alcohol (methanol): This poisonous alcohol made from wood is used as a *chemical solvent* (a liquid that dissolves other chemicals).

Isopropyl alcohol (rubbing alcohol): This poisonous alcohol is made from *propylene,* a petroleum derivative.

Denatured alcohol: This product is alcohol plus a chemical (denaturant) that makes it taste and smell bad so you won't drink it. Some denaturants are poisonous.

Check the spelling

Here's an interesting consumer note: Whiskey is spelled with an *e* if it's made in North America or Ireland, without an *e* — whisky — if it comes from another country (Scotland is the best example).

Why? Nobody knows for sure. But a reasonable assumption is that the Scots may simply have dropped the *e* to differentiate their distilled spirits from the spirits distilled in Ireland. When they journeyed to the United States, Irish immigrants brought their distillation methods and their *e* with them, so theirs became the name for whiskey made in America.

Distilled alcohol products

The second way to make an alcohol beverage is through *distillation.*

As with fermentation, yeasts are added to foods to make alcohol from sugars. But yeasts can't thrive in a place where the concentration of alcohol is higher than 20 percent. To concentrate the alcohol and separate it from the rest of the ingredients in the fermented liquid, distillers pour the fermented liquid into a *still,* a large vat with a wide columnlike tube on top. The still is heated so that the alcohol, which boils at a lower temperature than everything else in the vat, turns to vapor, which rises through the column on top of the still and is collected in containers, where it condenses back into a liquid.

Distilled alcohol, called *neutral spirits,* is the base for the alcohol beverages called spirits or distilled spirits: gin, rum, tequila, whiskey, and vodka. Brandy is a special product, a spirit distilled from wine. Fortified wines such as port and sherry are wines with spirits added.

The foods used to make beverage alcohol

Beverage alcohol can be made from virtually any carbohydrate food. The foods most commonly used are cereal grains, fruit, honey, molasses, and potatoes. All produce alcohol, but the alcohols have slightly different flavours and colours. Table 9-1 shows you which foods are used to produce the different kinds of alcohol beverages.

On its own, alcohol provides energy (7 calories per gram) but no nutrients, so distilled spirits, such as whiskey or plain, unflavoured vodka, serve up nothing but calories. Beer, wine, cider, and other fermented beverages, such as kumiss (fermented milk), contain some of the food from which they were made, so they contain small amounts of proteins and carbohydrates, vitamins, and minerals.

Table 9-1	Foods Used to Make Alcohol Beverages
Original Food	*Alcohol Beverage Produced*
Fruit and fruit juice	
Agave plant	Tequila
Apples	Hard cider
Grapes and other fruits	Wine
Grain	
Barley	Beer, various distilled spirits, kvass
Corn	Bourbon, corn whiskey, beer
Rice	Sake (a distilled product), rice wine
Rye	Whiskey
Wheat	Distilled spirits, beer
Others	
Honey	Mead
Milk	Kumiss (koumiss), kefir
Potatoes	Vodka
Sugar cane	Rum

How Much Alcohol Is in That Bottle?

No alcohol beverage is 100 percent alcohol. It's alcohol plus water, and — if it's a wine or beer — some residue of the foods from which it was made.

The label on every bottle of wine, beer, and spirits shows the alcohol content as *alcohol by volume* (ABV). ABV measures the amount of alcohol as a percentage of all the liquid in the container. For example, if your container holds 250 mL (8 ounces) of liquid and 25 mL (0.8 ounces) of that is alcohol, the product is 10 percent ABV — the alcohol content divided by the total amount of liquid.

By the way, right now, alcohol beverages are the only entries in the food and drink market sold without a Nutrition Facts label. There is debate about whether warning labels on the potential health effects of alcohol consumption are feasible or effective, but there are no plans to include a Nutrition Facts label.

Moving Alcohol through Your Body

Other foods must be digested before being absorbed by your cells, but alcohol flows directly through your body's membranes into your bloodstream, which carries alcohol to nearly every organ in your body. Here's a road map to show you the route travelled by the alcohol in every drink you take.

Flowing down the hatch from mouth to stomach

Alcohol is an *astringent;* it coagulates proteins on the surface of the lining of your mouth to make it "pucker." Some alcohol is absorbed through the lining of your mouth and throat, but most of the alcohol you drink spills into your stomach, where an enzyme called *gastric alcohol dehydrogenase* (ADH) begins to metabolize (digest) it.

How much alcohol dehydrogenase your body churns out is influenced by your ethnicity and your gender. For example, Asians, Native North Americans, and Inuits appear to secrete less alcohol dehydrogenase than do most Caucasians, and average women (regardless of ethnicity) make less ADH than average men. As a result, more unmetabolized alcohol flows from their tummies into their bloodstreams, and they're likely to become tipsy on smaller amounts of alcohol than would an average Caucasian male.

While you ponder that, the unmetabolized alcohol is flowing through your stomach walls into your bloodstream and on to your small intestine.

Stopping for a short visit at the energy factory

Most of the alcohol you drink is absorbed through the *duodenum* (small intestine), from which it flows through a large blood vessel (the portal vein) into your liver. There, an enzyme similar to gastric ADH metabolizes the alcohol, which is converted to energy by a coenzyme called *nicotinamide adenine dinucleotide* (NAD). NAD is also used to convert the glucose you get from other carbohydrates to energy; while NAD is being used for alcohol, glucose conversion grinds to a halt.

The normal, healthy liver can process about 14 grams (½ ounce) of pure alcohol — that's 170 to 340 grams (6 to 12 ounces) of beer, 240 grams (5 ounces) of wine, or 28 grams (1 ounce) of spirits — in an hour. The rest flows on to your heart.

Taking time out for air

As it enters your heart, alcohol reduces the force with which your heart muscle contracts. You pump out slightly less blood for a few minutes, blood vessels all over your body relax, and your blood pressure goes down temporarily. The contractions soon return to normal, but the blood vessels may remain relaxed and your blood pressure lower for as long as half an hour.

At the same time, alcohol flows in blood from your heart through your pulmonary vein to your lungs. Now you breathe out a tiny bit of alcohol every time you exhale, and your breath smells of liquor. Then the newly oxygenated, still alcohol-laden blood flows back through the pulmonary artery to your heart, and up and out through the *aorta* (the major artery that carries blood to your body).

Rising to the surface

In your blood, alcohol raises your level of high-density lipoproteins (HDLs), although not necessarily the specific *good* ones that carry cholesterol out of your body. (For more about lipoproteins, see Chapter 7.) Alcohol also makes blood less likely to clot, temporarily reducing your risk of heart attack and stroke.

Alcohol makes blood vessels expand, so more warm blood flows up from the centre of your body to the surface of the skin. You feel warmer for a while and, if your skin is fair, you may flush and turn pink. (Asians, who tend to make less alcohol dehydrogenase than do Caucasians, often experience a characteristic flushing when they drink even small amounts of alcohol.) At the same time, tiny amounts of alcohol ooze out through your pores, and your perspiration smells of alcohol.

Encountering curves in the road

Alcohol is a sedative. When it reaches your brain, it slows the transmission of impulses between nerve cells that control your ability to think and move. That's why your thinking may be fuzzy, your judgment impaired, your tongue twisted, your vision blurred, and your muscles rubbery.

When you drink, do you feel a sudden urge to urinate? Alcohol reduces your brain's production of *antidiuretic hormones,* chemicals that keep you from making too much urine. You may lose lots of liquid, plus vitamins and minerals. You also grow very thirsty, and your urine may smell faintly of alcohol. This cycle continues as long as you have alcohol circulating in your blood, or in other words, until your liver can manage to produce enough ADH to metabolize all the alcohol you've consumed. How long is that? Most people need an hour to metabolize the amount of alcohol in one drink (14 grams, or ½ ounce). But that's an average: Some people have alcohol circulating in their blood for up to three hours after taking a drink.

Alcohol and Health

Beverage alcohol has benefits as well as side effects. The benefits seem to be linked to what is commonly called *moderate drinking* — no more than one drink a day for a woman, two drinks a day for a man, consumed with food. The risks generally appear to flow from alcohol abuse.

Moderate drinking: Some benefits, some risks

Moderate amounts of alcohol reduce stress, so it isn't surprising that recent well-designed scientific studies on large groups of men and women suggest that moderate drinking is heart-healthy, that is, it protects the cardiovascular system (that's science talk for heart and blood vessels). Here are some findings about the cardiovascular and other benefits moderate drinking can provide:

- The American Cancer Society's Cancer Prevention Study 1 followed more than one million Americans in 25 states for 12 years to find that moderate alcohol intake had an "apparent protective effect on coronary heart disease." Translation: Men who drink moderately lower their risk of heart attack. The risk is 21 percent lower for men who have one drink a day than for men who never drink.

  A similar analysis of data for nearly 600,000 women in the long-running (Harvard) Nurses' Health Study shows that women who drink occasionally or have one drink a day are less likely to die of heart attack than those who don't drink at all.

- A 2003 study at Tulane University School of Public Health and Tropical Medicine shows that men who drink moderately (two drinks a day) also are less likely to die of clot-related stroke. But because alcohol reduces blood clotting, it increases the risk of *hemorrhagic* stroke (stroke caused by bleeding in the brain). Sorry about that.

- According to researchers at USDA's Agricultural Research Service (ARS) laboratory at Beltsville, Maryland, moderate drinking may lower a healthy older woman's risk of developing diabetes.

- Contrary to popular opinion, a 15-year, 1,700-person heart disease study at the Institute of Preventive Medicine, Kommunehospitalet in Copenhagen, Denmark, showed that older men and women who regularly consumed up to 21 drinks of wine a week were less likely than teetotalers to develop Alzheimer's disease and other forms of dementia. Similarly, a recent 12-year, 1,488-person survey at Johns Hopkins University in Maryland suggests that regular, moderate drinkers score better over time than teetotalers do on the Mini-Mental State Examination (MMSE), a standard test for memory, reasoning, and decision making.

That's the good news. Here's the bad news: The same studies that applaud the effects of moderate drinking on heart health are less reassuring about the relationship between alcohol and cancer. The American Cancer Society's Cancer Prevention Study 1 shows that people who take more than two drinks a day have a higher incidence of cancer of the mouth and throat (esophagus). In addition:

- Researchers at the University of Oklahoma say that men who drink five or more beers a day double their risk of rectal cancer.

- American Cancer Society statistics show a higher risk of breast cancer among women who have more than three drinks a week, but newer studies suggest this effect may apply only to older women using hormone replacement therapy.

The physical risks of alcohol abuse

Alcohol abuse is a term generally taken to mean drinking so much that it interferes with your ability to have a normal, productive life. The short-term effects of excessive drinking are well known to one and all, especially to men who may find that drinking too much decreases sexual desire and makes it impossible to . . . well . . . perform. (No evidence suggests that excessive drinking interferes with female orgasm.)

A lot and a little versus the middle

When scientists talk about the relationship between alcohol and heart disease, the word *J-curve* often pops up. What's a J-curve? A statistical graph in the shape of the letter J.

In terms of heart disease, the lower peak on the left of the J shows the risk among teetotalers, the high spike on the right shows the risk among those who drink too much, and the curve in the centre shows the risk in the moderate middle. In other words, the J-curve says that people who drink moderately have a lower risk of heart disease than people who drink too much or not at all.

That info's nice. This is better: According to a recent report from the Alberta Alcohol and Drug Abuse Commission, the J-curve may also describe the relationship between alcohol and stroke, alcohol and diabetes, alcohol and bone loss, and alcohol and longevity. The simple fact is that moderate drinkers appear to live longer, healthier lives than either teetotalers or alcohol abusers. Cheers!

Binge drinking: A behavioural no-no

Binge drinkers are "once-in-a-while alcoholics." They don't drink every day, but when they do indulge, they go so far overboard that they sometimes fail to come back up. In simple terms, binge drinking is downing very large amounts of alcohol in a short time, not for a pleasant lift but to get drunk. Binge drinkers may consume so much beer, wine, or spirits that the amount of alcohol in their blood rises to lethal levels, leading to death by alcohol poisoning. Got the picture? Binge drinking is not a sport. It's potentially fatal behaviour. Don't do it.

Excessive drinking can also make you feel terrible the next day. *The morning after* is not fiction. A hangover is a miserable physical fact:

- You're thirsty because you lost excess water through copious urination.

- Your stomach hurts and you're queasy because even small amounts of alcohol irritate your stomach lining, causing it to secrete extra acid and lots of *histamine*, the same immune system chemical that makes the skin around a mosquito bite red and itchy.

- Your muscles ache and your head pounds because processing alcohol through your liver requires an enzyme — nicotinamide adenine dinucleotide (NAD) — normally used to convert *lactic acid*, a by-product of muscle activity, to other chemicals that can be used for energy. The extra, unprocessed lactic acid piles up painfully in your muscles.

Alcoholism: An addiction disease

Alcoholics are people who can't control their drinking. Untreated alcoholism is a life-threatening disease that can lead to death from an accident or suicide (both are more common among heavy drinkers), from a toxic reaction (acute alcohol poisoning that paralyzes body organs, including the heart and lungs), from liver damage (cirrhosis), or from malnutrition.

Alcoholism makes it extremely difficult for your body to get essential nutrients. Here's why:

- Alcohol depresses appetite.

- An alcoholic may substitute alcohol for food, getting calories but no nutrients.

- Even when alcoholics eat, the alcohol in their tissues can prevent the proper absorption of vitamins (notably the B vitamins), minerals, and other nutrients. Alcohol may also reduce the alcoholic's ability to synthesize proteins.

No one knows exactly why some people are able to have a drink once a day or once a month or once a year, enjoy it, and move on, while others become addicted to alcohol. In the past, alcoholism has been blamed on heredity (bad genes), lack of willpower, or even a bad upbringing. But as science continues to unravel the mysteries of body chemistry, it's reasonable to expect that researchers will eventually come up with a rational scientific explanation for the differences between social drinkers and people who can't safely use alcohol. It just hasn't happened yet.

Who should not drink

No one should drink to excess. But some people shouldn't drink at all, not even in moderation. They include

- **People who plan to drive or do work that requires both attention and skill.** Alcohol slows reaction time and makes your motor skills — turning the wheel of the car, operating a sewing machine — less precise.

- **Women who are pregnant or who plan to become pregnant in the near future.** *Fetal alcohol syndrome* (FAS) is a collection of birth defects including low birth weight, heart defects, retardation, and facial deformities documented only in babies born to female alcoholics. No evidence links FAS to casual drinking — that is, one or two drinks during a pregnancy or even one or two drinks a week.

- **People who take certain prescription drugs or over-the-counter medication.** Alcohol makes some drugs stronger, increases the side effects of some drugs, and renders other drugs less effective. At the same time, some drugs make alcohol a more powerful sedative or slow down the elimination of alcohol from your body.

Table 9-2 shows some of the interactions known to occur between alcohol and some common prescription and over-the-counter drugs. This short list gives you an idea of the general interactions likely to occur between alcohol and drugs. But the list is far from complete, so if you're taking any kind of medication — over-the-counter or prescription — check with your doctor or pharmacist regarding the possibility of an interaction with alcohol.

Table 9-2	Drug and Alcohol Interactions
Drug	*Possible Interaction with Alcohol*
Analgesics (acetaminophen)	Increased liver toxicity
Analgesics (aspirin and other non-steroidal inflammatory drugs — NSAIDs)	Increased stomach bleeding; irritation

Drug	*Possible Interaction with Alcohol*
Antiarthritis drugs	Increased stomach bleeding; irritation
Antidepressants	Increased drowsiness/intoxication; high blood pressure (depends on the type of drug — check with your doctor)
Antidiabetes drugs	Excessively low blood sugar
Antihypertension drugs	Very low blood pressure
Antituberculosis medication (isoniazid)	Decreased drug effectiveness; higher risk of hepatitis
Diet pills	Excessive nervousness
Diuretics	Low blood pressure
Iron supplements	Excessive absorption of iron
Sleeping pills	Increased sedation
Tranquilizers	Increased sedation

James W. Long and James J. Rybacki. The Essential Guide to Prescription Drugs 1995 (New York: Harper Collins, 1995)

The power of purple (and peanuts)

Grape skin, pulp, and seeds contain *resveratrol,* a naturally occurring plant chemical that seems to reduce the risk of heart disease and some kinds of cancer. The darker the grapes, the higher the concentration of resveratrol.

Dark purple grape juice, for example, has more resveratrol than red grape juice, which has more resveratrol than white grape juice. Because wine is made from grapes, it, too, contains resveratrol (red wine has more resveratrol than white wine).

But you don't need to drink grape juice or wine to get resveratrol. You can simply snack on peanuts. Yes, peanuts. A 1998 analysis from the USDA Agricultural Research Service in Raleigh, North Carolina, showed that peanuts have 1.7 to 3.7 micrograms of resveratrol per gram of nuts. Compare that to the 0.7 micrograms of resveratrol in a glass of red grape juice or 0.6 to 8.0 micrograms of resveratrol per gram of red wine.

This fact may explain data from the long-running Harvard University/Brigham and Women's Hospital Nurses' Health Study, which shows that women who eat an ounce of nuts a day have a lower risk of heart disease. So let's see — wine, grape juice, peanuts … decisions, decisions.

Heeding Advice from the Sages: Moderation

Good advice is always current. The folks who wrote Ecclesiastes (a book in the Bible) centuries ago may have been speaking to you when they said, "Wine is as good as life to man if it be drunk moderately." And it's impossible to improve on this slogan from the Romans (actually, one Roman writer named Terence): "Moderation in all things." Hey, you can't get a message more direct — or more sensible — than that.

Chapter 10

Vigorous Vitamins

. . . .

In This Chapter

▶ Understanding the value of vitamins

▶ Revealing the best food sources for the vitamins you need

▶ Discovering the consequences of taking too many (or too few) vitamins

▶ Knowing when you may need extra vitamins

. . . .

*V*itamins are *organic chemicals,* substances that contain carbon, hydrogen, and oxygen. They occur naturally in all living things, plants and animals alike: flowers, trees, fruits, vegetables, chickens, fish, cows — and you.

Vitamins regulate a variety of bodily functions. They're essential for building body tissues such as bones, skin, glands, nerves, and blood. They assist in metabolizing (digesting) proteins, fats, and carbohydrates so that you can get energy from food. They prevent nutritional deficiency diseases, promote healing, and encourage good health.

This chapter is a guide to where the vitamins are, how you can add them to your diet, how to tell how much is more than enough of any specific vitamin, and ever so much more . . . maybe more than you really want to know.

Taking a Look at the Vitamins Your Body Needs

Your body needs at least 13 specific vitamins: vitamin A, vitamin D, vitamin E, vitamin K, vitamin C, and the members of the B vitamin family: thiamine (B1), riboflavin (B2), niacin (B3), pantothenic acid (B5), pyridoxine (B6), biotin, folate, and cobalamin (B12). And one unusual compound called choline has recently received some favourable mention (more about it in the "Choline" section later in this chapter). You need only minuscule quantities of vitamins for good health. In some cases, the Recommended Dietary Allowances (RDAs), determined by the National Research Council in the U.S., may be as small as several micrograms (1/1,000,000 — that's one one-millionth — of a gram).

The father of all vitamins: Casimir Funk

Vitamins are so much a part of modern life you may have a hard time believing they were first discovered less than a century ago. Of course, people have long known that certain foods contain something special. For example, the ancient Greek physician Hippocrates prescribed liver for night-blindness (the inability to see well in dim light). By the end of the 18th century (1795), British Navy ships carried a mandatory supply of limes or lime juice to prevent scurvy among the men, thus earning the Brits once and forever the nickname Limeys. Later on, the Japanese Navy gave its sailors whole grain barley to ward off beriberi.

Everyone knew these prescriptions worked, but nobody knew why — until 1912, when Casimir Funk

(1884–1967), a Polish biochemist working first in England and then in the U.S., identified "somethings" in food that he called *vitamines* (vita = life; amines = nitrogen compounds).

The following year, Funk and a fellow biochemist, Briton Frederick Hopkins, suggested that some medical conditions such as scurvy and beriberi were simply deficiency diseases caused by the absence of a specific nutrient in the body. Adding a food with the missing nutrient to one's diet would prevent or cure the deficiency disease.

Eureka!

Vitamins are either *fat soluble* or *water soluble,* meaning that they dissolve either in fat or in water. If you consume larger amounts of fat-soluble vitamins than your body needs, the excess is stored in body fat. Excess water-soluble vitamins are eliminated in urine.

Large amounts of fat-soluble vitamins stored in your body may cause problems (see the section "Fat-soluble vitamins" in this chapter). With water-soluble vitamins, your body simply shrugs its shoulders, so to speak, and urinates away most of the excess.

 Medical students often use mnemonic devices — memory joggers — to remember complicated lists of body parts and symptoms of diseases. Here's one you can use to remember which vitamins are fat soluble: "All Dogs Eat Kidneys." This saying helps us remember that vitamins A, D, E, and K are fat soluble. All the rest dissolve in water.

Fat-soluble vitamins

Vitamin A, vitamin D, vitamin E, and vitamin K are relatives that have two characteristics in common: All dissolve in fat, and all are stored in your fatty tissues. But like members of any family, they also have distinct personalities. One keeps your skin moist. Another protects your bones. A third keeps reproductive organs purring happily. And the fourth enables you to make special proteins.

Help! I'm turning orange

Because you store retinol in your liver, megadoses of preformed vitamin A can build up to toxic levels. Not so with carotenoids, which serve up a precursor of that vitamin. They aren't stored in the liver, so these red and yellow pigments in fruits and vegetables are safe even in very large amounts.

But that doesn't mean that excess carotenoids don't have side effects. Carotenoids, like retinoids, are stored in body fat. If you wolf down large quantities of carotenoid-rich foods like carrots and tomatoes every day, day after day, for several weeks, your skin — particularly the palms of your hands and the soles of your feet — will turn a nifty shade of dusty orange, brighter if your skin is naturally light, darker if it's naturally dark. It sounds fantastic, but it has actually happened to people eating two cups of carrots and two whole tomatoes a day for several months. When they cut down on the carrots and tomatoes, the colour faded.

Now, let's see … it's September 1, and you've been invited to a Halloween party. Maybe this year you'll go as a pumpkin. If you start packing in the carrots and tomatoes right now …

Which does what? Read on.

Vitamin A

Vitamin A is the moisturizing nutrient that keeps your skin and *mucous membranes* (the slick tissue that lines the eyes, nose, mouth, throat, vagina, and rectum) smooth and supple. Vitamin A is also the vision vitamin, a constituent of *11-cis retinol,* a protein in the *rods* (cells in the back of your eye that enable you to see even when the lights are low) that prevents or slows the development of age-related *macular degeneration,* or progressive damage to the retina of the eye, which can cause the loss of central vision (the ability to see clearly enough to read or do fine work). Finally, vitamin A promotes the growth of healthy bones and teeth, keeps your reproductive system humming, and encourages your immune system to churn out the cells you need to fight off infection.

Two chemicals provide vitamin A: retinoids and carotenoids. *Retinoids* are compounds whose names all start with *ret:* retinol, retinaldehyde, retinoic acid, and so on. These fat-soluble substances are found in several foods of animal origin: liver (again!) and whole milk, eggs, and butter. Retinoids give you *preformed* vitamin A, the kind of nutrient your body can use right away.

The second form of vitamin A is the *vitamin A precursor,* a chemical such as beta-carotene, a deep yellow carotenoid (pigment) found in dark green and bright yellow fruits and vegetables. Your body transforms a vitamin A precursor into a retinol-like substance. So far, scientists have identified at least 500 different carotenoids. Only 1 in 10 — about 50 altogether — is considered, like beta-carotene, to be a source of vitamin A.

Hand in hand: How vitamins help each other

All vitamins have specific jobs in your body. Some have partners. Here are some examples of nutrient cooperation:

- ✔ Vitamin E keeps vitamin A from being destroyed in your intestines.

- ✔ Vitamin D enables your body to absorb calcium and phosphorus.

- ✔ Vitamin C helps folate build proteins.

- ✔ Vitamin B1 works in digestive enzyme systems with niacin, pantothenic acid, and magnesium.

Taking vitamins with other vitamins may also improve body levels of nutrients. For example, in 1993, scientists at the National Cancer Institute and the U.S. Department of Agriculture (USDA) Agricultural Research Service gave one group of volunteers a vitamin E capsule plus a multivitamin pill; they gave a second group vitamin E alone; and they gave a third group no vitamins at all. The people getting vitamin E plus the multivitamin had the highest amount of vitamin E in their blood — more than twice as high as those who took plain vitamin E capsules.

Sometimes, one vitamin may even alleviate a deficiency caused by the lack of another vitamin. People who do not get enough folate are at risk of a form of anemia in which their red blood cells fail to mature. As soon as they get folate, either by injection or by mouth, they begin making new healthy cells. That's to be expected. What's surprising is that anemia caused by *pellagra*, the niacin deficiency disease, may also respond to folate treatment.

Isn't nature neat?

Traditionally, the recommended dietary allowances of vitamin A are measured in International Units (IU). However, because retinol is the most efficient source of vitamin A, the modern way to measure the RDA for vitamin A is as retinol equivalents, abbreviated as RE. One microgram (mcg) RE = 3.3 IU. However, many vitamin products still list the RDA for vitamin A in IUs.

Vitamin D

If you see the word "bones" or "teeth," what nutrient springs most quickly to mind? If you answer calcium, you're giving only a partial picture. True, calcium is essential for hardening teeth and bones. But no matter how much calcium you consume, without vitamin D, your body can't absorb and use the mineral. So vitamin D is vital for building — and holding — strong bones and teeth.

Researchers at the Bone Metabolism Laboratory at the Jean Mayer USDA Human Nutrition Research Center on Aging at Tufts University in Boston say vitamin D may also reduce the risk of tooth loss by preventing the inflammatory response that leads to periodontal disease, a condition that destroys the thin tissue (ligaments) that connects the teeth to the surrounding jawbone. Finally, a report in the February 2006 issue of *The American Journal of Public Health* suggests that taking 1,000 IU of vitamin D a day may cut in half a person's risk of developing some forms of cancer, including cancer of the colon, breast, and ovaries.

Vitamin D comes in three forms: calciferol, cholecalciferol, and ergocalciferol. *Calciferol* occurs naturally in fish oils and egg yolk. In Canada, it's added to margarines and milk. *Cholecalciferol* is created when sunlight hits your skin and ultraviolet rays react with steroid chemicals in body fat just underneath the skin. *Ergocalciferol* is synthesized in plants exposed to sunlight. Cholecalciferol and ergocalciferol justify vitamin D's nickname: the Sunshine Vitamin.

The RDA for vitamin D is measured either in International Units (IUs) or micrograms (mcg) of cholecalciferol: 10 mcg cholecalciferol = 400 IU vitamin D.

Vitamin E

Every animal, including you, needs vitamin E to maintain a healthy reproductive system, nerves, and muscles. Like B vitamins, vitamin E is a family of eight different molecules: four *tocopherols* and four *tocotrienols* (alpha, beta, gamma, and delta forms for each) of naturally occurring chemicals in vegetable oils, nuts, whole grains, and green leafy vegetables — your best natural sources of vitamin E.

Both tocopherols and tocotrienols are powerful antioxidants. *Antioxidants* prevent free radicals (incomplete pieces of molecules) from hooking up with other molecules or fragments of molecules to form toxic substances that can attack tissues in your body. In fact, nutrition scientists at Purdue University, in Indiana, released a study showing that vitamin E promotes bone growth by stopping free radicals from reacting with polyunsaturated fatty acids (see Chapter 7 for information on fats) to create molecules that interfere with the formation of new bone cells.

But some claims about E's heart health benefits are now considered iffy. True, a recent clinical trial at Cambridge University in England showed that taking 800 IU of vitamin E, two times the RDA, may reduce the risk of nonfatal heart attacks for people who already have heart disease. And, yes, a federal Women's Health Study in the U.S. found that older women taking 600 IU of vitamin E per day had a lower risk of heart attack and a lower risk of death from heart disease. But the Heart Outcomes Prevention Evaluation (HOPE) study showed no such benefits. In fact, people taking 400 IU per day of vitamin E were more likely to develop heart failure. No one (and no study) has found similar problems among those taking less vitamin E, say 100 IU per day. Whew.

One of the possible reasons for the confusion and conflicting results is that only one form of vitamin E was used in these studies: alpha tocopherol. In nature, all eight forms of the vitamins occur together, and the health benefits are most likely conferred when the whole vitamin is consumed in whole food. Vitamins, minerals, and other health-promoting properties of food work in concert with each other. So get your vitamin E by consuming rich whole foods.

The best sources of vitamin E are vegetables, oils, wheat germ, wheat germ oil, whole grain breads and cereals, nuts, and seeds. The RDA is expressed as milligrams *a-tocopherol equivalents* (abbreviated as *a-TE*).

Vitamin K

Vitamin K is a group of chemicals that your body uses to make specialized proteins found in blood *plasma* (the clear fluid in blood), such as prothrombin, the protein chiefly responsible for blood clotting. You also need vitamin K to make bone and kidney tissues. Like vitamin D, vitamin K is essential for healthy bones. Vitamin D increases calcium absorption; vitamin K activates at least three different proteins that take part in forming new bone cells. For example, a report on 888 men and women from the long-running Framingham (Massachusetts) Heart Study shows that people who consumed the least vitamin K each day had the highest incidence of broken bones. The same was true for a 1999 analysis of data from the Nurses' Health Study.

Vitamin K is found in dark green, leafy vegetables (cabbage, kale, lettuce, spinach, and turnip greens, including broccoli), cheese, liver, cereals, and fruits, but most of what you need comes from resident colonies of friendly bacteria in your intestines, an assembly line of busy bugs churning out the vitamin day and night.

Water-soluble vitamins

Vitamin C and the entire roster of B vitamins (thiamin, riboflavin, niacin, pantothenic acid, pyridoxine, folate, biotin, and cobalamin) are usually grouped together simply because they all dissolve in water.

The ability to dissolve in water is an important point, because that means large amounts of these nutrients can't be stored in your body. If you take in more than you need to perform specific bodily tasks, you will simply pee away all the excess. The good news is that these vitamins rarely cause side effects. The bad news is that you have to take enough of these vitamins every day to protect yourself against deficiencies.

Vitamin C

Vitamin C, which also is referred to as ascorbic acid, is essential for the development and maintenance of connective tissue (the fat, muscle, and bone framework of the human body). Vitamin C speeds the production of new cells in wound healing, is a powerful antioxidant, protects your immune system, helps you fight off infection, reduces the severity of allergic reactions, and plays a role in the syntheses of hormones and other body chemicals. For more on this important nutrient, see "A special case: The continuing saga of vitamin C," later in this chapter.

Thiamine (vitamin B1)

Call it thiamine. Call it B1. Just don't call it late for lunch (or any other meal). This sulphur *(thia)* and nitrogen *(amin)* compound, the first of the B vitamins to be isolated and identified, helps ensure a healthy appetite. It acts as a *coenzyme* (a substance that works along with other enzymes) essential to at least four different processes by which your body extracts energy from carbo-hydrates. It also helps maintain proper functioning of the heart, nervous system, and digestive system.

Although thiamine is found in every body tissue, the highest concentrations are in your vital organs — heart, liver, and kidneys.

The richest dietary sources of thiamine are unrefined cereals and grains, lean pork, beans, nuts, and seeds. In Canada, refined flours, stripped of their thiamine, are a nutritional reality, so many Canadians get most of their thiamine from breads and cereals enriched with additional B1.

Riboflavin (vitamin B2)

Riboflavin (vitamin B2), the second B vitamin to be identified, was once called "vitamin G." Its present name is a derivative of its chemical structure, a carbon-hydrogen-oxygen skeleton that includes *ribitol* (a sugar) attached to a *flavonoid* (a substance from plants that contains a pigment called flavone).

Like thiamine, riboflavin is a coenzyme. Without it, your body can't digest and use proteins, fats, and carbohydrates. In fact, it plays a key role in energy production. Like vitamin A, it protects the health of mucous membranes — the moist tissues that line the eyes, mouth, nose, throat, vagina, and rectum.

You get riboflavin from foods of animal origin (meat, fish, poultry, eggs, and milk), whole or enriched grain products, brewer's yeast, and dark green vegetables (like broccoli and spinach), as well as from legumes such as soybeans and kidney beans.

PQQ, a whole new itty-bitty vitamin?

The next time someone tells you to mind your *p*s and *q*s, don't take offense. The subject may be nutrition, not manners — pyrroloquinoline quinone (PQQ), the first new vitamin-like substance in more than half a century. The water-soluble compound, which is very similar to riboflavin and niacin, was identified at the University of Texas in 1979 and proposed as a new vitamin four years later by researchers at Tokyo's Institute of Physical and Chemical Research. It's widely available in plant foods such as green tea, green bell peppers, papaya, spinach, carrots, cabbage, and bananas. Animal studies show a connection between PQQ and an enzyme used by mammals to digest lysine, an amino acid found in proteins. Despite suggestions that it is truly a vitamin (absolutely essential for health), the jury is still out on this one. The molecule is essential for some bacteria, and maybe for mice. And you? Well, if you need it, you need very, very little. The amounts of other vitamins are measured in milligrams (thousandths of a gram) or micrograms (millionths of a gram). But PQQ is measured in nanograms (billionths of a gram) — 1/1,000,000,000. Which is about as itty-bitty as it gets.

Lemons, limes, oranges — and bacon?

Check the meat label. There it is, plain as day — vitamin C in the form of *sodium ascorbate* or *isoascorbate*.

The Food and Drug Administration (FDA) says it has to be there because vitamin C does for meat exactly what it does for your body: It prevents free radicals (incomplete pieces of molecules) from hooking up with each other to form damaging compounds, in this case *carcinogens*, substances that cause cancer.

Processed meats such as bacon and sausages are preserved with sodium nitrite, which protects the meat from *Clostridium botulinum*, a micro-organism that causes the potentially fatal food poisoning known as botulism.

On its own, sodium nitrite reacts at high temperatures with compounds in meat to form carcinogens called nitrosamines. But like the Lone Ranger, antioxidant vitamin C rides to the rescue, preventing the chemical reaction and keeping the sausage and bacon safe to eat. How's that for healthy eating, Kemo Sabe?

Niacin (vitamin B3)

Niacin is one name for a pair of naturally occurring nutrients, nicotinic acid and nicotinamide. Niacin is essential for proper growth, and like other B vitamins, it's intimately involved in enzyme reactions. In fact, it's an integral part of an enzyme that enables oxygen to flow into body tissues. Like thiamine, it gives you a healthy appetite and participates in the metabolism of sugars and fats.

Niacin is available either as a preformed nutrient or via the conversion of the amino acid tryptophan. Preformed niacin comes from meat; tryptophan comes from milk and dairy foods. Some niacin is present in grains, but your body can't absorb it efficiently unless the grain has been treated with lime — the mineral, not the fruit. This is a common practice in Central American and South American countries, where lime is added to cornmeal in making tortillas. In Canada, breads and cereals are routinely fortified with niacin. Your body easily absorbs the added niacin.

The term used to describe the niacin RDA is NE (niacin equivalent): 60 milligrams tryptophan = 1 milligram niacin = 1 niacin equivalent (NE).

Pyridoxine (vitamin B6)

Vitamin B6 is another multiple compound, this one comprising three related chemicals: pyridoxine, pyridoxal, and pyridoxamine. Vitamin B6, a component of enzymes that metabolizes proteins and fats, is essential for getting energy and nutrients from food. It helps balance sodium and potassium in the body and is involved in the production of neurotransmitters (chemicals the cells of the brain use to communicate with each other). It also helps lower blood levels of homocysteine (see Chapter 6), an amino acid produced when you digest proteins. Canada's Heart and Stroke Foundation Web site says the total evidence to date is that a high level of homocysteine is an independent (but not major) risk factor for atherosclerosis, and the *American Journal of Clinical Nutrition* reported in 2005 that a high homocysteine level may be associated with an age-related decline in memory. Some follow-up studies have shown no reduction in the risk of heart disease and no improvement in memory in those who reduce their blood levels of homocysteine, so we'll have to wait for more evidence. The general rule of thumb is still to follow a healthy balanced diet to reduce your risk of heart disease.

The best food sources of vitamin B6 are liver, chicken, fish, pork, lamb, milk, eggs, unmilled rice, whole grains, soybeans, potatoes, beans, nuts, seeds, and dark green vegetables such as turnip greens. In Canada, bread and other products made with refined grains have added vitamin B6.

Folate

Folate, or folic acid, is an essential nutrient for human beings and other *vertebrates* (animals with backbones). Folate takes part in the synthesis of DNA, the metabolism of proteins, and the subsequent synthesis of amino acids used to produce new body cells and tissues. Folate is vital for normal growth and wound healing. Pregnant women need an adequate supply of the vitamin so they can create new maternal tissue as well as fetal tissue. In addition, an adequate supply of folate dramatically reduces the risk of spinal cord birth defects. Beans, dark green leafy vegetables, liver, yeast, and various fruits are excellent food sources of folate, and all multivitamin supplements must now provide 400 mcg of folate per dose.

Cobalamin (vitamin B12)

Vitamin B12 (cyanocobalamin) makes healthy red blood cells. Vitamin B12 protects *myelin,* the fatty material that covers your nerves and enables you to transmit electrical impulses (messages) between nerve cells. These messages make it possible for you to see, hear, think, move, and do all the things a healthy body does each day. In 2005, the *Canadian Medical Association Journal* reported that low blood levels of B12 in older people are linked to higher levels of homocysteine (a minor risk factor for heart disease; see "Pyridoxine [vitamin B6]").

Vitamin B12 is unique. First, it's the only vitamin that contains a mineral, cobalt. (Cyanocobalamin, a cobalt compound, is commonly used as "vitamin B12" in vitamin pills and nutritional supplements.) Second, it's a vitamin that can't be made by higher plants (the ones that give us fruits and vegetables). Like vitamin K, vitamin B12 is made by beneficial bacteria living in your small intestine. Meat, fish, poultry, milk products, and eggs are good sources of vitamin B12. Grains don't naturally contain vitamin B12, but like other B vitamins, it's added to grain products in Canada.

Biotin

Biotin is a B vitamin, a component of enzymes that ferry carbon and oxygen atoms between cells. Biotin helps you metabolize fats and carbohydrates and is essential for synthesizing the fatty acids and amino acids you need for healthy growth. And it seems to prevent a buildup of fat deposits that may interfere with the proper functioning of your liver and kidneys. (No, biotin won't keep fat from settling in more visible places, such as your hips.)

The best food sources of biotin are liver, egg yolk, yeast, nuts, and beans. If your diet doesn't give you all the biotin you need, bacteria in your gut will synthesize enough to make up the difference. No RDA exists for biotin, but the Food and Nutrition Board has established an Adequate Intake (AI), which means a safe and effective daily dose.

Pantothenic acid (vitamin B5)

Pantothenic acid, another B vitamin, is vital to enzyme reactions that enable you to use carbohydrates and create steroid biochemicals such as hormones. Pantothenic acid also helps stabilize blood sugar levels; it defends against infection and protects *hemoglobin* (the protein in red blood cells that carries oxygen through the body), as well as nerve, brain, and muscle tissue. You get pantothenic acid from meat, fish, poultry, eggs, legumes such as beans, whole grain cereals, and fortified grain products. As with biotin, the Food and Nutrition Board has established an AI for pantothenic acid.

Choline

Choline is not a vitamin, a mineral, a protein, a carbohydrate, or a fat, but it is an essential nutrient and is usually lumped in with the B vitamins, so heeeeere's choline!

In 1998, 138 years after this nutrient first was identified, the Institute of Medicine (IOM) finally declared it essential for human beings. The IOM had good reasons for doing so. Choline keeps body cells healthy. It's used to make *acetylcholine,* a chemical that enables brain cells to exchange messages. It protects the heart and lowers the risk of liver cancer. And new research at the University of North Carolina (Chapel Hill) shows that choline plays a role in developing and maintaining the ability to think and remember, at least among rat pups and other beasties born to lab animals that were given choline supplements while pregnant. Follow-up studies showed that prenatal choline supplements helped the animals grow bigger brain cells.

True, no one knows whether this would also be true for human pups, er, babies, but some researchers advise pregnant women to eat a varied diet, because getting choline from basic stuff like eggs, meat, and milk is so easy.

IOM's Food and Nutrition Board, the group that sets the RDAs, has established an AI (Adequate Intake) for choline.

Getting Your Vitamins

One reasonable set of guidelines for good nutrition is the list of Recommended Dietary Allowances (RDAs) established by the National Research Council's Food and Nutrition Board. The RDAs present safe and effective doses for healthy people.

You can find the chart of RDAs for adults (ages 19 and up) in Chapter 4. It's very, very long, with RDAs for ten different groups of people (men, women, old, young) for 25 specific vitamins and minerals, plus choline.

Meanwhile, Table 10-1 is the easy alternative: It gives you the RDAs for adult men and women (ages 19 to 50), plus a quick, no-brainer guide to food portions that provide at least 25 percent of the RDAs of vitamins for healthy adult men and women ages 25 to 50.

Photocopy this chart. Pin it on your fridge. Tape it to your organizer or appointment book. Stick it in your wallet. Think of it as the truly simple way to see how easy it is to eat healthy.

Table 10-1	**Servings That Provide at Least 25 Percent of the RDA**
Food	*Serving = 25 Percent of the RDA*
VITAMIN A	**RDA: Women 4,000 IU, Men 5,000 IU***
Breads, cereals, grains	
Oatmeal — instant, fortified	575 mL (2⅓ cups)
Cold cereal	30 mL (2 tablespoons)
Fruits	
Apricots (dried, cooked)	125 mL (½ cup)
Cantaloupe (raw)	125 mL (½ cup)
Mango (raw)	½ medium
Vegetables	
Carrots, kale, peas and carrots, sweet red pepper (all cooked)	125 mL (½ cup)
Meat, poultry, fish	
Liver — chicken, turkey, diced	125 mL (½ cup)

(continued)

Table 10-1 *(continued)*

Food	Serving = 25 Percent of the RDA
Dairy products	
Milk — low-fat, skim	500 mL (2 cups)
VITAMIN D	RDA: Women 5 mcg or 200 IU, Men 5 mcg or 200 IU
Meat, poultry, fish	
Salmon (canned)	42 grams (1(½ ounces)
Tuna (canned)	56 grams (2 ounces)
Dairy products	
Eggs	3 medium
Milk — enriched	250 mL (1 cup)
VITAMIN E	RDA: Women 15 mg a-TE, Men 15 mg a-TE
Breads, cereals, grains	
Cold cereal	30 mL (2 tbsp)
Wheat germ — plain	30 mL (2 tbsp)
Fruits	
Apricots, peaches (canned)	250 mL (1 cup)
Vegetables	
Greens — dandelion, mustard, turnip (cooked)	250 mL (1 cup)
Meat, poultry, fish	
Shrimp	85 grams (3 ounces)
Other	
Almonds, hazelnuts, filberts	30 mL (2 tbsp)
Peanut butter	30 mL (2 tbsp)
Sunflower seeds	30 mL (2 tbsp)
VITAMIN C	RDA: Women 75 mg, Men 90 mg**
Breads, cereals, grains	
Cold cereal	30 mL (2 tbsp)

Food	Serving = 25 Percent of the RDA
Fruits	
Cantaloupe, diced	125 mL (½ cup)
Grapefruit	½ medium
Mango (raw)	½ medium
Orange	1 medium
Strawberries	125 mL (½ cup)
Grape, orange, or tomato juice	50 mL (¼ cup)
Vegetables	
Asparagus, broccoli, Brussels	125 mL (½ cup) sprouts, kale, kohlrabi, snow peas (cooked), sweet peppers
Sweet potato	1 medium
Meat, poultry, fish	
Liver — beef, pork	85 grams (3 ounces)
THIAMIN (VITAMIN B1)	**RDA: Women 1.1 mg, Men 1.2 mg**
Breads, cereals, grains	
Bagel, English muffin, roll	2 whole
Bread	4 slices
Farina, grits	125 mL (½ cup)
Oatmeal — instant, fortified	75 mL (⅓ cup)
Fruits	
Cantaloupe, honeydew melon	250 mL (1 cup)
Vegetables	
Corn, peas, peas and carrots (cooked)	250 mL (1 cup)
Meat, poultry, fish	
Ham — roast, smoked, cured, lean	85 grams (3 ounces)
Liver — beef, pork	85 grams (3 ounces)
Pork — all varieties except sausage	85 grams (3 ounces)

(continued)

Table 10-1 *(continued)*

Food	Serving = 25 Percent of the RDA
Other	
Sunflower seeds (hulled, unroasted)	30 mL (2 tbsp)
RIBOFLAVIN (VITAMIN B2)	**RDA: Women 1.1 mg, Men 1.3 mg**
Breads, cereals, grains	
Bagel, English muffin, pita	2 whole
Cold cereal	30 mL (2 tbsp)
Meat, poultry, fish	
Liver — beef, calf, pork	85 grams (3 ounces)
Liver — chicken, turkey	125 mL (½ cup), diced
Liverwurst	28 grams (1 ounce)
Dairy products	
Milk — all varieties	500 mL (2 cups)
Yogourt — low-fat, non-fat	250 mL (1 cup)
NIACIN	**RDA: Women 14 mg NE, Men 16 mg NE**
Breads, cereals, grains	
Bagel, bran muffin, English muffin, pita, roll	2 whole
Cold cereal — fortified	30 mL (2 tbsp)
Meat, poultry, fish	
Lamb, pork, veal — lean	85 grams (3 ounces)
Liver — beef, calf, pork	85 grams (3 ounces)
Chicken half-breast (no skin)	85 grams (3 ounces)
Mackerel, mullet, salmon, swordfish	85 grams (3 ounces)
Other	
Peanuts, peanut butter	60 mL (4 tbsp)
VITAMIN B6	**RDA: Women 1.3 mg, Men 1.3 mg**
Breads, cereals, grains	
Oatmeal — instant, fortified	75 mL (⅓ cup)

Food	Serving = 25 Percent of the RDA
Cold cereal	30 mL (2 tbsp)
Fruits	
Banana (raw)	1 medium
Prunes (dried, cooked)	250 mL (1 cup)
Vegetables	
Plantain (boiled)	1 medium
Meat, poultry, fish	
Chicken half-breast (roasted, no skin)	85 grams (3 ounces)
Lamb chop — lean only	1
Liver — beef	85 grams (3 ounces)
FOLATE	**RDA: Women 400 mcg, Men 400 mcg**
Breads, cereals, grains	
Whole wheat English muffin, pita	2 whole
Cold cereal	30 mL (2 tbsp)
Vegetables	
Asparagus, beets, broccoli, Brussels sprouts, cauliflower, Chinese cabbage, creamed corn, spinach (cooked)	250 mL (1 cup)
Beans — black-eyed peas, lentils, red kidney (dry, cooked)	125 mL (½ cup)
Greens — mustard, turnip (cooked)	250 mL (1 cup)
Meat, poultry, fish	
Liver — beef, calf, pork	85 grams (3 ounces)
VITAMIN B12	**RDA: Women 2.4 mcg, Men 2.4 mcg**
Meat, poultry, fish	
Beef, pork, lamb, veal	85 grams (3 ounces)
Liver — beef, calf, pork	85 grams (3 ounces)
Liver — chicken, turkey	125 mL (½ cup), diced

(continued)

Table 10-1 *(continued)*

Food	Serving = 25 Percent of the RDA
Catfish, crabmeat, croaker, lobster, mackerel, mussels, oysters, scallops, swordfish, trout, tuna	85 grams (3 ounces)
Dairy products	
Eggs	2 large
Milk — whole, low-fat, skim	500 mL (2 cups)
Yogourt	500 mL (2 cups)
CHOLINE	**Adequate Intake: Women 425 mg, Men 550 mg**
Fruits	
Grape juice (canned)	250 mL (1 cup)
Vegetables	
Cauliflower (cooked)	250 mL (1 cup)
Potato (baked)	1 medium
Meat, poultry, fish	
Beef (cooked)	85 grams (3 ounces)
Liver (cooked) — beef	85 grams (3 ounces)
Dairy	
Eggs	1 large
Milk — whole	250 mL (1 cup)
Other	
Peanut butter	30 mL (2 tbsp)

* Although these remain the "official" RDAs, newer recommendations are 900 mcg RE/3,000 IU per day for men and 700 mcg RE/2,300 IU per day for women (the IU amounts are rounded off).
** The Food and Nutrition Board is debating whether to raise the RDA for vitamin C to 200 mg for both men and women.
"Good Sources of Nutrients" (Washington D.C.: U.S. Department of Agriculture/Human Nutrition Service, 1990); "Nutritive Value of Food" (Washington D.C.: U.S. Department of Agriculture, 1991)

Too Much or Too Little: Avoiding Two Ways to Go Wrong with Vitamins

RDAs are broad enough to prevent vitamin deficiencies and avoid the side effects associated with very large doses of some vitamins. If your diet doesn't meet these guidelines, or if you take very large amounts of vitamins as supplements, you may be in for trouble.

Vitamin deficiencies

The good news is that vitamin deficiencies are rare among people who have access to a wide variety of foods and know how to put together a balanced diet. For example, the only people likely to experience a vitamin E deficiency are premature and/or low–birth weight infants and people with a metabolic disorder that keeps them from absorbing fat. A healthy adult may go as long as ten years on a vitamin E–deficient diet without developing any signs of a problem.

Aha, you say, but what's this subclinical deficiency I hear so much about?

Nutritionists use the term *subclinical deficiency* to describe a nutritional deficit not yet far enough advanced to produce obvious symptoms. In lay terms, however, the phrase has become a handy explanation for common but hard-to-pin-down symptoms such as fatigue, irritability, nervousness, emotional depression, allergies, and insomnia. And it's a dandy way to increase the sale of nutritional supplements.

Simply put, the RDAs protect you against deficiency. If your odd symptoms linger even after you take reasonable amounts of vitamin supplements, probably something other than a lack of any one vitamin is to blame. Don't wait until your patience or your bank account has been exhausted to find out. Get a second opinion as soon as you can. Table 10-2 lists the symptoms of various vitamin deficiencies.

Table 10-2	Vitamin Alert: What Happens When You Don't Get the Vitamins You Need
A Diet Low in This Vitamin	*May Produce These Signs of Deficiency*
Vitamin A	Poor night vision; dry, rough, or cracked skin; dry mucous membranes including the inside of the eye; slow wound healing; nerve damage; reduced ability to taste, hear, and smell; inability to perspire; reduced resistance to respiratory infections

(continued)

Table 10-2 (continued)

A Diet Low in This Vitamin	May Produce These Signs of Deficiency
Vitamin A	Poor night vision; dry, rough, or cracked skin; dry mucous membranes including the inside of the eye; slow wound healing; nerve damage; reduced ability to taste, hear, and smell; inability to perspire; reduced resistance to respiratory infections
Vitamin D	In children: rickets (weak muscles, delayed tooth development, and soft bones, all caused by the inability to absorb minerals without vitamin D) In adults: osteomalacia (soft, porous bones that fracture easily)
Vitamin E	Inability to absorb fat
Vitamin K	Blood fails to clot
Vitamin C	Scurvy (bleeding gums; tooth loss; nosebleeds; bruising; painful or swollen joints; shortness of breath; increased susceptibility to infection; slow wound healing; muscle pains; skin rashes)
Thiamin (vitamin B1)	Poor appetite; unintended weight loss; upset stomach; gastric upset (nausea, vomiting); mental depression; an inability to concentrate
Riboflavin (vitamin B2)	Inflamed mucous membranes, including cracked lips, sore tongue and mouth, burning eyes; skin rashes; anemia
Niacin	Pellagra (diarrhea; inflamed skin and mucous membranes; mental confusion and/or dementia)
Vitamin B6	Anemia; convulsions similar to epileptic seizures; skin rashes; upset stomach; nerve damage (in infants)
Folate	Anemia (immature red blood cells)
Vitamin B12	Pernicious anemia (destruction of red blood cells, nerve damage, increased risk of stomach cancer attributed to damaged stomach tissue, neurological/psychiatric symptoms attributed to nerve cell damage)
Biotin	Loss of appetite; upset stomach; pale, dry, scaly skin; hair loss; emotional depression; skin rashes (in infants younger than 6 months)

Big trouble: Vitamin megadoses

Can you get too much of a good thing? Darn right, you can. Some vitamins are toxic when taken in very large amounts — popularly known as *megadoses*. How much is a megadose? Nobody knows for sure. The general consensus, however, is that a megadose is several times the RDA, but the term is vague — the dictionary says it's "a very large dose," and who could get more vague than that?

- ✔ Megadoses of vitamin A (as retinol) may cause symptoms that make you think you have a brain tumour. Taken by a pregnant woman, megadoses of vitamin A may damage the fetus.

- ✔ Megadoses of vitamin D may cause kidney stones and hard lumps of calcium in soft tissue (muscles and organs).

- ✔ Megadoses of niacin (sometimes used to lower cholesterol levels) can damage liver tissue.

- ✔ Megadoses of vitamin B6 can cause (temporary) damage to nerves in arms, legs, fingers, and toes.

But here's an interesting fact: With one exception, the likeliest way to get a megadose of vitamins is to take supplements (see Chapter 5 for more on supplements). It's pretty much impossible for you to cram down enough food to overdose on vitamins D, E, K, C, and all the Bs. Did you notice the exception? Right: vitamin A. Liver and fish liver oils are concentrated sources of pre-formed vitamin A (retinol), the potentially toxic form of vitamin A. Liver contains so much retinol that early twentieth century explorers to the South Pole made themselves sick on seal and whale liver. Cases of vitamin A toxicity also have been reported among children given daily servings of chicken liver. (See Table 10-3 for more on vitamin A toxicity, this time from supplements.) On the other hand, even very large doses of vitamin E, vitamin K, thiamin (vitamin B1), riboflavin (vitamin B2), folate, vitamin B12, biotin, and pantothenic acid appear safe for human beings. Table 10-3 lists the effects of vitamin overdoses.

Table 10-3	Amounts and Effects of Vitamin Overdoses for Healthy People
Vitamin	*Overdose and Possible Effect*
Vitamin A	15,000 to 25,000 IU retinol a day for adults (2,000 IU or more for children) may lead to liver damage, headache, vomiting, abnormal vision, constipation, hair loss, loss of appetite, low-grade fever, bone pain, sleep disorders, and dry skin and mucous membranes. A pregnant woman who takes more than 10,000 IU a day doubles her risk of giving birth to a child with birth defects.

(continued)

Table 10-3 *(continued)*

Vitamin	Overdose and Possible Effect
Vitamin D	2,000 IU a day can cause irreversible damage to kidneys and heart. Smaller doses may cause muscle weakness, headache, nausea, vomiting, high blood pressure, retarded physical growth in children, mental retardation in children, and fetal abnormalities.
Vitamin E	Large amounts (more than 400 to 800 IU a day) may cause upset stomach or dizziness.
Vitamin C	1,000 mg or more may cause upset stomach or diarrhea.
Niacin	Doses higher than the RDA raise the production of liver enzymes and blood levels of sugar and uric acid, leading to liver damage and an increased risk of diabetes and gout.
Vitamin B6	Continued use of 50 mg or more a day may damage nerves in arms, legs, hands, and feet. Some experts say the damage is likely to be temporary; others say it may be permanent.
Choline	Very high doses (14 to 37 times the adequate amount) have been linked to vomiting, salivation, sweating, low blood pressure, and — ugh! — fishy body odour.

You may not have to go sky-high on vitamin A to run into trouble. In January 2003, new data from a long-running (30-year) study at University Hospital in Uppsala (Sweden) suggested that taking a multivitamin with normal amounts of vitamin A may weaken bones and raise the risk of hip fractures by as much as 700 percent, a conclusion supported by data released in 2004 from the long-running Nurses' Health Study. A high blood level of retinol — from large amounts of vitamin A in food or supplements — apparently inhibits special cells that usually make new bone, revs up cells that destroy bone, and interferes with vitamin D's ability to help you absorb calcium. Of course, confirming studies are needed, but you can bet the debate about lowering the amount of A in your favourite supplement will be vigorous. The new recommendations for vitamin A are 700 RE/2,300 IU for women and 900 RE/3,000 IU for men, but many popular multivitamins still contain 750 to 1500 RE/2,500 to 5,000 IU. Oops?

Exceeding the RDAs: Taking Extra Vitamins as Needed

Who needs extra vitamins? Maybe you. The RDAs are designed to protect healthy people from deficiencies, but sometimes the circumstances of your life (or your lifestyle) mean that you need something extra. Are you taking medication? Do you smoke? Are you on a restricted diet? Are you pregnant? Are you a nursing mother? Are you approaching menopause? Answer yes to any of these questions, and you may need larger amounts of vitamins than the RDAs provide.

I'm taking medication

Many valuable medicines interact with vitamins. Some drugs increase or decrease the effectiveness of vitamins; some vitamins increase or decrease the effectiveness of drugs. For example, a woman who's using birth control pills may absorb less than the customary amount of the B vitamins. For more about vitamin and drug interactions, see Chapter 25.

A special case: The continuing saga of vitamin C

In 1970, chemist Linus Pauling published *Vitamin C and the Common Cold,* a small book (just about 100 pages) made weightier by the fact that Pauling had not one, but two Nobel prizes on his shelf — one for chemistry and one for peace. Ever since, people have been fighting over Pauling's message that very large doses of vitamin C — called *gram doses* because they provide more than 1,000 milligrams (1 gram) — prevent or cure the common cold, or his later (unfounded) claim that these doses may also cure advanced cancer.

Over the past decade, the argument has switched to vitamin C's reputed ability to protect heart health. For example, an April 2004 report in the *Journal of the American College of Nutrition* said vitamin C could lower blood levels of CRP, an inflammation-related protein that increases the risk of heart disease. University of California, Berkeley, researchers gave 160 healthy adult volunteers either 500 milligrams of vitamin C, or a mixture of antioxidant nutrients, or a look-alike pill with no nutrients once a day for two months. In the end, the folks who got the vitamin C experienced a 24 percent drop in CRP blood levels versus a statistically insignificant 4.7 percent for the cocktail and no change at all for those on the placebo. Not surprisingly, UC epidemiologists thought vitamin C would become an important aid to heart health.

On the other hand, a small study found possible evidence that vitamin C may not be all it's cracked up to be if you're taking medicines to knock down your "bad" cholesterol and boost the "good" kind. As the American Heart Association (AHA) Council on Nutrition, Physical Activity and Metabolism points out, when 20 volunteers in an HDL-atherosclerosis treatment study were given vitamin C supplements along with their anti-cholesterol meds, they ended up with lower-than-expected levels of heart healthy, high-density lipoproteins (HDLs). This is only one small study, however, and to date there is no conclusive evidence, and no recommendation to stop taking vitamin C. The debate continues.

I'm a smoker

It's a fact — you probably have abnormally low blood levels of vitamin C. More trouble: Chemicals from tobacco smoke create more free radicals in your body. Even the National Research Council, which is tough on vitamin overdosing, says that regular smokers need to take about 66 percent more vitamin C — up to 100 mg a day — than nonsmokers.

I never eat animals

On the other hand, if you're nuts for veggies but follow a vegan diet — one that shuns all foods from animals (including milk, cheese, eggs, and fish) — you simply cannot get enough vitamin D without taking supplements. Vegans also benefit from extra vitamin C because it increases their ability to absorb iron from plant food. (Vegans frequently don't get and absorb enough iron.) And vitamin B12–enriched grains or supplements are a must to supply the nutrient found only in fish, poultry, milk, cheese, and eggs. As well, vegans need to be sure they're getting enough zinc; animal sources are best, and the higher fibre intake of vegetarian diets can interfere with zinc absorption.

I'm pregnant

Keep in mind that "eating for two" means you're the sole source of nutrients for the growing fetus, not that you need to double the amount of food you eat. If you don't get the vitamins you need, neither will your baby.

For an expecting mother, the RDAs for many nutrients are the same as those for women who aren't pregnant. But when you're pregnant, you need extra

- ✔ **Vitamin D:** Every smidgen of vitamin D in a newborn's body comes from his or her mom. If the mother doesn't have enough D, neither will the baby. Are vitamin pills the answer? Yes. And no. The qualifier is how many pills, because although too little vitamin D can weaken a developing fetus, too much can cause birth defects. That's why, until new recommendations for vitamin D are issued, the second important *d*-word is "doctor." As in, check with yours to see what's right for you.

- ✔ **Vitamin E:** To create all that new tissue (the woman's as well as the baby's), a pregnant woman needs two extra a-TE each day, the approximate amount in one egg.

- ✔ **Vitamin C:** The level of vitamin C in your blood falls as your vitamin C flows across the placenta to your baby, who may — at some point in the pregnancy — have vitamin C levels as much as 50 percent higher than yours. So you need an extra 10 milligrams of vitamin C each day (you can get it by eating 125 mL or ½ cup of cooked zucchini, or two stalks of asparagus).

✔ **Riboflavin (vitamin B2):** To protect the baby against structural defects such as cleft palate or a deformed heart, a pregnant woman needs an extra 0.3 milligrams of riboflavin each day (slightly less than 30 mL or 2 tablespoons of ready-to-eat cereal).

✔ **Folate:** Folate protects the child against cleft palate and neural tube (spinal cord) defects. As many as 4 of every 10,000 babies born each year in Canada have a neural tube defect, for example spina bifida, because their mothers didn't get enough folate to meet the RDA standard. The accepted increase in folate for pregnant women has been 200 micrograms (slightly more than the amount in 250 mL or one cup of orange juice). But new studies show that taking 400 micrograms of folate before becoming pregnant and through the first two months of pregnancy significantly lowers the risk of giving birth to a child with cleft palate. Taking 400 micrograms of folate each day through an entire pregnancy reduces the risk of a neural tube defect.

✔ **Vitamin B12:** To meet the demands of the growing fetus, a pregnant woman needs an extra 0.2 micrograms of vitamin B12 each day (85 grams or 3 ounces of roast chicken).

I'm breast-feeding

You need extra vitamin A, vitamin E, thiamin, riboflavin, and folate to produce sufficient quantities of nutritious breast milk, about 750 mL (3 cups) each day. You need extra vitamin D, vitamin C, and niacin as insurance to replace the vitamins you lose — that is, the ones you transfer to your child in your milk.

I'm approaching menopause

Information about the specific vitamin requirements of older women is as hard to find as, well, information about the specific vitamin requirements of older men. It's enough to make you wonder what's going on with the people who set the RDAs. Don't they know that everyone gets older? Right now, all anybody can say for sure about the nutritional needs of older women is that as they age, women require extra calcium to stem the natural loss of bone that occurs when they reach menopause and their production of the female hormone estrogen declines. They may also need extra vitamin D to enable their bodies to absorb and use calcium. Gender bias alert! No similar studies are available for older men. But adding vitamin D supplements to calcium supplements increases bone density in older people. The current RDA for vitamin D is set at 5 micrograms or 200 IU for all adults, but the new AI (Adequate Intake) for vitamin D is 10 micrograms or 400 IU for people ages 51 to 70 and 15 micrograms or 600 IU or more for people 71 and older. Some researchers suggest that even these amounts may be too low to guarantee maximum calcium absorption. Because of the increased need for vitamin D as we grow older, the latest revision of Canada's Food Guide recommends that everyone older than 50 take a daily vitamin D supplement of 10 micrograms, or 400 IU, every day.

Large doses (more than 50 mcg or 2,000 IU per day) of vitamin D should be avoided at this time as it can be toxic.

I have very light skin or very dark skin

Sunlight — yes, plain old sunlight — transforms fats just under the surface of your skin to vitamin D. So getting what you need should be a cinch, right? Not necessarily. Getting enough vitamin D from sunlight is hard to do when you have very light skin and avoid the sun for fear of skin cancer. Even more diffi-cult is getting enough vitamin D when you have very dark skin, which acts as a kind of natural sunblock. When Centers for Disease Control and Prevention researchers surveyed the vitamin D status of more than 2,000 African-American and Caucasian women ages 15 to 49, they found low body levels of vitamin D in 42 percent of the African-American women and 4.2 percent of the Caucasian women. Based on these numbers, Boston University researchers suggest that the Recommended Dietary Amount for adults who don't get enough sunlight may be as much as four times the current recommended amount. Check this out with your doctor; it's very important news for women who are or hope to be pregnant and need extra vitamin D (check back a few paragraphs for this information).

The situation is especially precarious in Canada. The opportunity to make vitamin D from sunlight is limited because of *latitude* (the distance from the equator). Essentially we only have from mid-April or so to mid-October to make this very important vitamin. UVB, the ultraviolet rays responsible for the production of vitamin D, wanes during the fall and isn't present in suffi-cient amounts in the winter to make vitamin D. The situation gets worse as you move farther north.

Very few foods contain naturally occurring vitamin D. Exceptions are fatty fish such as salmon and sardines. Fortified food sources in Canada include milk, some yogourts made from fortified milks (be sure to check the labels), and margarines. It's a good idea to get extra vitamin D from a supplement — especially during the winter. The 10 micrograms, or 400 IU, found in multivita-mins is safe for most adults.

Chapter 11

Mighty Minerals

· ·

· ·

Minerals are *elements,* substances composed of only one kind of atom. They're inorganic (translation: They don't contain the carbon, hydrogen, and oxygen atoms found in all organic compounds, including vitamins.). Minerals occur naturally in nonliving things such as rocks and metal ores. Although minerals also are present in plants and animals, they're imported: Plants get minerals from soil; animals get minerals by eating plants.

Most minerals have names reflecting the places where they're found or characteristics such as their colour. For example, the name *calcium* comes from *calx,* the Greek word for "lime" (chalk), where calcium is found; *chlorine* comes from *chloros,* the Greek word for "greenish-yellow," which just happens to be the colour of the mineral. Other minerals, such as americium, curium, berkelium, californium, fermium, and nobelium, are named for where they were found or to honour an important scientist.

This chapter tells you which minerals your body requires to stay in tiptop shape, where to find these minerals in food, and precisely how much of each mineral a healthy person needs.

Taking Inventory of the Minerals You Need

Think of your body as a house. Vitamins (read all about them in Chapter 10) are like tiny little maids and butlers, scurrying about to turn on the lights and make sure that the windows are closed to keep the heat from escaping. Minerals play two roles:

- ✔ They're active in many metabolic reactions such as protein metabolism, energy production, nerve transmission (communication between different parts of the body), and muscle contraction, and are a part of many *enzymes* (protein structures that enable many metabolic reactions to occur).
- ✔ They're part of the structural components of the body, such as bones and teeth.

Think of minerals as the mortar and bricks that strengthen the frame of the house, and as the current that keeps the lights running.

Minerals compose about 4 percent of a person's body weight, with most of that found in the skeleton. For example, if a person weighs 65 kg (143 pounds), then 2.6 kg (5.7 pounds) of that would be from the total mineral content. Calcium and phosphorus make up about 75 percent of the average adult body's mineral content.

Nutritionists classify the minerals essential for human life as either major minerals (including the principal electrolytes — see Chapter 13) or trace elements. *Major minerals* (also known as *macrominerals*) and *trace elements* are both minerals. The difference between them, nutritionally speaking, is how much you have in your body and how much you need to take in to maintain a steady supply. How a mineral is classified — major or minor — isn't an indication of its importance to your health. A deficiency or suboptimal intake of either one can have detrimental effects.

Your body stores varying amounts of minerals, but keeps more than 5 grams (about ⅙ of an ounce) of each of the major minerals and principal electrolytes on hand; you need to consume more than 100 milligrams a day of each major mineral to maintain a steady supply and to make up for losses. You store less than 5 grams of each trace element and need to take in less than 100 milligrams a day to stay even.

Some minerals interact with other minerals or with medical drugs. For example, calcium binds tetracycline antibiotics into compounds your body can't break apart so that the antibiotic moves out of your digestive tract, unabsorbed and unused. That's why your doctor warns you off milk and dairy products when you're taking this medicine. For more about interactions between minerals and medicines, turn to Chapter 25.

Introducing the major minerals

The following major minerals are essential for human beings:

✔ Calcium

✔ Phosphorus

✔ Magnesium

✔ Sodium

✔ Potassium

✔ Chloride

Note: Sodium, potassium, and chloride, also known as the principal electrolytes, are covered in Chapter 13.

Although sulphur is a mineral found in the human body and is an essential nutrient for human beings, it's almost never included in nutritional books and/or charts. Why? Because it's an integral part of all proteins. Any diet that provides adequate protein also provides adequate sulphur. (For more on proteins, bookmark this page and turn to Chapter 6. After you've checked out proteins, come on back to look at the major minerals in minute detail.)

An elementary guide to minerals

The early Greeks thought that all material on Earth was constructed of a combination of four basic elements: earth, water, air, and fire. Wrong. Centuries later, alchemists looking for the formula for precious metals, such as gold, decided that the essential elements were sulphur, salt, and mercury. Wrong again.

In 1669, a group of German chemists isolated phosphorus, the first mineral element to be accurately identified. After that, things moved a bit more swiftly. By the end of the 19th century, scientists knew the names and chemical properties of 82 elements. Today, we have identified 112 elements.

The classic guide to chemical elements is the periodic table, a chart devised in 1869 by Russian chemist Dmitri Mendeleev (1834–1907), for whom mendelevium was named. The table was revised by British physicist Henry Moseley (1887–1915), who came up with the concept of *atomic numbers,* numbers based on the number of *protons* (positively charged particles) in an elemental atom.

The periodic table is a clean, crisp way of characterizing the elements, and if you are now or ever were a chemistry, physics, or premed student, you can testify firsthand to the joy (maybe that's not the best word?) of memorizing the information it provides.

Calcium

When you step on the scale in the morning, you can assume that about 1.36 kg (3 pounds) of your body weight is calcium, most of it packed into your bones and teeth.

Calcium is also present in extracellular fluid (the liquid around body cells), where it performs the following duties:

- Regulating fluid balance by controlling the flow of water in and out of cells
- Enabling cells to send messages back and forth to one to another
- Keeping muscles moving smoothly and preventing cramping
- Helping blood clot

An adequate amount of calcium is important for controlling high blood pressure — and not only for the person who takes the calcium directly. At least one study shows that when a pregnant woman gets a sufficient amount

Calcium: The bone team player

The toe bone's connected to the foot bone. The foot bone's connected to the ankle bone. The ankle bone's connected to the knee bone. And what holds them together all the way up to the head bone is connected to your diet.

Like all body tissues, bones are constantly being remodelled. Old bone cells break down, and new ones are born. Specialized cells called *osteoclasts* start the process by boring tiny holes into solid bone so that other specialized cells, called *osteoblasts*, can refill the open spaces with fresh bone. At that point, crystals of calcium, the best-known dietary bone builder, glom onto the network of new bone cells to harden and strengthen the bone.

Calcium begins its work on your bones while you're still in your mother's womb. But it's not the only mineral at play. You should also think zinc. Based on a survey of 242 pregnant women in Peru, where zinc deficiency is common, Johns Hopkins researchers found that babies born to women who got prenatal supplements

with iron, folic acid, and zinc had longer, stronger leg bones than did babies born to women who got the same supplement minus the zinc.

After you're born, calcium continues to build your bones, but only with the help of vitamin D, which produces a calcium-binding protein that enables you to absorb the calcium in the milk Mummy feeds you. To make sure you get your D, virtually all milk sold in Canada is fortified with the vitamin. And because you may outgrow your taste for milk but never outgrow your need for calcium, calcium supplements for adults frequently include vitamin D.

But vitamin D isn't milk's only contribution. Remember the iron in the Peruvian prenatal supplements? It isn't there by accident. Iron increases the production of collagen, the most important protein in bone. Milk contains lactoferrin (lacto = milk; ferri = iron), an iron-binding compound that stimulates the production of the cells that promote bone growth.

When researchers at the University of Auckland in New Zealand added lactoferrin from cow's milk to a dish of osteoblasts, the bone cells grew more quickly. When they injected lactoferrin into the skulls of five lab mice, the bone at the site of the injection also grew faster, leading the team to suggest in the journal *Endocrinology* that lactoferrin may play a role in treating osteoporosis.

No surprise to the Department of Nutrition Sciences at the University of Arizona, where a study done with scientists from the University of Arkansas and Columbia University shows that women in their 40s, 50s, and 60s who get about 18 milligrams of iron a day have stronger, denser bones than women who get less iron. What makes this intriguing is that 18 milligrams a day is more than double the current RDA (8 milligrams) for older women.

But the iron/calcium dance is a balancing act. In your body, iron and calcium appear to compete to see which one gets absorbed. So the extra iron works only for women who get about 800 to 1,200 milligrams of calcium a day — women who get less and women who get more don't seem to benefit from extra iron.

Finally, please note that the word *bones* begins with *b* — as in vitamin B12. The female sex hormone estrogen preserves bone; the male sex hormone testosterone builds new bone. As people age and their supply of sex hormones diminishes, they lose bone faster than they can replace it. One complicating factor may be low levels of vitamin B12. A report in the *Journal of Clinical Endocrinology and Metabolism* says researchers at the University of California, San Francisco, found that women with lower levels of this vitamin also have less dense hip bones.

So to protect your bones, you need calcium, zinc, iron, and vitamins D and B12, all found most abundantly in milk, cheese, eggs, and red meat. Which sounds like a cardiologist's nutritional high-fat, high-cholesterol nightmare — unless you edit the menu to read: low-fat milk, low-fat cheese, one egg per day but unlimited egg whites, and lean beef. Way to go.

of calcium, her baby's blood pressure stays lower than average for at least the first seven years of life, meaning a lower risk of developing high blood pressure later on.

Your best food sources of calcium are milk and other dairy products, plus fish with bones, such as canned sardines and salmon. Calcium also is found in almonds, sesame seeds, tofu made with calcium salts (calcium sulphate), calcium-fortified orange juice, and calcium-fortified soy and rice beverages. Calcium is present in dark green, leafy vegetables (bok choy, kale, broccoli, collards, and mustard greens), but the calcium in some of these plant foods, such as spinach, almonds, and sesame, is bound into compounds that are less easily absorbed by your body.

Phosphorus

Like calcium, phosphorus is essential for strong bones and teeth. For tiptop performance, you need just over two-thirds as much phosphorus as calcium. Like calcium, phosphorus is a major player when it comes to the amount in your body. About 700 to 800 grams (about 1.5 to 1.7 pounds) of your body weight is phosphorus, and about 85 percent of all phosphorus is found in your bones and teeth. Phosphorus also enables a cell to transmit the *genetic code* (genes and chromosomes that carry information about your special characteristics) to the new cells created when a cell divides and reproduces. In addition, phosphorus

- ✔ Helps maintain the pH balance of blood (that is, keeps it from being too acidic or too alkaline)
- ✔ Is vital for metabolizing carbohydrates, synthesizing proteins, and ferrying fats and fatty acids among tissues and organs
- ✔ Is part of *myelin*, the fatty sheath that surrounds and protects each nerve cell

Phosphorus is in almost everything you eat, but the best sources are high-protein foods such as meat, fish, poultry, eggs, cheese, and milk. These foods provide more than half the phosphorus in a nonvegetarian diet; grains, nuts, seeds, and dry beans also provide respectable amounts.

Magnesium

Your body uses magnesium to make body tissues, especially bone. The adult human body has about 28 g (one ounce) of magnesium, and about 60 percent of it is in the bones, with muscle making up the next-largest reservoir, about 27 percent. Magnesium also is part of more than 300 different enzymes that trigger chemical reactions throughout your body. You use magnesium to

- ✔ Move nutrients in and out of cells
- ✔ Send messages between cells
- ✔ Transmit the genetic code (genes and chromosomes) when cells divide and reproduce
- ✔ Help insulin to be released from the pancreas

An adequate supply of magnesium also is heart-healthy because magnesium helps convert food to energy using less oxygen. Additionally, higher dietary intakes of magnesium-rich foods are associated with lower rates of diabetes, which is most likely due to magnesium's role in carbohydrate metabolism.

The best sources of magnesium are whole grains and dark green fruits and vegetables (magnesium is part of *chlorophyll,* the green pigment in plants), whole seeds, nuts, and legumes (such as lentils, chickpeas, and kidney beans).

Sodium

Sodium has gotten a bad rap for sure; however, sodium is an essential nutrient. It is a very abundant mineral making up about 0.15 percent of total body weight, most of which is found outside of the cells. You may think that because there is a lot of sodium in the body, your requirements are equally high. This isn't true because the kidneys are very efficient at keeping sodium in the body as needed. In fact, only 500 mg or 0.2 ml (about one-fifth of a teaspoon) of sodium is required to maintain sodium balance. Sodium is involved in nerve transmission. As well it

✔ Helps muscles to contract to move the body

✔ Enables a pumplike mechanism to move nutrients into cells

✔ Is involved in water balance

A lot of sodium can be lost in sweat; anywhere between 600 and 1,000 mg per litre of sweat. This becomes very important for those involved in high-intensity sports where a lot of sweating occurs, especially in warmer climates or during warmer seasons such as late spring and summer. It can also occur in cooler climates where perspiration is increased because the body is covered with sports equipment. Because there is a lot of sodium present in our food supply, this amount of sodium can be replaced with food, and special considerations such as salt tablets are not necessary.

Potassium

Potassium is mostly found inside the cells of the body with relatively smaller amounts in the blood. Most (90 percent) of the potassium that is consumed is absorbed, unlike other minerals that are absorbed to a lesser extent. Contrary to popular belief, unlike sodium, potassium is not lost in sweat in large amounts (about 40 mg per litre of sweat, or the equivalent to that which is found in 15 ml [1 tablespoon] of orange juice). Potassium helps to maintain a healthy fluid balance in the body, and also

✔ Is important in nerve transmission

✔ Is involved in muscle contraction, including regulating heart function

✔ Helps to convert glucose (blood sugar) into glycogen (fuel for muscles)

✔ Helps to reduce blood pressure

Potassium is in everything that you eat, as it is stored in the cells of both animals and plants. So while bananas may be the first food that comes to mind when you think of potassium, there is as much potassium in 250 ml (1 cup) of yogourt or 115 g (4 ounces or the size of a computer mouse) of beef.

Introducing the trace elements

Trace elements also are minerals, but they're present in much, much smaller amounts. That's why they are called *trace elements* or *trace minerals.* You need just a trace. Get it? Good! Trace elements include

✔ Iron

✔ Zinc

✔ Iodine

✔ Selenium

✔ Copper

✔ Manganese

✔ Fluoride

✔ Chromium

✔ Molybdenum

✔ Cobalt

Step up to meet and greet the trace elements.

Iron

Iron is an essential constituent of hemoglobin and myoglobin, two proteins that store and transport oxygen. You find hemoglobin in red blood cells (it's what makes them red). Myoglobin (myo = muscle) is in muscle tissue. Iron also is part of various enzymes.

Your best food sources of iron are organ meats (liver, heart, kidneys), red meat, chicken, fish (especially sardines, tuna, salmon, and halibut), egg yolks, and oysters. These foods contain heme (heme = blood) iron, a form of iron that your body can easily absorb.

Whole grains, wheat germ, raisins, nuts, seeds, prunes and prune juice, and potato skins contain nonheme iron. Because plants contain substances called *phytates,* which bind this iron into compounds, your body has a hard time getting at the iron. Eating plant foods with meat or with foods that are rich in vitamin C (like tomatoes or citrus fruits) increases your ability to split away the phytates and use the iron in the plant foods.

Zinc

Zinc protects nerve and brain tissue, bolsters the immune system, is needed for *taste acuity* (the ability to taste food), and is essential for healthy growth. Zinc is part of the enzymes (and hormones such as insulin) that metabolize food, and you can fairly call it the macho male mineral. Zinc is probably the most versatile mineral in the body. It is involved in more than 200 enzymatic reactions, including helping the liver to break down alcohol after it is ingested and in the digestion of dietary protein. It helps in wound healing and DNA synthesis, and it aids in the growth and maintenance of bone. Truly a star player.

The largest quantities of zinc in the male human body are in the testes, where it's used in making a continuous supply of *testosterone,* the hormone a man needs to produce plentiful amounts of healthy, viable sperm. Without enough zinc, male fertility falters. So, yes, the old wives' tale is true: Oysters — a rich source of zinc — are useful for men. By the way, women also need zinc . . . just not as much as men do. How much is that? Aha! Check Table 11-1 or leaf back to Chapter 4.

Other good sources of zinc are meat, liver, and eggs. There is plenty of zinc in nuts, beans, miso, pumpkin and sunflower seeds, whole-grain products, and wheat germ. But the zinc in plants, like the iron in plants, occurs in compounds that your body absorbs less efficiently than the zinc in foods from animals.

Iodine

Iodine is a component of the thyroid hormones thyroxine and triiodothyronine, which help regulate cell activities. These hormones increase cellular reactions and regulate overall metabolic rate. They're also essential for protein synthesis, tissue growth (including the formation of healthy nerves and bones), and reproduction.

The best natural sources of iodine are seafood and plants grown near the ocean, but most Canadians are most likely to get the iodine they need from iodized salt (plain table salt with iodine added). And here's an odd nutritional note: You may get substantial amounts of iodine from milk. Are the cows consuming iodized salt? No. The milk is processed and stored in machines and vessels kept clean and sanitary with iodates and *iodophors,* iodine-based disinfectants. Tiny trace amounts get into the products sent to the stores. Iodates are also used as dough conditioners (additives that make dough more pliable), so you're also likely to find some iodine in most bread sold in supermarkets.

Selenium

Selenium was identified as an essential human nutrient in 1979 when Chinese nutrition researchers discovered that people with low body stores of selenium were at increased risk of *Keshan disease,* a disorder of the heart muscle with symptoms that include rapid heartbeat, enlarged heart, and (in severe cases) heart failure, a consequence most common among young children and women of childbearing age.

How does selenium protect your heart? One possibility is that it works as an antioxidant in tandem with vitamin E. A second possibility, raised by U.S. Department of Agriculture studies with laboratory rats, is that it prevents viruses from attacking heart muscle.

Here's some exciting news: The results of a four-year study involving 1,312 patients previously treated for skin cancer strongly suggest that daily doses of selenium in amounts 3.8 times the current Recommended Dietary Allowance (RDA) (55 micrograms) may reduce the incidence of cancers of the lung, prostate, colon, and rectum. The University of Arizona study was designed to see whether taking selenium lowered the risk of skin cancer. It didn't. But among the patients who got selenium rather than a placebo, researchers recorded 45 percent fewer lung cancers, 58 percent fewer colon and rectal cancers, 63 percent fewer prostate cancers, and a 50 percent lower death rate from cancer overall. A follow-up study will determine whether these results hold up.

Selenium is the mineral found in the enzyme glutathione peroxidase, a powerful antioxidant. In fact, selenium's role as an antioxidant is unique because selenium acts as an antioxidant as part of an enzyme complex but also on its own. Its actions are very close to those of vitamin E, and if needed, selenium can substitute for vitamin E as an antioxidant. Each is a part of two separate but overlapping antioxidant systems — their roles are synergistic, and they work better together than on their own.

Although fruits and vegetables grown in selenium-rich soils are themselves rich in this mineral, the best source of selenium is brazil nuts, hands down. One gram or six to eight nuts have about 540 mcg of selenium, or almost ten times the RDA. The next best sources are seafood and fish, meat and organ meats (liver, kidney), eggs, and dairy products.

Copper

Copper is a mineral found in several enzymatic antioxidants that deactivate *free radicals* (pieces of molecules that can link up to form compounds that damage body tissues). Copper also helps the body use iron and is involved in the production of hemoglobin. Additionally, copper may play a role in slowing the aging process by decreasing the incidence of *protein glycation,* a reaction in which sugar molecules (gly = sugar) hook up with protein molecules in your bloodstream, twist the protein molecules out of shape, and make them unusable. Protein glycation may result in bone loss, high cholesterol, cardiac abnormalities, and a slew of other unpleasantries. In people with diabetes, excess protein glycation may also be one factor involved in complications such as loss of vision.

In addition, copper

- Promotes the growth of strong bones
- Protects the health of nerve tissue
- Prevents hair from turning grey prematurely

But, no no, a thousand times, no: Large amounts of copper absolutely, and we repeat, *absolutely* will not turn grey hair back to its original colour. Besides, megadoses of copper are potentially toxic.

You can get the copper you need from organ meats (such as liver and heart), seafood, poultry, nuts, dark green leafy vegetables, and dried beans, including cacao beans (the beans used to make chocolate).

Manganese

Most of the manganese in your body is in glands (pituitary, mammary, pancreas), organs (liver, kidneys, intestines), and bones. Manganese is an essential constituent of the enzymes that metabolize carbohydrates and synthesize fats (including cholesterol). Manganese is important for a healthy reproductive system. During pregnancy, manganese speeds the proper growth of fetal tissue, particularly bones and cartilage.

You get manganese from whole grains, cereal products, fruits, and vegetables. Tea is also a good source of manganese.

Fluoride

Fluoride is the form of fluorine (an element) found in drinking water. Your body stores fluoride in bones and teeth. Although researchers still have some questions about whether fluoride is an essential nutrient, it's clear that it hardens dental enamel, reducing your risk of getting cavities. In addition, some nutrition researchers suspect (but cannot prove) that some forms of fluoride strengthen bones; rates of osteoporosis are reduced in areas with naturally occurring or added fluoride in drinking water.

Small amounts of fluoride are in all soil, water, plants, and animal tissues. You also get a steady supply of fluoride from fluoridated drinking water.

Chromium

Very small amounts of *trivalent chromium,* a digestible form of the very same metallic element that decorates your car and household appliances, are essential for several enzymes that help metabolize fat.

Chromium is also a necessary partner for glucose tolerance factor (GTF), a group of chemicals that enables insulin (an enzyme from the pancreas) to regulate your use of glucose, the end product of metabolism and the basic fuel for every body cell (see Chapter 8). In a recent joint study by the USDA and Beijing Medical University, adults with non-insulin-dependent diabetes who took chromium supplements had lower blood levels of sugar, protein, and cholesterol, which are all good signs for people with diabetes. In a related study, chromium reduced blood pressure in laboratory rats bred to develop hypertension (high blood pressure), a common complication in diabetes.

Right now, little information exists about the precise amounts of chromium in specific foods. Nonetheless, brewer's yeast, calves' liver, cheese, whole-grain breads and cereals, wheat germ, and broccoli are regarded as valuable sources of this trace element.

Molybdenum

Molybdenum (pronounced mo-*lib*-de-num) is part of several enzymes that metabolize proteins. You get molybdenum from beans, leafy vegetables, and whole-grain breads and cereals. Cows eat grains, so milk and cheese have some molybdenum. Molybdenum also leeches into drinking water from surrounding soil. The molybdenum content of plants and drinking water depends entirely on how much molybdenum is in the soil.

Cobalt

Cobalt is a component of vitamin B12 (cobalamin). It's essential for *erythropoiesis* (the formation of red blood cells). Your body stores cobalt in the liver and kidneys. Cobalt can also substitute in times of need for manganese or zinc in various metabolic reactions. Because of its central role in the formation of vitamin B12, any deficiency in cobalt is ultimately a deficiency in B12, so replacing this vitamin alleviates any cobalt deficiency. Dietary sources of cobalt are the same as for vitamin B12, with organ meats (liver, kidney, and heart) being the best. Other sources include beef, pork, chicken, and seafood, as well as fermented soy.

Getting the Minerals You Need

Table 11-1 is a handy guide to foods that provide the minerals and trace elements your body needs. This chart is the easy way to figure out which foods (and how much) provide at least 25 percent of the RDA for healthy adults ages 25 to 50.

No muss, no fuss, no calculators. Just photocopy these pages and stick them on the fridge. What an easy way to eat right! Wait! One more important note: When you see "men" or "women" in the chart, it means "men and women ages 25 to 50" — unless otherwise noted.

Table 11-1 Get Your Minerals Here! — Foods and Serving Sizes	
Food	**Serving**
CALCIUM and PHOSPHORUS	**RDA: Calcium — men and women 1,000 mg** **RDA: Phosphorus — men and women 700 mg**
Breads, cereals, grains	
Bran muffin, English muffin	2 whole
Vegetables	
Broccoli, spinach, turnip greens (cooked)	250 mL (1 cup)
Dairy products	
Natural Gruyère, Romano, Swiss, Parmesan cheeses	28 grams (1 ounce)
Processed Cheddar or Swiss cheeses	42 grams (1½ ounces)

Food	Serving
Natural blue, brick, Camembert, feta, Gouda, Monterey, mozzarella, Muenster, provolone, Roquefort cheeses	56 grams (2 ounces)
Ricotta cheese	125 mL (½ cup)
Ice cream/ice milk	250 mL (1 cup)
Milk — all varieties, including chocolate	250 mL (1 cup)
Yogourt — all varieties	250 mL (1 cup)
Other	
Tofu	125 mL (½ cup), cubed
MAGNESIUM	**RDA: Men 400–420 mg,* women 310–320 mg***
Breads, cereals, grains	
Bread — whole wheat	4 slices
Bran muffin, English muffin, pita — whole wheat	2 whole
Cold cereal	62 mL (¼ cup)
Vegetables	
Artichoke	2 medium
Black-eyed peas, chickpeas, soybeans, white beans (dried, cooked)	250 mL (1 cup)
Dairy products	
Milk — chocolate, made with skim milk	500 mL (2 cups)
Yogourt — plain nonfat	500 mL (2 cups)
Other	
Nuts and seeds	30 mL (2 tbsp.)
Tofu	125 mL (½ cup), cubed
IRON	**RDA: Men 8 mg, women 18 mg, 8 mg***
Breads, cereals, grains	
Bagel, bran muffin, pita	2 whole
Farina, oatmeal — instant, fortified	235 mL (⅓ cup)
Cold cereal	30 mL (⅛ cup)

(continued)

Table 11-1 *(continued)*

Food	*Serving*
Fruits	
Apricots (dried, cooked)	250 mL (1 cup)
Vegetables	
Black-eyed peas, chickpeas, lentils, red and white beans (dried, cooked)	250 mL (1 cup)
Soybeans (cooked)	125 mL (½ cup)
Meat, poultry, fish	
Liver — beef, pork	85 grams (3 ounces)
Liver — chicken, turkey	225 grams (8 ounces), diced
Clams (raw) — meat only	85–113 grams (3–4 ounces)
Oysters (raw) — meat only	28–56 grams (1–2 ounces)
Other	
Pine nuts, seeds — pumpkin or squash	60 mL (4 tbsp)
ZINC	**RDA: Men 11 mg, women 8 mg**
Breads, cereals, grains	
Cold cereals — fortified	56 grams (2 ounces)
Meat, poultry, fish	
Beef — all varieties, lean	85 grams (3 ounces)
Lamb — all varieties, lean	85 grams (3 ounces)
Tongue (braised)	85 grams (3 ounces)
Veal — roast, lean only	85 grams (3 ounces)
Chicken (no skin)	2 legs
Oysters	85 grams (3 ounces)
Dairy products	
Yogourt — all varieties	500 mL (2 cups)
Other	
Seeds — pumpkin or squash	60 grams (4 tbsp)

Food	Serving
COPPER	*AI (Adequate Intake): Men and women 900 mg*
Breads, cereals, grains	
Barley (cooked)	235 mL (⅓ cup)
Bran muffin, English muffin, pita	2 whole
Fruits	
Prunes (dried, cooked)	250 mL (1 cup)
Vegetables	
Black-eyed peas, lentils(dried, cooked), soybeans (cooked)	250 mL (1 cup)
Meat, poultry, fish	
Liver — beef, calf	85 grams (3 ounces)
Liver — chicken, turkey	113 grams (4 ounces, diced)
Crabmeat, lobster, oysters, shrimp	85 grams (3 ounces)
Other	
Almonds, Brazil nuts, cashews, hazelnuts/ filberts, peanuts, pistachios, walnuts, mixed nuts	60 mL (4 tbsp)
Seeds — pumpkin, sesame, squash, sunflower	60 mL (4 tbsp)

*The lower numbers are for people age 19–30; the higher numbers, for people age 31+.
Good Sources of Nutrients (Washington, D.C.: U.S. Department of Agriculture/Human Nutrition Service, 1990); Nutritive Value of Food (Washington, D.C.: USDA, 1991); DRI reports 1998–2004

Did you notice something missing from this list? Right you are. There are no entries for the essential trace elements chromium, fluoride, iodine, molybdenum, and selenium, because a healthful, varied diet provides sufficient quantities of these nutrients. Iodized salt and fluoridated water are extra insurance.

Overdoses and Underdoses: Too Much and Too Little

The Recommended Dietary Allowances (RDAs) and Adequate Intakes (AIs) for minerals and trace elements are generous — large enough to prevent deficiency but not so large that they trigger toxic side effects. (Read more about RDAs and AIs in Chapter 4.)

Avoiding mineral deficiency

What happens if you don't get enough minerals and trace elements? Some minerals, such as phosphorus and magnesium, are so widely available in food that deficiencies are rare to non-existent. No nutrition scientist has yet been able to identify a naturally occurring deficiency of sulphur, manganese, chromium, or molybdenum in human beings who follow a sensible diet. Most drinking water contains adequate fluoride, and Canadians get so much copper (can it be from chocolate bars?) that deficiency is practically unheard of in Canada.

But other minerals are more problematic:

- **Calcium:** Without enough calcium, a child's bones and teeth don't grow strong and straight, and an adult's bones will weaken. Calcium is a team player. To protect against deficiency, you also need adequate amounts of vitamin D, the nutrient that allows you to absorb the calcium you get from food or supplements. Milk fortified with vitamin D (see Chapter 10) has done much to eliminate rickets.

- **Iron:** *Iron deficiency anemia* is not just an old advertising slogan. Lacking sufficient iron, your body can't make the hemoglobin it requires to carry energy-sustaining oxygen to every tissue. As a result, you're often tired and feel weak. Mild iron deficiency may also inhibit intellectual performance. In one Johns Hopkins study, high school girls attained higher verbal, memory, and learning test scores when they took supplements providing recommended dietary amounts of iron.

 Check with your doctor before downing iron supplements or cereals fortified with 100 percent of your daily iron requirement. Hemochromatosis, a common but often-undiagnosed genetic defect affecting 1 in every 250 Canadians, can lead to *iron overload,* an increased absorption of the mineral linked to arthritis, heart disease, and diabetes, as well as an increased risk of infectious diseases and cancer (viruses and cancer cells thrive in iron-rich blood).

- **Zinc:** An adequate supply of zinc is vital for making testosterone and healthy sperm. Men who don't get enough zinc may be temporarily infertile. Zinc deprivation can make you lose your appetite and your ability to taste food. It may also weaken your immune system, increasing your risk of infections. Wounds heal more slowly when you don't get enough zinc. That includes the tissue damage caused by working out. In plain language: If you don't get the zinc you need, your charley horse may linger longer. And, yes, zinc may fight the symptoms of the common cold. To date, several studies have confirmed that sucking on lozenges containing one form of zinc (zinc gluconate) shortens a cold — by a day or two. Others show no differences. Your choice.

These results are for adults, not children, and the zinc tablets are meant just for the several days of your cold. To find out more about zinc excess, see the following section, "Knowing how much is too much."

✔ **Iodine:** A moderate iodine deficiency leads to *goiter* (a swollen thyroid gland) and reduced production of thyroid hormones. A more severe deficiency early in life may cause a form of mental and physical retardation called *cretinism.*

✔ **Selenium:** Not enough selenium in your diet? Watch out for muscle pain or weakness. To protect against selenium problems, make sure that you get plenty of vitamin E. Some animal studies show that a selenium deficiency responds to vitamin E supplements, and a vitamin E deficiency responds to selenium supplements (they each help to regenerate the other if one is lacking).

Knowing how much is too much

Like some vitamins, some minerals are potentially toxic in large doses:

✔ **Calcium:** Though clearly beneficial in amounts higher than the current RDAs, calcium is not problem free:

- Constipation, bloating, nausea, and intestinal gas are common side effects among healthy people taking supplements equal to 1,500 to 4,000 milligrams of calcium a day.

- Doses higher than 4,000 milligrams a day may be linked to kidney damage.

- Megadoses of calcium can bind with iron and zinc, making it harder for your body to absorb these two essential trace elements.

✔ **Phosphorus:** Too much phosphorus can lower your body's store of calcium.

✔ **Magnesium:** Megadoses of magnesium appear safe for healthy people (you'll know if you're taking too much when you start to have loose stools and/or diarrhea; some laxatives are magnesium based), but if you have kidney disease, the magnesium overload can cause weak muscles, breathing difficulty, irregular heartbeat, and/or cardiac arrest (your heart stops beating).

✔ **Iron:** Overdosing on iron supplements can be deadly, especially for young children. The lethal dose for a young child may be as low as 3 grams (3,000 milligrams) elemental iron at one time. This is the amount in 60 tablets with 50 milligrams elemental iron each. For adults, the lethal dose is estimated to be 200 to 250 milligrams elemental iron per kilogram (2.2 pounds) of body weight. That's about 13,600 milligrams for a 68 kg (150-pound) person — the amount you'd get in 292 tablets with 50 milligrams elemental iron each.

- **Zinc:** Moderately high doses of zinc (up to 25 milligrams a day) may slow your body's absorption of copper. Doses 27 to 37 times the RDA (11 mg/males; 8 mg/females) may interfere with your immune function and make you more susceptible to infection, the very thing normal doses of zinc protect against. Gram doses (2,000 milligrams/2 grams) of zinc cause symptoms of zinc poisoning: vomiting, gastric upset, and irritation of the stomach lining.

- **Iodine:** Overdoses of iodine cause exactly the same problems as iodine deficiency: goiter. How can that be? When you consume very large amounts of iodine, the mineral stimulates your thyroid gland, which swells in a furious attempt to step up its production of thyroid hormones. This reaction may occur among people who eat lots of dried seaweed for long periods of time.

- **Selenium:** In China, nutrition researchers have linked doses as high as 5 milligrams of selenium a day (90 times the RDA) to thickened but fragile nails, hair loss, and perspiration with a garlicky odour. In the United States, a small group of people who had accidentally gotten a supplement that mistakenly contained 27.3 milligrams selenium (436 times the RDA) fell victim to *selenium intoxication* — fatigue, abdominal pain, nausea and diarrhea, and nerve damage. The longer they used the supplements, the worse their symptoms were.

- **Fluoride:** Despite decades of argument, no scientific proof exists that the fluorides in drinking water increase the risk of cancer in human beings. But there's no question that large doses of fluoride — which you're unlikely to consume unless you drink well or groundwater that has high amounts of fluoride — cause fluorosis (brown patches on your teeth), brittle bones, fatigue, and muscle weakness. Over long periods of time, high doses of fluoride may also cause *outcroppings* (little bumps) of bone on the spine.

  Fluoride levels higher than 6 milligrams a day are considered hazardous.

- **Molybdenum:** Doses of molybdenum two to seven times the Adequate Intake (AI) (45 micrograms) may increase the amount of copper you excrete in urine.

Exceeding the RDAs: People who need extra minerals

If your diet provides enough minerals to meet the RDAs, you're in pretty good shape most of the time. But a restrictive diet, the circumstances of your reproductive life, and just plain getting older can increase your need for minerals. Here are some scenarios.

I'm looking for an iron supplement. What's this "ferrous" stuff?

The iron in iron supplements comes in several different forms, each one composed of elemental iron (the kind of iron your body actually uses) coupled with an organic acid that makes the iron easy to absorb.

The iron compounds commonly found in iron supplements are:

✔ Ferrous citrate (iron plus citric acid)

✔ Ferrous fumarate (iron plus fumaric acid)

✔ Ferrous gluconate (iron plus a sugar derivative)

✔ Ferrous lactate (iron plus lactic acid, an acid formed in the fermentation of milk)

✔ Ferrous succinate (iron plus succinic acid)

✔ Ferrous sulphate (iron plus a sulphuric acid derivative)

In your stomach, these compounds dissolve at different rates, yielding different amounts of elemental iron. So supplement labels list the compound, and the amount of elemental iron it provides, like this:

Ferrous gluconate 300 milligrams

Elemental iron 34 milligrams

This tells you that the supplement has 300 milligrams of the iron compound ferrous gluconate, which gives you 34 milligrams of usable elemental iron. If the label just says "iron," that's shorthand for elemental iron. The elemental iron number is what you look for in judging the iron content of a vitamin/mineral supplement.

You're a strict vegetarian

Vegetarians who pass up fish, meat, and poultry must get their iron either from fortified grain products such as breakfast cereals and commercial breads, or naturally from foods such as seeds, nuts, blackstrap molasses, raisins, prune juice, potato skins, green leafy vegetables, tofu, miso, or brewer's yeast. Because iron in plant foods is bound into compounds that are difficult for the human body to absorb, iron supplements are pretty much standard fare.

Vegans — vegetarians who avoid all foods from animals, including dairy products — have a similar problem getting the calcium they need. Calcium is in vegetables, but it, like iron, is bound into hard-to-absorb compounds. So vegans need calcium-rich substitutes. Good food choices are soybean milk fortified with calcium, orange juice with added calcium, and tofu processed with calcium sulphate.

You live inland, away from the ocean

Now here's a story of 20th-century nutritional success. Seafood and plants grown near the ocean are exposed to iodine-rich seawater. Freshwater fish, plants grown far from the sea, and the animals that feed on these fish and plants are not exposed to iodine. So people who live inland and get all their food from local gardens and farms cannot get the iodine they need from food.

American savvy and technology rode to the rescue in 1924 with the introduction of iodized salt, which was later introduced in Canada. Then came refrigerated railroad cars and trucks to carry food from both coasts to every inland city and state. Together, modern salt and efficient shipment virtually eliminated goiter, the iodine deficiency disease, in the U.S. Nonetheless, millions of people worldwide still suffer from chronic iodine deficiency.

You're a man

Just as women lose iron during menstrual bleeding, men lose zinc at ejaculation. Men who are extremely active sexually may need extra zinc. The trouble is, no one has ever written down standards for what constitutes "extremely active." Check this one out with your doctor.

Men who take a daily supplement of 200 micrograms of selenium seem to cut their risk of prostate cancer by two-thirds. The selenium supplement also produces an overall drop in cancer mortality, plus a significantly lower risk of colon cancer and lung cancer in both men and women.

You're a woman

The average woman loses about 10 to 15 ml (2 to 3 teaspoons) of blood during each menstrual period, a loss of 1.4 milligrams of iron. Women whose periods are very heavy lose more blood and more iron. It may be impossible to get the iron you need from a diet providing fewer than 2,000 calories a day, so you may develop a mild iron deficiency. To remedy this, some doctors prescribe a daily iron supplement.

Women who use an intrauterine device (IUD) may also be given a prescription for iron supplements because IUDs irritate the lining of the uterus and cause a small but significant loss of blood and iron.

You're pregnant

The news about pregnancy is that women may not need extra calcium. This finding, released late in 1998, is so surprising that it probably pays to stay tuned for more — and definitely check with your own doctor. Meanwhile, pregnant women still need supplements to build not only fetal tissues but also new tissues and blood vessels in their own bodies. Animal studies suggest (but don't prove) that you may also need extra copper to protect nerve cells in the fetal brain. Nutritional supplements for pregnant women are specifically formulated to provide the extra nutrients they need, primarily folic acid, vitamin D, and iron.

You're breast-feeding

Nursing mothers need extra calcium, phosphorus, magnesium, iron, zinc, and selenium to protect their own bodies while producing nutritious breast milk. The same supplements that provide extra nutrients for pregnant women will meet a nursing mother's needs.

Wow — You think that was a hot flash?

Then you need extra calcium. Both men and women produce the sex hormones testosterone and estrogen, although men make proportionately more testosterone, and women more estrogen. Testosterone builds bone; estrogen preserves it.

At menopause, a woman's production of estrogen drops precipitously, and her bones rapidly become less dense. As men age and their testosterone levels drop, they're also at risk of losing bone tissue, but the loss is less rapid and dramatic than a woman's.

For both men and women, severe loss of bone density can lead to osteoporosis and an increased risk of bone fractures, a condition more common among women of Caucasian and Asian ancestry. Estrogen supplements can help a woman maintain bone tissue, but taking the hormone may have serious side effects, including an increased risk of breast cancer.

Twenty years ago, nutritionists thought it impossible to stop age-related loss of bone density — that your body ceased to absorb calcium when you passed your mid-20s. Today, medications such as alendronate (Fosamax) protect an aging woman's bones without estrogen's potentially harmful effects. Increasing your consumption of calcium plus vitamin D may also be helpful, whatever your gender. But a study released in February 2006 says the value of extra calcium may not be as high as once believed. Stay tuned for more on this one.

Calcium supplements: What kind of calcium is in that pill?

Calcium-rich foods give you calcium paired with natural organic acids, a combination that your body easily digests and absorbs.

The form of calcium most commonly found in supplements, however, is calcium carbonate, the kind of calcium that occurs naturally in limestone and oyster shells.

Calcium carbonate is a versatile compound. Not only does it build strong bones and teeth, it also neutralizes stomach acid and relieves heartburn. Calcium carbonate antacids can be used as calcium supplements. They're nutritionally sound and generally cost less than products designed solely as nutritional supplements.

Some calcium supplements contain compounds that mix calcium with an organic acid. Calcium lactate is calcium plus lactic acid, the combination that occurs naturally in milk. Calcium citrate is calcium plus citric acid, an acid found in fruits.

These compounds are easier to digest, but they're sometimes more expensive than calcium carbonate products. Calcium carbonate is nearly half calcium, a very high percentage. But unless your stomach is very acidic, it's hard for your digestive system to break the compound open and get at the elemental calcium (the kind of calcium your body can use). You can increase your absorption of calcium from calcium carbonate by taking the tablets with meals.

Because different calcium compounds yield different amounts of elemental calcium, the label lists both the calcium compound and the amount of elemental calcium provided, like this:

Calcium carbonate, 500 milligrams, providing 200 milligrams elemental calcium.

Whenever you see the word *calcium* alone, it stands for *elemental calcium.*

The human body absorbs calcium most efficiently in amounts of 500 milligrams or less. You get more calcium from one 500-milligram calcium tablet twice a day than one 1,000-milligram tablet. If the 1,000-milligram tablets are a better buy, break them in half.

Warning: Not all antacids double as dietary supplements. Antacids containing magnesium or aluminum compounds are safe for neutralizing stomach acid, but they won't work as supplements. In fact, just the opposite is true. Taking magnesium antacids reduces your absorption of calcium, and taking aluminum antacids reduces your absorption of phosphorus. Because manufacturers sometimes change the ingredients in their products without notice, you always need to read the product label. Never assume an antacid can double as a calcium supplement.

Chapter 12

Phabulous Phytochemicals

• •

• •

*J*ust when you think you have a handle on a big issue like nutrition, the Folks in Charge of Everything toss something new on the table.

A new word has started showing up in nutrition articles and reports. The word is *phytochemicals,* a five-syllable mouthful meaning chemicals from plants. The word has becoming so engrained in nutrition vernacular that finding a nutrition junkie who hasn't heard of phytochemicals is difficult. But what people are hearing has turned around a bit.

Phytochemicals (chemicals manufactured only in plants) produce many of the beneficial effects associated with a diet that includes lots of fruits, vegetables, beans, and grains. This chapter gives you a brief summary of the nature of phytochemicals, tells you where to find them, and explains how they work.

Phytochemicals Are Everywhere

Did you take French literature in high school or university? If your answer is no, you may as well skip to the third sentence in the paragraph that follows. But if your answer's yes, then you're probably familiar with Molière's *The Bourgeois Gentleman.* The bourgeois gentleman is a lovable but pompous character who's surprised to discover he's been speaking prose all his life without knowing it.

Your relationship with phytochemicals is probably something like that. You've been eating them all your life without knowing it. The following are all phytochemicals:

- *Carotenoids,* the pigments that make fruits and vegetables orange, red, and yellow (dark green vegetables and fruits like kiwi contain these pigments, too, but green chlorophyll masks the carotenoids' colours)

- *Thiocyanates,* the smelly sulphur compounds that make you turn up your nose at the aroma of boiling cabbage

- *Daidzein* and *genistein,* hormone-like compounds in many fruits and vegetables, abundant in soy

- Dietary fibre

These chemicals perform beneficial housekeeping chores in your body. They

- Keep your cells healthy

- Help prevent the formation of *carcinogens* (cancer-producing substances)

- Reduce cholesterol levels

- Help move food through your intestinal tract

The undeniable value of phytochemicals is one reason Health Canada, through its publication *Eating Well with Canada's Food Guide,* urges you to have at least seven servings of fruits and vegetables and several servings of grains every day.

Did you notice that no minerals appear in the list of phytochemicals? The omission is deliberate. Plants don't manufacture minerals; they absorb them from the soil. Therefore, minerals aren't phytochemicals.

Perusing the Different Kinds of Phytochemicals

The most interesting phytochemicals in plant foods appear to be antioxidants, hormone-like compounds, and enzyme-activating sulphur compounds. Each group plays a specific role in maintaining health and reducing your risk of certain illnesses.

Antioxidants

Antioxidants are named for their ability to prevent a chemical reaction called *oxidation,* which enables molecular fragments called *free radicals* to join together, forming potentially carcinogenic (cancer-causing) compounds in your body.

Antioxidants also slow the normal wear-and-tear on body cells, so some researchers noted that a diet rich in plant foods (fruits, vegetables, grains, and beans) seems likely to reduce the risk of heart disease and may reduce the risk of some kinds of cancer. For example, consuming lots of lycopene (the red carotenoid in tomatoes) has been linked to a lower risk of prostate cancer — as long as the tomatoes are mixed with a dab of oil, which makes the lycopene easy to absorb.

However (you knew this was coming, right?), recent studies show that although a diet rich in fruits and veggies is healthful, stuffing yourself with the antioxidant vitamins A, beta carotene, and C has ab-so-lute-ly no effect on the risk of heart disease. Thousands and thousands of different antioxidants exist in the foods we eat. Although nutrition researchers may have an idea of which ones carry the most clout, they may be missing the finer details on how these nutrients really do their job. As well, nutrients in isolation, as they are found in supplements, may not act the same way they act when they come from food. It appears more and more that nutrients from food work in concert with each other in their ability to promote health.

Hormone-like compounds

Many plants contain compounds that behave like *estrogens,* the female sex hormones. Because only animal bodies can produce true hormones, these plant chemicals are called *hormone-like compounds* or *phytoestrogens* (plant estrogen). Seems fair.

The three kinds of phytoestrogens are

- ✔ Isoflavones, in fruits, vegetables, and beans
- ✔ Lignans, in grains
- ✔ Coumestans, in sprouts and alfalfa

The most-studied phytoestrogens are the isoflavones known as *daidzein* and *genistein* (found in soy), two compounds with a chemical structure similar to *estradiol,* which is the estrogen produced by mammalian ovaries.

Like natural or synthetic estrogens, daidzein and genistein hook onto sensitive spots, called estrogen receptors, in reproductive tissue (breast, ovary, uterus, prostate). But phytoestrogens have weaker estrogenic effects than natural or synthetic estrogens. It takes about 100,000 molecules of daidzein or genistein to produce the same estrogenic effect as one molecule of estradiol. Every phytoestrogen molecule that hooks onto an estrogen receptor displaces a stronger estrogen molecule. As a result, researchers suggested that consuming isoflavone-rich foods such as soy products may provide post-menopausal women with the benefits of estrogen (stronger bones and relief from hot flashes) without the higher risk of reproductive cancers (of the breast, ovary, or uterus) associated with hormone replacement therapy (HRT). The theory was supported by the fact that the incidence of breast and uterine cancer, heart disease, osteoporosis, and menopausal discomfort is lower in countries where soy — a primary source of phytoestrogens — is a significant part of the diet.

However, recent animal and human studies offer conflicting evidence. On the one hand, these studies

- Raise questions about the safety of phytoestrogen-rich foods for women with hormone-sensitive tumours

- Show that phytoestrogen may stimulate tumour growth in animals whose ovaries have been removed

- Demonstrate that isoflavone-rich foods have only modest effects on preserving bone and relieving hot flashes at menopause

- Indicate that large amounts of soy protein (20 g for example) in the diet only modestly reduce LDL cholesterol, and have little to no effect on raising HDL cholesterol (see Chapter 7).

On the other hand, including isoflavone-rich soy foods such as tofu, miso, tempeh, soy milk, soy flour, and soy protein in a healthful diet

- Reduces your overall intake of saturated fats, which are known to raise the LDL cholesterol

- Provides a good source of plant-based, omega-3 fats and antioxidants

- Helps people feel full longer so they can stick to a lower-calorie diet to manage weight loss

Bottom line? According to the International Food Information Council, "Further clinical studies will continue to increase understanding of the role of soy in maintaining and improving health." We couldn't have said it better.

Sulphur compounds

Slide an apple pie in the oven, and soon the kitchen fills with a yummy aroma that makes your mouth water and your digestive juices flow. But boil some cabbage and — yuck! What is that awful smell? It's sulphur, the same chemical you smell in rotten eggs.

Cruciferous vegetables (named for the Latin word for "cross," in reference to their *x*-shaped blossoms) — such as broccoli, Brussels sprouts, cauliflower, kale, kohlrabi, mustard seed, radishes, rutabaga, turnips, and watercress — all contain stinky sulphur compounds, such as *sulphoraphane glucosinolate (SGS), glucobrassicin, gluconapin, gluconasturtin, neoglucobrassicin,* and *sinigrin.* These compounds seem to tell your body to rev up its production of enzymes that inactivate and help eliminate carcinogens.

These smelly sulphurs may be one reason people who eat lots of cruciferous veggies generally have a lower risk of cancer. In animal studies at Johns Hopkins University School of Medicine, rats given chemicals known to cause breast tumours were less likely to develop tumours when they were given broccoli sprouts, a food that's unusually high in sulphoraphane. In 2005, a human trial conducted in China by researchers from Johns Hopkins, Qidong Liver Cancer Institute, Jiao Tong University (Shanghai), and the University of Minnesota Cancer Center showed that the sulphoraphane-rich sprouts appear to help the body defang aflatoxins produced by moulds that grow on grains such as rice. *Aflatoxins,* which damage cells and raise the risk of cancer, may be linked to the high incidence of stomach and liver cancer in China. Further studies are in the planning phases. (But of course.)

Dietary fibre

Dietary fibre is a special bonus found only in plant foods. You can't get it from meat or fish or poultry or eggs or dairy foods.

Soluble dietary fibre, such as the pectins in apples and the gums in beans, mops up cholesterol and lowers your risk of heart disease. Insoluble dietary fibre, such as the cellulose in fruit skins and the bran of grains such as wheat, oat, or barley, bulks up stool and prevents constipation, moving things more quickly through your gut so there's less time for food to create substances thought to trigger the growth of cancerous cells. (Turn to Chapter 4 to find out how much dietary fibre you need each day and to Chapter 8 to read everything you ever wanted to know about dietary fibre — maybe even more.)

Phorecasting the Phuture of Phytochemicals

Phytochemical research is serious stuff that eventually should enable people to identify biochemical reactions that trigger — or prevent — specific medical conditions.

While you're waiting for final analyses, the best nutrition advice is to dig into those veggies, fruits, and grains — and turn to Chapter 13 to find out why you need to wash them down with plenty of cold, clear water.

Chapter 13

Water Works

*Y*our body is mostly (50 to 70 percent) water. Exactly how much water depends on how old you are and how much muscle and fat you have. Muscle tissue has more water than fat tissue. Because the average male body has proportionately more muscle than the average female body, it also has more water. For the same reason — more muscle — a young body has more water than an older one.

You definitely won't enjoy the experience, but if you have to, you can live without food for weeks at a time, getting subsistence levels of nutrients by digesting your own muscle and fat. But water's different. Without it, you'll die in a matter of days — more quickly in a place warm enough to make you perspire and lose water more quickly.

This chapter clues you in on why water is so important, not to mention how you can manage to keep your body's water level, well, *level.*

Investigating the Many Ways Your Body Uses Water

Water is a solvent. It dissolves other substances and carries nutrients and other material (such as blood cells) around the body, making it possible for every organ to do its job. You need water to

✔ Digest food, dissolving nutrients so that they can pass through the intestinal cell walls into your bloodstream, and move food along through your intestinal tract

- Carry waste products out of your body
- Provide a medium in which biochemical reactions such as metabolism (digesting food, producing energy, and building tissue) occur
- Send electrical messages between cells so that your muscles can move, your eyes can see, your brain can think, and so on
- Regulate body temperature — cooling your body with moisture (perspiration) that evaporates on your skin
- Lubricate your moving parts

Maintaining the Right Amount of Water in Your Body

As much as three-quarters of the water in your body is in *intracellular fluid,* the liquid inside body cells. The rest is in *extracellular fluid,* which is all the other body liquids, such as

- Interstitial fluid (the fluid between cells)
- Blood plasma (the clear liquid in blood)
- Lymph (a clear, slightly yellow fluid collected from body tissues that flows through your lymph nodes and eventually into your blood vessels)
- Bodily secretions, for example sweat, seminal fluid, and vaginal fluids
- Urine

A healthy body has just the right amount of fluid inside and outside each cell, a situation medical folk call *fluid balance.* Maintaining your fluid balance is essential to life. If too little water is inside a cell, it shrivels and dies. If there's too much water, the cell bursts.

A balancing act: The role of electrolytes

Your body maintains its fluid balance through the action of substances called *electrolytes,* which are mineral compounds that, when dissolved in water, become electrically charged particles called *ions.*

Many minerals, including calcium, phosphorus, and magnesium, form compounds that dissolve into charged particles. But nutritionists generally use the term *electrolyte* to describe sodium, potassium, and chlorine. The most familiar electrolyte is the one found on every dinner table: sodium chloride — plain old table salt. (In water, its molecules dissolve into two ions: one sodium ion and one chloride ion.)

Fluoridated water: The real Tooth Fairy

Except for the common cold, dental cavities are the most common human medical problem.

You get cavities from *mutans streptococci,* bacteria that live in dental plaque. The bacteria digest and ferment carbohydrate residue on your teeth, leaving acid that eats away at the mineral surface of the tooth. This eating away is called *decay.* When the decay gets past the enamel to the softer pulp inside of the tooth, your tooth hurts. And you head for the dentist even though you hate it so much you'd almost rather put up with the pain. But *almost* doesn't count, so off you go.

Brushing and flossing help prevent cavities by cleaning your teeth so that bacteria have less to feast on. Another way to reduce your susceptibility to cavities is to drink *fluoridated water* — water containing the mineral fluorine.

Fluoride — the form of fluorine found in food and water — combines with other minerals in teeth and makes the minerals less soluble (harder to dissolve). You get the most benefit by drinking water containing 1 part fluoride to every 1 million parts water (1 ppm) from the day you're born until the day you get your last permanent tooth, usually around age 11 to 13.

Some drinking water, notably in the American Southwest, is fluoridated naturally when it flows through rocks containing fluorine. Sometimes so much fluoride is in this water that it causes a brownish spotting (or mottling), which occurs while teeth are developing and accumulating minerals. This effect doesn't occur with drinking water artificially supplemented with fluoride at the approved standard of one part fluoride to every million parts of water.

Because fluorides concentrate in bones, some people believe that drinking fluoridated water raises the risk of bone cancers, but no evidence to support this claim has ever been found in human beings. However, in 1990, a U.S. Public Health Service National Toxicology Program (NTP) study of the long-term effects of high fluoride consumption on laboratory rats and mice added fuel to the fire: Four of the 1,044 laboratory rats and mice fed high doses of fluoride for two years developed *osteosarcoma,* a form of bone cancer.

The study sent an immediate *frisson* (shiver) of fear through the health community, but within a year, federal officials reviewing the study issued an opinion endorsing the safety and effectiveness of fluoridated water.

Here's why: First, the number of cancers among the laboratory animals was low enough to have occurred simply by chance. Second, the cancers occurred only in male rats; no cases were reported in female rats or in mice of either sex. Finally, the amount of fluorides the animals ingested was 50 to 100 times higher than what you get in drinking water. To get as much fluoride as those rats did, human beings would have to drink more than 380 226-gram (8-ounce) glasses of fluoridated water a day.

Today, about 40 percent of Canadians have access to adequately fluoridated public water supplies. The result is 33 to 50 percent less dental caries in Canadian children and a lifelong reduction in cavities among the adults of these communities.

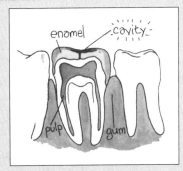

Under normal circumstances, the fluid inside your cells has more potassium than sodium and chloride. The fluid outside is just the opposite: more sodium and chloride than potassium. The cell wall is a *semipermeable membrane;* some things pass through, but others don't. Water molecules and small mineral molecules flow through freely, unlike larger molecules such as proteins.

The process by which sodium flows out and potassium flows in to keep things on an even keel is called the *sodium pump.* If this process stopped, sodium ions would build up inside your cells. Sodium attracts water; the more sodium there is inside the cell, the more water flows in. Eventually, the cell would burst and die. The sodium pump, regular as a clock, prevents this imbalance from happening so you can move along, blissfully unaware of those efficient electric ions.

Dehydrating without enough water and electrolytes

Drink more water than you need, and your healthy body simply shrugs its shoulders, so to speak, urinates more copiously, and readjusts the water level. It's hard for a healthy person on a normal diet to drink himself or herself to death on water.

But if you don't get enough water, your body lets you know pretty quickly.

The first sign is thirst, that unpleasant dryness in your mouth caused by the loss of water from cells in your gums, tongue, and cheeks. The second sign is reduced urination.

Reduced urination is a protective mechanism triggered by *ADH,* a hormone secreted by the hypothalamus, a gland at the base of your brain. The initials are short for *antidiuretic hormone.* Remember, a diuretic is a substance that increases urine production. ADH does just the opposite, helping your body conserve water rather than eliminate it.

If you don't heed these signals, your tissues will begin to dry out. In other words, you're dehydrating, and if you don't — or can't — get water, you won't survive.

Getting the Water You Need

Because you don't store water, you need to take in a new supply every day, enough to replace what you lose when you breathe, perspire, urinate, and defecate. On average, this needed amount adds up to 1,500 to 3,000 millilitres (50 to 100 ounces; 6 to 12.5 cups) a day. Here's where the water goes:

What else do those electrolytes do?

In addition to keeping fluid levels balanced, sodium, potassium, and chloride (the form of chlorine found in food) ions create electrical impulses that enable cells to send messages back and forth between themselves so you can think, see, move, and perform all the bioelectrical functions that you take for granted.

Sodium, potassium, and chloride are also major minerals (see Chapter 11) and essential nutrients. Like other nutrients, they're useful in these bodily processes:

✔ Sodium helps digest proteins and carbohydrates and keeps your blood from becoming too acidic or too alkaline.

✔ Potassium is used in digestion to synthesize proteins and starch and is a major constituent of muscle tissue.

✔ Chloride is a constituent of hydrochloric acid, which breaks down food in your stomach. It's also used by white blood cells to make *hypochlorite,* a natural antiseptic.

✔ 850 to 1,200 millilitres (28 to 40 ounces) are lost in breath and perspiration.

✔ 600 to 1,600 millilitres (20 to 53 ounces) are lost in urine.

✔ 50 to 200 millilitres (1.6 to 6.6 ounces) are lost in feces.

Toss in some extra ounces for a safe margin, and you get the current recommendations that women age 19 and up consume about 2.7 litres (11 cups) of water a day, and men age 19 and up about 3.7 litres (15 cups). But not all that water must come in a cup from the tap. About 15 percent of the water that you need is created when you digest and metabolize food. The end products of digestion and metabolism are carbon dioxide (a waste product that you breathe out of your body) and water composed of hydrogen from food and oxygen from the air that you breathe. The rest of your daily water comes directly from what you eat and drink. You can get water from, well, plain water. Eight 280-gram (10-ounce) glasses give you 2,400 millilitres, approximately enough to replace what your body loses every day, so everyone from athletes to couch potatoes knows that a healthy body needs eight full glasses of water a day. Or at least they thought they knew, but then Dartmouth Medical School kidney specialist Heinz Valtin turned off the tap.

Yes, the National Research Council's Food and Nutrition Board says each of us needs about 1 millilitre (ml) of water for each calorie of food we consume. On a 2,000-calorie-a-day diet, that's a little more than 2 litres (about 74 fluid ounces), or slightly more than nine 250-mL (8-ounce) glasses a day. Fair enough, Valtin said, but who says that it all has to come from, well, water? His report in the *American Journal of Physiology* (2003) points out that some of the water you require is right there in your food. Fruits and vegetables are

---

How does water know where to go?

Osmosis is the principle that governs how water flows through a semipermeable membrane (one that lets only certain substances pass through) such as the one surrounding a body cell.

Here's the principle: Water flows through a semipermeable membrane from the side where the liquid solution is least dense to the side where it's denser. In other words, the water, acting as if it has a mind of its own, tries to equalize the densities of the liquids on both sides of the membrane.

How does the water know which side is more dense? Now that one's easy: Wherever the sodium content is higher. When more sodium is inside the cell, more water flows in to dilute it. When more sodium is in the fluid outside the

cell, water flows out of the cell to dilute the liquid on the outside.

Osmosis explains why drinking seawater doesn't hydrate your body. When you drink seawater, liquid flows out of your cells to dilute the salty solution in your intestinal tract. The more you drink, the more water you lose. When you drink seawater, you're literally drinking yourself into dehydration.

Of course, the same thing happens — though certainly to a lesser degree — when you eat salted pretzels or nuts. The salt in your mouth makes your saliva saltier. This draws liquid out of the cells in your cheeks and tongue, which feel uncomfortably dry. You need . . . a drink of water!

---

full of water. Lettuce, for example, is 90 percent water. Beverages such as milk, juice, tea, and coffee all contribute to your daily intake of water. Furthermore, you get water from foods that you'd never think of as water sources: hamburger (more than 50 percent), cheese (the softer the cheese, the higher the water content — Swiss cheese is 38 percent water; skim milk ricotta, 74 percent), a plain, hard bagel (29 percent water), milk powder (2 percent), and even butter and margarine (10 percent). Only oils have no water.

In other words (actually in Valtin's words), a healthy adult in a temperate climate who isn't perspiring heavily can get enough water simply by drinking only when he or she is thirsty. Gulp.

Not all liquids are equally liquefying. The alcohol in beer, wine, and spirits is a *diuretic,* a chemical that makes you urinate more copiously. Although alcohol beverages provide water, they also increase its elimination from your body — which is why you feel thirsty the morning after you've had a glass or two of wine. And when you feel thirsty, what do you do? Drink some water.

Caffeinated beverages such as tea and coffee were once thought to be diuretic and dehydrating. While it's true that caffeine can stimulate urination, the amount of water in tea and coffee more than offsets any potential increase in water loss caused by drinking these beverages.

Taking in Extra Water and Electrolytes As Needed

In Canada, most people regularly consume much more sodium than they need. In fact, some people who are sodium sensitive may end up with high blood pressure that can be lowered if they reduce their sodium intake. For more about high blood pressure, check out *High Blood Pressure For Dummies* (published by Wiley) by Alan L. Rubin, M.D.

Potassium and chloride are found in so many foods that here, too, a dietary deficiency is a rarity. In fact, the only recorded case of chloride deficiency was among infants given a formula liquid from which the chloride was inadvertently omitted.

Death by dehydration: Not a pretty sight

Every day, you lose an amount of water equal to about 4 percent of your total weight. If you don't take in enough water to replace what you lose naturally by breathing, perspiring, urinating, and defecating, warning signals go off loud and clear.

Early on, when you've lost just a little water, equal to about 1 percent of your body weight, you feel thirsty. If you ignore thirst, it grows more intense.

When water loss rises to about 2 percent of your weight, your appetite fades. Your circulation slows as water seeps out of blood cells and blood plasma. And you experience a sense of emotional discomfort, a perception that things are, well, not right.

By the time your water loss equals 4 percent of your body weight (a little more than 2 kilograms, or 5 pounds for a 59-kilogram or 130-pound woman; 3 kilograms or 7 pounds for a 77-kilogram or 170-pound man), you're slightly nauseated, your skin is flushed, and you're very, very tired. With less water circulating through your tissues, your hands and feet tingle, your head aches, your temperature rises, you breathe more quickly, and your pulse quickens.

After this, things begin spiralling downhill. When your water loss reaches 10 percent of your body weight, your tongue swells, your kidneys start to fail, and you're so dizzy that you can't stand on one foot with your eyes closed. In fact, you probably can't even try: Your muscles are in spasm.

When you lose enough water to equal 15 percent of your body weight, you're deaf and pretty much unable to see out of eyes that are sunken and covered with stiffened lids. Your skin has shrunk, and your tongue has shriveled.

When you've lost water equal to 20 percent of your body weight, you've had it. You're at the limit of your endurance. Deprived of life-giving liquid, your skin cracks, and your organs grind to a halt. And — sorry about this — so do you. *Ave atque vale,* as the Romans say. Or as the Romans say when in the U.S.A, Canada, Great Britain, Australia, or any place where English is the mother tongue: "Hail and Farewell."

When ginger ale won't cut it

Serious dehydration calls for serious medicine, such as the World Health Organization's handy-dandy, two-tumbler electrolyte replacement formula.

Wait! Stop! If you're reading this while lying in bed exhausted by some variety of *turista,* the traveller's diarrhea acquired from impure drinking water, do not make the formula without absolutely clean glasses, washed in bottled water. Better yet, get paper cups.

Now here's what you need:

Glass No. 1

250 mL (8 ounces) orange juice

A pinch of salt

2 mL (½ teaspoon) sweetener (honey, corn syrup)

Glass No. 2

250 mL (8 ounces) boiled or bottled or distilled water

1 mL (¼ teaspoon) baking soda

Take a sip from one glass, then the other, and continue until finished. If diarrhea continues, contact your doctor.

In 2004, the Adequate Intake (AI) for sodium, potassium, and chloride were set at one-size-fits-all averages for a healthy adult age 19 to 50 weighing 70 kilograms (154 pounds; see Chapter 4 for more on AI):

- ✔ **Sodium:** 1,500 milligrams
- ✔ **Potassium:** 4,700 milligrams
- ✔ **Chloride:** 2,300 milligrams

Most Canadians get much more sodium and chloride as a matter of course, and sometimes you actually need extra water and electrolytes. The next sections tell you when.

You're sick to your stomach

Repeated vomiting or diarrhea drains your body of water and electrolytes. Similarly, you also need extra water to replace the liquid lost in perspiration when you have a high fever.

When you lose enough water to be dangerously dehydrated, you also lose the electrolytes you need to maintain fluid balance, regulate body temperature, and trigger dozens of biochemical reactions. Plain water doesn't replace those electrolytes. Check with your doctor for a drink that will hydrate your body without upsetting your tummy.

You're exercising or working hard in a hot environment

When you're warm, your body perspires. The moisture evaporates and cools your skin so that blood circulating up from the centre of your body to the surface is cooled. The cooled blood returns to the centre of your body, lowering the temperature (your *core temperature*) there, too.

If you don't cool your body down, you continue to lose water. If you don't replace the lost water, things can get dicey because not only are you losing water, you're also losing electrolytes. The most common cause of temporary sodium, potassium, and chloride depletion is heavy, uncontrolled perspiration.

Deprived of water and electrolytes, your muscles cramp, you're dizzy and weak, and perspiration, now uncontrolled, no longer cools you. Your core body temperature begins rising, and without relief — air conditioning or a cool shower, plus water, ginger ale, or fruit juice — you may progress from heat cramps to heat exhaustion to heat stroke. The latter is potentially fatal.

But — and it's a big one — drinking *too much* water while exercising can also be hazardous to your health. Flooding your body with liquid dilutes the sodium in your bloodstream and may make your brain and other body tissues swell, a condition known as *hyponaturemia,* or "water intoxication." The New Rule from the American College of Sports Medicine is to drink just enough water to maintain your body weight while working out. How much is that? Step on a scale before exercising. Exercise for an hour. Step back on the scale. You need 1 litre of water to replace every kilogram lost in your one hour's exercise. Lose one kilogram, drink 1 litre (4 cups) of water. Lose ½ kilogram, drink half a litre (2 cups). That was easy!

You're on a high-protein diet

You need extra water to eliminate the nitrogen compounds in protein. This is true of infants on high-protein formulas and adults on high-protein weight-reducing diets. See Chapter 6 to find out why too much protein may be harmful.

Water is water. Or is it?

Chemically speaking, water's an odd duck. It's the only substance on Earth than can exist as a liquid (water) and a solid (ice) — but not a bendable plastic. No, snow is not plastic water. It's a grouping of solids (ice crystals).

Water may be hard or soft, but these terms have nothing to do with how the water feels on your hand. They describe the liquid's mineral content:

✔ *Hard water* has lots of minerals, particularly calcium and magnesium. This water rises to the Earth's surface from underground springs, usually picking up calcium carbonate as it moves up through the ground.

✔ *Soft water* has fewer minerals. In nature, soft water is surface water, the runoff from rain-swollen streams or rainwater that falls directly into reservoirs. *Water softeners* are products that attract and remove the minerals in water.

What you get at the supermarket is another thing altogether:

✔ *Distilled water* is tap water that has been *distilled*, or boiled until it turns to steam, which is then collected and condensed back into a liquid free of impurities, chemicals, and minerals. The name may also be used to describe a liquid produced by *ultrafiltration*, a process that removes everything from the water except water molecules. Distilled water is very important in chemical and pharmaceutical processing. You'll appreciate the fact that it doesn't clog your iron; makes clean, clear ice cubes; and serves as a flavour-free mixer or base for tea and coffee.

✔ *Mineral water* is spring water. Because it has a higher mineral content, it's naturally alkaline and sometimes referred to as *hard water*. This makes it a natural antacid and a mild diuretic (a substance that increases urination). The term *spring water* is used to describe water from springs nearer to the Earth's surface, so it has fewer mineral particles and what some people describe as a "cleaner taste" than hard water.

✔ *Still water* is spring water that flows up to the surface on its own. *Sparkling water* is pushed to the top by naturally occurring gases in the underground spring. So, you ask, what's the big difference? Sparkling water has bubbles; still water doesn't.

✔ *Springlike* or *spring fresh* are terms designed to make something sound more highfalutin than it really is. These products aren't spring water; they're probably filtered tap water.

You're taking certain medications

Because some medications interact with water and electrolytes, always ask whether you need extra water and electrolytes whenever your doctor prescribes the following medications:

✔ **Diuretics:** They increase the loss of sodium, potassium, and chloride.

✔ **Neomycin (an antibiotic):** It binds sodium into insoluble compounds, making it less available to your body.

✔ **Colchicine (an antigout drug):** It lowers your absorption of sodium.

You have high blood pressure

In 1997, when researchers at Johns Hopkins analyzed the results of more than 30 studies dealing with high blood pressure, they found that people taking daily supplements of 2,500 mg (2.5 grams) of potassium were likely to have blood pressure several points lower than people not taking the supplements. Ask your doctor about this one, and remember: Food is also a good source of potassium. One whole banana has up to 470 milligrams of potassium, one cup of dates has 1,160 milligrams, and one cup of raisins has 1,239 milligrams.

Part III
Healthy Eating

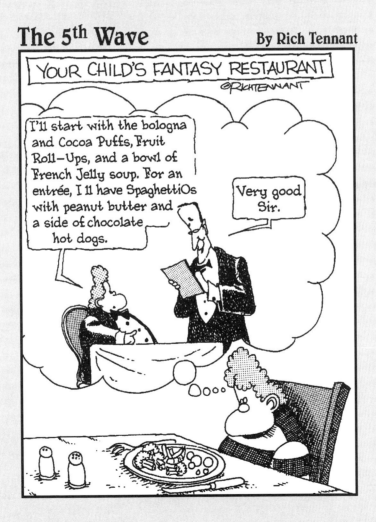

In this part . . .

You find out how to put foods together to build a healthy diet right here. The chapters in this part are chock full of guidelines and strategies based on Canada's Food Guide, the Official Word on making selections that enhance your body while pleasing your palate. And, oh yes, there's an explanation of why you get hungry and why you find some foods more appetizing than others — an important factor in creating a nutritious diet. (Hey, if it doesn't taste good, why would you want to eat it?)

Chapter 14

Why You Eat When You Eat

*B*ecause you need food to live, your body is no slouch at letting you know that it's ready for breakfast, lunch, dinner, and maybe a few snacks in between. This chapter explains the signals your body uses to get you to the table, to the drive-through of your favourite restaurant, or to the vending machine down the hall.

Understanding the Difference between Hunger and Appetite

People eat for two main reasons. The first reason is hunger; the second is appetite. Hunger and appetite are *not* synonyms. In fact, hunger and appetite are entirely different processes.

Hunger is the need for food. It is

- ✔ A physical reaction that includes chemical changes in your body related to a naturally low level of glucose in your blood several hours after eating

- ✔ An instinctive, protective mechanism that makes sure your body gets the fuel it requires to function reasonably well

Appetite is the desire for food. It is

- ✔ A sensory or psychological reaction (looks good! smells good!) that stimulates an involuntary physiological response (salivation, stomach contractions)
- ✔ A conditioned response to food (see the sidebar on Pavlov's dogs)

The practical difference between hunger and appetite is this: When you're hungry, you eat one hot dog. After that, your appetite may lead you to eat two more hot dogs just because they look appealing or taste good.

In other words, appetite is the basis for the familiar saying: "Your eyes are bigger than your stomach." Not to mention the well-known advertising slogan: "Bet you can't eat just one." Hey, these guys know their customers.

Refuelling: The Cycle of Hunger and Satiety

Your body does its best to create cycles of activity that parallel a 24-hour day. Like sleep, hunger occurs at pretty regular intervals, although your lifestyle may make it difficult to follow this natural pattern — even when your stomach loudly announces it's empty!

Pavlov's performing puppies

Ivan Petrovich Pavlov (1849–1936) was a Russian physiologist who won the Nobel Prize in physiology/medicine in 1904 for his research on the digestive glands. Pavlov's Big Bang, though, was his identification of respondent conditioning — a fancy way of saying that you can train people to respond physically (or emotionally) to an object or stimulus that simply reminds them of something they love or hate.

Pavlov tested respondent conditioning on dogs. He began by ringing a bell each time he offered food to his laboratory dogs so that the dogs learned to associate the sound of the bell with the sight and smell of food.

Then he rang the bell without offering the food, and the dogs responded as though food were on tap — salivating madly, even though the dish was empty.

Respondent conditioning applies to many things other than food. For example, it can make a winning Olympic athlete teary at the sight of the flag that represents his or her country. Food companies are great at using respondent conditioning to encourage you to buy their products: When you see a picture of a deep, dark, rich chocolate bar, doesn't your mouth start to water, and . . . hey, come back! Where are you going?

Recognizing hunger

The clearest signals that your body wants food, right now, are the physical reactions from your stomach and your blood that let you know it's definitely time to put more food in your mouth and — eat!

Growling and rumbling: Your stomach speaks

An empty belly has no manners. If you do not fill it right away, your stomach will issue an audible — sometimes embarrassing — call for food. This rumbling signal is called a *hunger pang*.

Hunger pangs actually are plain old muscle contractions. When your stomach's full, these contractions and their continual waves down the entire length of the intestine — known as *peristalsis* — move food through your digestive tract (see Chapter 2 for more about digestion). When your stomach's empty, the contractions just squeeze air, and that makes noise.

This phenomenon first was observed in 1912 by a physiologist named Walter B. Cannon. (Cannon? Rumble? Could anyone make this up?) Cannon convinced a fellow researcher to swallow a small balloon attached to a thin tube connected to a pressure-sensitive machine. Then Cannon inflated and deflated the balloon to simulate the sensation of a full or empty stomach. Measuring the pressure and frequency of his volunteer's stomach contractions, Cannon discovered that the contractions were strongest and occurred most frequently when the balloon was deflated and the stomach empty. Cannon drew the obvious conclusion: When your stomach is empty, you feel hungry.

Getting that empty feeling

Every time you eat, your pancreas secretes *insulin,* a hormone that enables you to move blood sugar (glucose) out of the blood and into cells where it's needed for various chores. *Glucose* is the basic fuel your body uses for energy. (See Chapter 8.) As a result, the level of glucose circulating in your blood rises and then declines naturally, producing a vague feeling of emptiness, and perhaps weakness, that prompts you to eat. Most people experience the natural rise and fall of glucose as a relatively smooth pattern that lasts about four hours.

Knowing when you're full

The satisfying feeling of fullness after eating is called *satiety,* the signal that says, okay, hold the hot dogs, I've had plenty, and I need to push back from the table.

As nutrition research and the understanding of brain functions have become more sophisticated, scientists have discovered that your *hypothalamus,* a small gland on top of the *brain stem* (the part of the brain that connects to the top of the spinal cord), seems to house your appetite controls in an area of the brain that makes hormones and other chemicals that control hunger and appetite (see Figure 14-1). For example, the hypothalamus releases neuropeptide Y (NPY), a chemical that latches onto brain cells, which then send out a signal: More food!

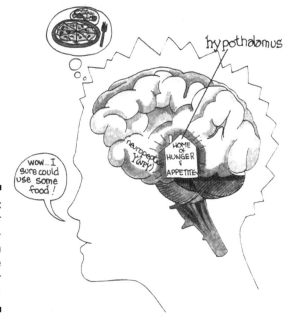

Figure 14-1:
Your hypothalamus is in charge of your appetite!

Other body cells also play a role in making your body say, "I'm full." In 1995, researchers at Rockefeller University discovered a gene in *fat cells* (the body cells that store fat) that directs the production of a hormone called *leptin* (from the Greek word for *thin*). Leptin appears to tell your body how much fat you have stored, thus regulating your hunger (need for food to provide fuel). Leptin also reduces the hypothalamus's secretion of NPY, the hormone that signals hunger. When the Rockefeller folks injected leptin into specially bred fat mice, the mice ate less, burned food faster, and lost significant amounts of weight.

Eventually, researchers hope that this kind of information can lead to the creation of safe and effective drugs to combat obesity.

What meal is this, anyway?

Breakfast and lunch leave no doubt. The first comes right after you wake up in the morning; the second, in the middle of the day, sometime around noon.

But when do you eat dinner? And what about supper?

According to _Webster's New International Dictionary of the English Language_ (2nd edition, 1941 — 15 pounds, including the new binding Carol put on when the old one crumbled after she dropped the darned thing on its spine once too often), dinner is the main meal of the day, usually eaten around midday, although (get this) some people, "especially in cities," have their dinner between 6 p.m. and 8 p.m. — which probably makes it their supper, because Webster's calls that a meal you eat at the end of the day.

In other words, dinner is lunch except when it's supper. Help!

Beating the four-hour hungries

Throughout the world, the cycle of hunger (namely, of glucose rising and falling) prompts a feeding schedule that generally provides four meals during the day: breakfast, lunch, _tea_ (a mid-afternoon meal), and supper.

In Canada, a three-meal-a-day culture forces people to fight their natural rhythm by going without food from lunch at noon to supper at 6 p.m. or later. The unpleasant result is that when glucose levels decline around 4 p.m., and people in other countries are enjoying afternoon tea, many Canadians get really testy and try to satisfy their natural hunger by grabbing the nearest food, usually a high-fat, high-calorie snack.

In 1989, David Jenkins, M.D., Ph.D., and Tom Wolever, M.D., Ph.D., of the University of Toronto, set up a "nibbling study" designed to test the idea that if you even out digestion — by eating several small meals rather than three big ones — you can spread out insulin secretion and keep the amount of glucose in your blood on an even keel all day long.

The theory turned out to be right. People who ate five or six small meals rather than three big ones felt better and experienced an extra bonus: lower cholesterol levels. After two weeks of nibbling, the people in the Jenkins–Wolever study showed a 13.5 percent lower level of low-density lipoproteins (LDL) than people who ate exactly the same amount of food divided into three big meals. As a result, many diets designed to help you lose weight or control your cholesterol (What? You haven't got a copy of

Controlling Cholesterol For Dummies? Impossible!) now emphasize a daily regimen of several small meals rather than the basic big three. Smart cookies. Low-fat, low-cholesterol, low-cal, of course.

Maintaining a healthy appetite

The best way to deal with hunger and appetite is to find out how to recognize and follow your body's natural cues.

If you're hungry, eat — in reasonable amounts that support a realistic weight. The key is to stop eating when you're satisfied and not stuffed. Appetite has the potential to work against you by encouraging you to eat more food, because the food looks and tastes good, resulting in an excess of calories consumed. Doug always tries to encourage people to undereat at meal- and snack-time, then wait to see if they're hungry in a few hours. If so, then nibble some more. (Confused about how much you should weigh? Check out the weight table in Chapter 3.) And remember: Nobody's perfect. Make one day's indulgence guilt free by reducing your calorie intake proportionately over the next few days. A little give here, a little take there, and you'll stay on target overall.

Responding to Your Environment on a Gut Level

Your physical and psychological environments definitely affect appetite and hunger, sometimes leading you to eat more than normal, sometimes less.

Baby, it's cold outside

You're more likely to feel hungry when you're in a cool place than you are when you're in a warm one. And you're more likely to want high-calorie dishes in cold weather than in hot weather. Just think about the foods that tempt you in winter — stews, roasts, thick soups — versus those you find pleasing on a simmering summer day — salads, chilled fruit, simple sandwiches.

This difference is no accident. Food gives you calories. Calories keep you warm. Making sure that you get what you need, your body even processes food faster when it's cold out. Your stomach empties more quickly as food speeds along through the digestive tract, which means those old hunger pangs show up sooner than expected, which, in turn, means that you eat more and stay warmer and . . . well, you get the picture.

Exercising more than your mouth

Everybody knows that working out gives you a big appetite, right? Well, everybody's wrong (it happens all the time). Yes, people who exercise regularly are likely to have a healthy (read: normal) appetite, but they're rarely hungry immediately after exercising because

- ✔ Exercise pulls stored energy — glucose and fat — out of body tissues, so your glucose levels stay steady and you don't feel hungry.

- ✔ Exercise slows the passage of food through the digestive tract. Your stomach empties more slowly, and you feel fuller longer.

  Caution: If you eat a heavy meal right before heading for the gym or the stationary bike in your bedroom, the food sitting in your stomach may make you feel stuffed. Sometimes, you may develop cramps. Or — as *Heartburn & Reflux For Dummies* (Wiley) explains — heartburn. Ouch.

- ✔ Exercise (including mental exertion) reduces anxiety. For some people, that means less desire to reach for a snack.

Nursing your appetite back to health

Severe physical stress or trauma — a broken bone, surgery, a burn, a high fever — reduces appetite and slows the natural contractions of the intestinal tract. If you eat at times like this, the food may back up in your gut or even stretch your bowel enough to tear it. In such situations, intravenous feeding — fluids with nutrients sent through a needle directly into a vein — give you nutrition without irritation.

Taking medicine, changing your appetite

Taking some medicines may make you more (or less) likely to eat. Some drugs used to treat common conditions affect your appetite. When you use these medicines, you may find yourself eating more (or less) than usual. This side effect is rarely mentioned when doctors hand out prescriptions, perhaps because it isn't life threatening and usually disappears when you stop taking the drug.

Some examples of appetite uppers are certain antidepressants (mood elevators), antihistamines (allergy pills), diuretics (drugs that make you urinate more frequently), steroids (drugs that fight inflammation), and tranquilizers (calming drugs). Appetite reducers include some antibiotics, anti-cancer drugs, anti-seizure drugs, blood pressure medications, and cholesterol-lowering drugs.

Of course, not every drug in a particular class of drugs (for example, anti-biotics or antidepressants) has the same effect on appetite. For example, the antidepressant drug amitriptyline (Elavil) increases your appetite and may cause weight gain; another antidepressant drug, fluoxetine (Prozac), usually does not.

The fact that a drug affects appetite is almost never a reason to avoid using it. But knowing that a relationship exists between the drug and your desire for food can be helpful. Plain common sense dictates that you ask about possible drug/appetite interactions whenever your doctor prescribes a drug for you. If the drug package the pharmacist gives you doesn't come with an insert, ask for one. Read the fine print about side effects and other interesting details — such as the direction to avoid drinking alcohol or driving or using heavy machinery.

Looking at Appetite Anomalies: Eating Disorders

An eating disorder is a psychological illness that leads you to eat either too much or too little. Indulging in a hot fudge sundae once in a while is not an eating disorder. Neither is dieting for three weeks so that you can fit into last year's dress this New Year's Eve.

The difference between normal indulgence and normal dieting to lose weight versus an eating disorder is that the first two are acceptable, healthy behaviours, while an eating disorder is a potentially life-threatening illness that requires immediate medical attention.

Eating too much

Although many recent studies document an alarming worldwide increase in obesity, particularly among young children, not everyone who is larger or heavier than the current Canadian ideal has an eating disorder. Human bodies come in many different sizes, and some healthy people are just naturally larger or heavier than others. An eating disorder may be present, though, when a person

- ✔ Continually confuses the desire for food (appetite) with the need for food (hunger)

- ✔ Restricts his or her eating and/or starts to avoid types of food or groups of food, such as fats or carbohydrates, or suddenly adopts a new way of eating, such as vegetarianism (To be clear, vegetarianism is a valid and nutritionally sound way to eat, but many people with eating disorders have used this as a way to legitimize restrictive eating and to avoid food.)

✔ Starts to develop anxiety about putting on weight or being fat

✔ Withdraws from situations that include food or eating with others

✔ Is preoccupied with dieting, counting calories, or monitoring his or her body weight

✔ Who has access to a normal diet experiences psychological distress when denied food

✔ Uses food to relieve anxiety provoked by what he or she considers a scary situation — a new job, a party, ordinary criticism, or a deadline

Traditionally, doctors have found that treating obesity successfully is difficult (see Chapter 3). However, recent research suggests that some people overeat in response to irregularities in the production of chemicals that regulate satiety (the feeling of fullness). This research may open the path to new kinds of drugs that can control extreme appetite, thus reducing the incidence of obesity-related disorders such as arthritis, diabetes, high blood pressure, and heart disease.

Bingeing, purging, and starving: Unhealthy relationships with food

Some people relieve their anxiety not by eating but by refusing to eat or by regurgitating food after they've eaten it. The first kind of behaviour is called anorexia nervosa; the second, bulimia.

Anorexia nervosa (voluntary starvation), the eating disorder that sidelined Mary-Kate Olsen in 2004, is virtually unknown in places where food is hard to come by. It seems to be an affliction of affluence, most likely to strike the young and well-to-do. It's nine times more common among women than among men.

Many doctors who specialize in treating people with eating disorders suggest that anorexia nervosa may be an attempt to control one's life by rejecting a developing body. In other words, by starving themselves, anorexic girls avoid developing breasts and hips, and anorexic boys avoid developing the broad wedge-shape adult male body. By not growing wide, both hope to avoid growing up.

Left untreated, anorexia nervosa can end in death by starvation.

A second form of eating disorder is *bulimia*. Unlike people with anorexia, individuals with bulimia don't refuse to eat. In fact, they may often binge (consume enormous amounts of food in one sitting: a whole chicken, several pints of ice cream, a whole loaf of bread).

But bulimic people don't want to keep the food they eat in their bodies. They may use laxatives to increase defecation, but the more common method they use for getting rid of food is regurgitation. Bulimic people may simply retire to the bathroom after eating and stick their fingers into their throats to make themselves throw up. Or they may use *emetics* (drugs that induce vomiting). Either way, danger looms.

The human body is not designed for repeated stuffing followed by regurgitation. Bingeing may dilate the stomach to the point of rupture; constant vomiting may severely irritate or even cause tears in the lining of the esophagus (throat). In addition, the continued use of large quantities of emetics may result in a life-threatening loss of potassium, which could trigger an irregular heartbeat or heart failure, factors that contributed to the 1983 death of singer Karen Carpenter, an anorexic/bulimic who — at one point in her disease — weighed only 80 pounds but still saw herself as overweight. One symptom of anorexia and bulimia is the inability to look in a mirror and see yourself as you really are. Even at their most skeletal, people with these eating disorders perceive themselves as grossly fat.

As you can see, eating disorders are life-threatening conditions. But they can be treated. If you (or someone you know) experience any of the signs or symptoms just described, the safest course is to seek immediate medical advice and treatment. For more information about eating conditions, contact the National Eating Disorders Information Centre, ES 7-421, 200 Elizabeth St, Toronto, ON M5G 2C4; phone 1-866-NEDIC-20 (1-866-633-4220); e-mail `nedic@uhn.on.ca`; Web site `www.nedic.ca`.

Chapter 15

Why You Like the Foods You Like

....

....

*N*utritionally speaking, *taste* is the ability to perceive flavours in food and beverages. *Preference* is appreciation of one food and distaste of another. Decisions about taste are physical reactions that depend on specialized body organs called taste buds. Although your culture has a decided influence on what you think is good to eat, decisions about food preferences may also depend on your genes, your medical history, and your personal reactions to specific foods.

Tackling Taste: How Your Brain and Tongue Work Together

Your *taste buds* are sensory organs that enable you to perceive different flavours in food — in other words, to taste the food you eat.

Taste buds (also referred to as *taste papillae*) are not flowers. They're tiny bumps on the surface of your tongue (see Figure 15-1). Each one contains groups of receptor cells that anchor an antenna-like structure called a *microvillus*, which projects up through a gap (or pore) in the centre of the taste bud, sort of like a thread sticking through the hole in a Life Savers candy. (For more about the microvilli and how they behave in your digestive tract, see Chapter 2.)

The microvilli in your taste buds transmit messages from flavour chemicals in the food along nerve fibres to your brain, which translates the messages into perceptions: "Oh, wow, that's good," or "Man, that's awful."

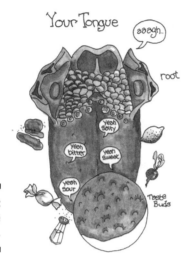

Figure 15-1:
Your tongue
up close.

The four (maybe five) basic flavours

Your taste buds definitely recognize four basic flavours: *sweet, sour, bitter,* and *salty.* Some people add a fifth basic flavour to this list. It's called *umami,* a Japanese word describing richness or a savoury flavour associated with certain amino acids such as glutamates — there is more about monosodium glutamate (MSG) later in this section — and soy products such as tofu.

Early on, scientists thought that everyone had specific taste buds for specific flavours: sweet taste buds for sweets, sour taste buds for sour, and so on. However, the prevailing theory today is that groups of taste buds work together so that flavour chemicals in food link up with chemical bonds in taste buds to create patterns that you recognize as sweet, sour, bitter, and salty. The technical term for this process is *across-fibre pattern theory of gustatory coding.* Receptor patterns for the fave four (sweet, sour, bitter, salty) have been tentatively identified, but the pattern for umami remains elusive.

Flavours are not frivolous. They're one of the factors that enable you to enjoy food. In fact, flavours are so important that MSG is used to make food taste better. MSG, most often found in food prepared in Chinese restaurants, stimulates brain cells. People who are sensitive to MSG may actually develop *Chinese restaurant syndrome,* which is characterized by tight facial muscles, headache, nausea, and sweating caused by overbouncy brain cells. Very large doses of MSG given to lab rats have been lethal, and the compound is banned from baby food. However, no real evidence indicates that a little MSG is a problem for people who aren't sensitive to it. Which leaves only one question: How does MSG work? Does it enhance existing flavours or simply add that umami flavour on its own? Believe it or not, right now nobody knows. Sorry about that.

Your health and your taste buds

Some illnesses and medicines alter your ability to taste foods. The result may be partial or total *ageusia* (the medical term for loss of taste). Or you may experience *flavour confusion* — meaning that you mix up flavours, translating sour as bitter, or sweet as salty, or vice versa.

Table 15-1 lists some medical conditions that affect your sense of taste.

Table 15-1	These Things Make Tasting Food Difficult
This Condition	*May Lead to This Problem*
A bacterial or viral infection of the tongue	Secretions that block your taste buds
Injury to the mouth, nose, or throat	Damage to the nerves that transmit flavour signals
Radiation therapy to the mouth and throat	Damage to the nerves that transmit flavour signals

Tricking your taste buds

Combining foods can short-circuit your taste buds' ability to identify flavours correctly. For example, when you sip wine (even an apparently smooth and silky one), your taste buds say, "Hey, that alcohol's sharp." Take a bite of

The nose knows — and the eyes have it

Your nose is important to your sense of taste. Just like the taste of food, the aroma of food stimulates sensory messages. Think about how you sniff your brandy before drinking and how the wonderful aroma of baking bread warms the heart and stirs the soul — not to mention the salivary glands. When you can't smell, you can't really taste. As anyone who's ever had a cold knows, when your nose is stuffed and your sense of smell is deadened, almost everything tastes like plain old cotton. Don't have a cold? You can test this theory by closing your eyes, pinching your nostrils shut, and having someone put a tiny piece of either a raw onion or a fresh apple into your mouth. Bet you can't tell which is which without looking — or sniffing!

Food colour is also an important clue to what you'll enjoy eating. Repeated studies show that when testers change the expected colour of foods, people find them (the foods, not the testers) less appealing. For example, blue mashed potatoes and green beef lose to plain old white mashed potatoes and red meat every time.

cheese first, and the wine tastes smoother (less acidic) because the cheese's fat and protein molecules coat your receptor cells so the acidic wine molecules cannot connect.

A similar phenomenon occurs during serial wine tastings (tasting many wines, one after another). Try two equally dry, acidic wines, and the second seems mellower because acid molecules from the first one fill up space on the chemical bonds that perceive acidity. Drink a sweet wine after a dry one, and the sweetness often is more pronounced.

Here's another way to fool your taste buds: Eat an artichoke. The meaty part at the base of the artichoke leaves contains *cynarin,* a sweet-tasting chemical that makes any food you taste after the artichoke taste sweeter.

Determining Deliciousness

When it comes to deciding what tastes good, all human beings and most animals have four things in common: They like sweets, crave salt, go for the fat, and avoid the bitter (at least at first).

These choices are rooted deep in biology and evolution. In fact, you can say that whenever you reach for something you consider good to eat, the entire human race — especially your own individual ancestors — reaches with you.

Listening to your body

Here's something to chew on: The foods that taste good — sweet foods, salty foods, fatty foods — are essential for a healthy body.

✔ Sweet foods are a source of quick energy because their sugars can be converted quickly to glucose, the molecule that your body burns for energy. (Check out Chapter 8 for an explanation of how your body uses sugars.)

Better yet, sweet foods make you feel good. Eating them tells your brain to release natural painkillers called *endorphins.* Sweet foods may also stimulate an increase in blood levels of *adrenaline,* a hormone secreted by the adrenal glands. Adrenaline sometimes is labelled the *fight-or-flight hormone* because it's secreted more heavily when you feel threatened and must decide whether to stand your ground — *fight* — or hurry away — *flight.*

✔ Salt is vital to life. As Chapter 13 explains, salt enables your body to maintain its fluid balance and to regulate chemicals called *electrolytes,* which give your nerve cells the power they need to fire electrical charges that energize your muscles, pump up your organs, and transmit messages from your brain.

✔ Fatty foods are even richer in calories (energy) than sugars. So the fact that you want them most when you're very hungry comes as no surprise. (Chapter 2 and Chapter 7 explain how you use fats for energy.)

✔ Which fatty food you want may depend on your sex. Several studies suggest that women like their fats with sugar — Hey, where's the chocolate? Men, on the other hand, seem to prefer their fat with salt — Bring on the fries!

Loving the food you're with: Geography and taste

Marvin Harris was an anthropologist with a special interest in the history of food. In a perfectly delightful book called *Good to Eat: Riddles of Food and Culture* (Simon & Schuster, 1986), Harris posed this interesting situation:

Suppose you live in a forest where someone has pinned $20 and $5 bills to the upper branches of the trees. Which will you reach for? The $20 bills, of course. But wait. Suppose that only a couple of $20 bills are pinned to branches among millions and millions of $5 bills. Does that change the picture? You betcha.

Searching for food is hard work. You don't want to spend so much time and energy searching for food that you end up using more calories than the food you find can provide. Substitute "chickens" for $20 bills and "large insects" for $5 bills, and you can see why people who live in places where insects far outnumber chickens spend their time and energy picking off the plentiful high-protein bugs rather than chasing after the occasional chicken — although they wouldn't turn it down if it fell into the pot.

So, you may say that Harris's first rule of food choice is that people tend to eat and enjoy what is easily available, which explains the differences in cuisine in different parts of the world.

Here's a second rule: For a food to be appealing (good to eat), it must be both nutritious and relatively easy or economical to produce.

Creepy crawly nutrients

Who's to say grilled grasshopper is less appetizing than a lobster? After all, both have long skinny bodies and plenty of legs. But the difference is in the nutrients: The bug beats the lobster hands (legs?) down.

Food 3.5 oz	Protein (g)	Fat (g)	Carbohydrates (g)	Iron (mg)
Water Beetle	19.8	8.3	2.1	13.6
Red Ant	13.9	3.5	2.9	5.7
Cricket	12.9	5.5	5.1	9.5
Small Grasshopper	20.6	6.1	3.9	5.0
Large Grasshopper	14.3	3.3	2.2	3.0
Lobster	22	<1	<1	0.4
Blue crab	20	<1	0	0.8

USDA and Iowa State University
(www.ent.iastate.edu/misc/insectnutrition.html)

A food that meets one test but not the other is likely to be off the list. For example:

- The human stomach cannot extract nutrients from grass. So even though grass grows here, there, and everywhere, under ordinary circumstances, grass never ends up in your salad.

- Cows are harder to raise than plants, especially under the hot South Asian sun; pigs eat what people do, so they compete for your food supply. In other words, although they're highly nutritious, sometimes neither the cow nor the pig is economical to produce. This anthropological explanation is a reasonable argument for why some cultures have prohibited the use of pigs and cows as food.

Taking offense to tastes

Virtually everyone instinctively dislikes bitter foods, at least at first tasting. This dislike is a protective mechanism. Bitter foods are often poisonous, so disliking stuff that tastes bitter is a primitive but effective way to keep you from eating potentially toxic food.

According to Linda Bartoshuk, Ph.D., professor of surgery (otolaryngology — ear, nose, and throat) at the Yale University School of Medicine, about two-thirds of all human beings carry a gene that makes them especially sensitive to bitter flavours. This gene may have given their ancestors a leg up in surviving their evolutionary food trials.

People with this gene can taste very small concentrations of a chemical called phenylthiocarbamide (PTC). Because PTC is potentially toxic, Dr. Bartoshuk tests for the trait by having people taste a piece of paper impregnated with 6-n-propylthiouracil, a thyroid medication whose flavour and chemical structure are similar to PTC. People who say the paper tastes bitter are called *PTC tasters*. People who taste only paper are called *PTC nontasters*.

If you're a PTC taster, you're likely to find the taste of saccharin, caffeine, the salt substitute potassium chloride, and the food preservatives sodium benzoate and potassium benzoate really nasty. The same is true for the flavour chemicals common to cruciferous vegetables — members of the mustard family, including broccoli, Brussels sprouts, cabbage, cauliflower, and radishes.

No such ambivalence exists among people who've gotten truly sick — we're talking nausea and vomiting here — after eating a specific food. When that happens, you'll probably come to like its flavour less. Sometimes, says psychologist Alexandra W. Logue, author of *The Psychology of Eating and Drinking*, your revulsion may be so strong that you'll never try the food again — even when you know that what actually made you sick was something else entirely, like riding a roller coaster just before eating, or having the flu, or taking a drug whose side effects upset your stomach.

If you're allergic to a food or have a metabolic problem that makes digesting it hard for you, you may eat the food less frequently, but you'll enjoy it as much as everyone else does. For example, people who cannot digest lactose, the sugar in milk, may end up gassy every time they eat ice cream, but they still like the way the ice cream tastes.

Does it matter whether you like your food? Yes, of course, it does. The simple act of putting food into your mouth needs to stimulate the flow of saliva and the secretion of enzymes that you need to digest the food. Some studies suggest that if you really like your food, your pancreas may release as much as 30 times its normal amount of digestive enzymes.

However, if you truly loathe what you're eating, your body may refuse to take it in. No saliva flows; your mouth becomes so dry that you may not even be able to swallow the food. If you do manage to choke it down, your stomach muscles and your digestive tract may convulse in an effort to be rid of the awful stuff.

Changing the Menu: Adapting to Exotic Foods

New foods are an adventure. As a rule, people may not like a new food the first time around, but in time — and with patience — what once seemed strange can become just another dish at dinner.

Learning to like unusual foods

Exposure to different people and cultures often expands your taste horizons. Some taboos — horsemeat, snake, dog — may simply be too emotion laden to be overcome. Others with no emotional baggage fall to experience. Most people hate very salty, very bitter, very acidic, or very slippery foods such as caviar, coffee, wine, beer, Scotch whisky, and oysters on first taste, but many later learn to enjoy them.

Coming to terms with these foods can be both physically and psychologically rewarding:

- Many bitter foods, such as coffee and unsweetened chocolate, are relatively mild stimulants that temporarily improve mood and physical performance. They're also a rich source of antioxidants, as are vegetables and fruit.

- Strongly flavoured foods, such as salty caviar, offer a challenge to the taste buds.

- Foods such as oysters, which may seem totally disgusting the first time you see or taste them, are symbols of wealth or worldliness. Trying them implies a certain sophistication in the way you face life.

Happily, an educated, adventurous sense of taste can be a pleasure that lasts as long as you live. Professional tea tasters, wine tasters, and others (maybe you?) who have developed the ability to recognize even the smallest differences among flavours continue to enjoy their gift well into old age. Although your sense of taste declines as you grow older, you can keep it perking as long as you supply the stimuli in the form of tasty, well-seasoned food.

In other words, as they say about adult life's other major sensory delight, "Use it or lose it."

Stirring the stew: The culinary benefits of immigration

If you're lucky enough to live in a place that attracts many immigrants, your dining experience is flavoured by the favourite foods of other people (meaning the foods of other cultures). Canadian cooking literally bubbles with contributions from every group that's ever stepped ashore.

Table 15-2 lists some of the foods and food combinations characteristic of specific ethnic/regional cuisines. Imagine how few you might sample living in a place where everybody shares exactly the same ethnic, racial, or religious backgrounds. Just thinking about it is enough to make me want to stand up and shout, "Hooray for diversity at the dinner table!" (Check out Figure 15-2 for the visuals!)

Table 15-2	Geography and Food Preference
If Your Ancestors Came From	*You're Likely to Be Familiar with This Flavour Combination*
Central and Eastern Europe	Sour cream and dill or paprika
China	Soy sauce plus wine and ginger
Germany	Meat roasted in vinegar and sugar
Greece	Olive oil and lemon
India	Cumin and curry
Italy	Tomatoes, cheese, and olive oil
Japan	Soy sauce plus rice wine and sugar
Korea	Soy sauce plus brown sugar, sesame, and chili
Mexico	Tomatoes and chili peppers
Middle Europe	Milk and vegetables
Puerto Rico	Rice and fish
West Africa	Peanuts and chili peppers

A.W. Logue, The Psychology of Eating and Drinking, 2nd edition (New York: W.H. Freeman and Company, 1991)

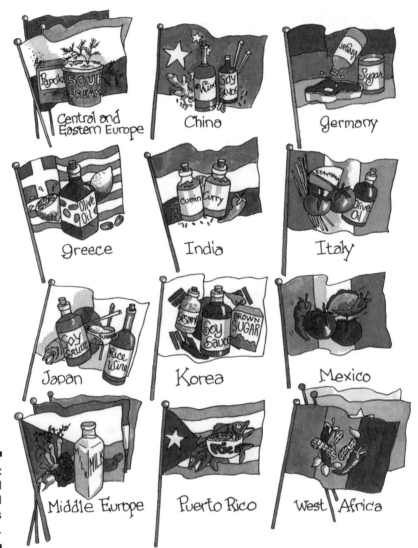

Figure 15-2:
Ethnic and regional cuisines abound.

Of course, enjoying other people's foods doesn't mean you don't have your own special treats. Table 15-3 is a flag waver: a list of Canadian taste sensations and flavours. Canadian cuisine varies from coast to coast, with regional differences. Many flavours and dishes have been influenced by immigrants who came over to help build the country. Canadian cuisine is best described as a fusion or blending of traditional recipes and flavours with those that are abundant in Canada. Particularly Canadian ingredients include wild berries (blueberries, raspberries, strawberries, and cranberries), wild game (bison, duck, caribou, and salmon), maple syrup, wild rice, mushrooms, and honey.

Table 15-3	Foods and Flavours from Canada
This Food Item	*Has Its Roots Here*
Nanaimo Bars	Nanaimo, BC (recipe origin unknown but a well-loved Canadian dessert popularized in Nanaimo, BC)
Butter Tarts	Northern Ontario (earliest recipe dates to 1915; the classic butter tart was a staple of pioneer cooking)
Maple Syrup	Northeastern North America (but is hugely popular in Canada, which produces 80 percent of the world's maple syrup)
Figgy Duff	Newfoundland (a traditional pudding made by combining flour, butter, sugar, and raisins, then boiling in a bag)
Dragon's Breath	Nova Scotia (a regional soft blue cheese)
Poutine	Quebec (French fries with cheese curds covered with gravy)
Ice Wine	Although invented in Germany, it was perfected in the Niagara Peninsula (wine produced from grapes that are left on the vines into winter)

Chapter 16

What Is a Healthful Diet?

The Heart and Stroke Foundation of Canada says to limit your consumption of fats and cholesterol. The Canadian Cancer Society says to eat more vegetables, fruit, and fibre. Health Canada says to watch out for fats, sugar, and salt. The Canadian Diabetes Association says to eat regular meals so your blood sugar stays even. The Food Police say if it tastes good, forget it!

Health Canada has incorporated virtually all but the "tastes good, forget it" rules into *Eating Well with Canada's Food Guide*. They've even added some advisories of their own. Before you begin reading this chapter, make sure you have a couple bookmarks or something else to hold your place — the material here often refers to information in other chapters, so you may have to skip back and forth.

What Is Canada's Food Guide?

Canada's Food Guide, created by Health Canada, is a blueprint to healthy eating. It is a rigorously scientifically proven eating pattern that outlines both the amount and type of food that people need to achieve and maintain health. It does this by putting the theory of nutrition and health into an eating pattern based on practical food choices. First published in 1942 as *Canada's Official Food Rules,* the guide and its guidelines have been irregularly updated over the decades.

The most recent version was published in early 2007. In this new Food Guide, Health Canada introduced a new, more comprehensive set of guidelines that includes more guidance on making quality choices with respect to nutrient content. *Eating Well with Canada's Food Guide* is the reader-friendly document that explains the Guide (which makes it the guide to the Guide, which makes this the guide to the guide to the Guide — whew!).

Although *Eating Well with Canada's Food Guide* is a short pamphlet, it packs in a lot of information. Health Canada's Food Guide Web site, `www.hc-sc. gc.ca/fn-an/food-guide-aliment/index_e.html`, has even more material for you to read. In this chapter, we've covered the high points in three handy sections: "Controlling Your Weight," "Making Smart Food Choices," and "Advice for Different Ages and Stages."

Controlling Your Weight

During the past two decades, as the number of overweight Canadians has bounced upward like a rubber ball, the incidence of obesity-related conditions such as Type 2 diabetes, high blood pressure, and heart disease also has risen.

The challenge (as always) is to set, reach, and maintain a healthful weight. Three aspects of healthy weight management centre around a nutrient-dense diet within an appropriate caloric range, a healthy weight, and physical activity.

Getting the most nutritious calories

Some foods provide lots of nutrients per calorie. Some don't. The former are called "nutrient-dense foods." The latter aren't.

As you may expect, Canada's Food Guide recommends choosing foods that are nutrient-dense to meet your requirements for vitamins and minerals and to provide your body with just the right amount of calories each day, while limiting the amount of:

- Foods high in saturated fat
- Foods high in trans fats
- Foods high in cholesterol
- Foods with added sugar
- Foods with added salt
- Alcohol beverages

In other words, stick to a balanced diet. No surprise there. And for a list of superstar foods, check out Chapter 28, which is — this *is* a surprise! — titled "Twelve Superstar Foods."

Managing your weight

To reach and keep a healthful weight, follow a few realistic rules:

- **Evaluate your weight.** The best test of who's actually overweight is the *Body Mass Index (BMI),* a measure of body fat versus body lean mass (in other words, muscle) that can be used to predict health outcomes. Because BMI is limited and doesn't apply to everyone (it does not apply to pregnant women, growing children, or those who are highly muscular, for example), it is best to consider your waist circumference (WC) as well rather than just focusing on BMI alone. This is also an invaluable predictor of health outcomes. You can read all about BMI and WC in Chapter 3. So if you haven't already done so, turn back to Chapter 3 and read, read, read, but come right back here when you're done.

- **If you need to lose weight, do so gradually.** Forget the "lose 13.5 kg (30 pounds) in 30 days" jazz. Because it's unrealistic for a person to put on 15 kg (30+ pounds) in two months, it is just as unrealistic to try and take it off in the same time frame. In reality, it goes something like this: Someone will wake up one day and say to themselves, "Gosh, I used to weight 15 kg less about five years ago." Just as weight gain is gradual, effective and sustained weight loss occurs when it is done slowly as well. Depending on how much weight you have to lose, your long-term goal needs to be losing about 10 percent of your total weight over a six-month period. Losing 0.2 to 0.9 kg (½ to 2 pounds) a week is a safe and practical way of doing so.

- **Encourage healthy weight in children.** One unhappy fact is that overweight kids tend to become overweight adults. Helping children stick to a healthy weight pays large dividends down the road of life.

- **Check with your doctor before starting a weight-loss diet.** This advice is most important for women who are pregnant or nursing, for children, and for anyone — young or old — who has a chronic disease and/or is on medication.

Being physically active

When you take in more calories from food than you use up running your body systems (heart, lungs, brain, and so forth) and doing a day's physical work, you end up storing the extra calories as body fat. In other words, you gain weight. The reverse also is true. When you spend more energy in a day than you take in as food, you pull the extra energy you need out of stored fat and you lose weight.

I'm no mathematician, but I can reduce this principle to two simple equations in which E stands for *energy* (in calories), > stands for *greater than*, < stands for *less than*, and W stands for the change in *weight:*

$$\text{If } E_{in} > E_{out} : E_{total} = +W$$
$$\text{If } E_{in} < E_{out} : E_{total} = -W$$

It ain't Einstein's theory of relativity, but you get the picture!

For real-life examples of how the *energy-in, energy-out theory* works, stick your bookmark in this page and go to Table 3-1 in Chapter 3 to find out how to calculate the number of calories a person can consume each day without pushing up the poundage. Even being mildly active increases the number of calories you can wolf down without gaining weight. The more strenuous the activity, the more plentiful the calorie allowance. Suppose that you're a 25-year-old man who weighs 64 kg (140 pounds). The formula in Table 3-1 shows that you require 1,658 calories a day to run your body systems. Clearly, you need more calories for doing your daily physical work, simply moving around, or exercising.

The 2007 Food Guide recommends specific amounts of *added activity* — anything that's above and beyond the basic activities of daily living — in order to help maintain a healthy weight and to reduce the risk of chronic disease. The goal is to build in activity above and beyond what you do for day-to-day living. How much should you do?

- ✔ Most people will benefit from 30 minutes of moderate physical activity — such as a brisk walk — per day.

- ✔ To prevent gradual weight gain, you'll need 30 to 60 minutes of moderate-to-vigorous-intensity activity several days a week.

- ✔ To take weight off, you'll really need to get at least 60 minutes of daily moderate physical activity.

- ✔ Children and youth should get at least 90 minutes a day to help prevent weight gain.

- ✔ To reach true physical fitness, your regimen should include cardiovascular conditioning (anything that breaks a sweat like biking, jogging, spinning, hockey, basketball, fast swimming, and so on), stretching exercises (yoga, Pilates, tai chi, or classic stretching) for flexibility, and resistance exercises (weight/strength training) or calisthenics for muscle strength and endurance.

Not everybody can — or should — run right out and start chopping down trees or throwing touchdown passes to control his or her weight. In fact, if you have gained a lot of weight recently, have been overweight for a long time, haven't exercised in a while, or have a chronic medical condition, you need to check with your doctor before starting any new regimen. (*Caution:* Avoid any gym that puts you right on the floor without first checking your vital signs — heartbeat, respiration, and so forth.)

Other reasons to exercise

Weight control is a good reason to step up your exercise level, but it isn't the only one. Here are four more:

✔ **Exercise increases muscles.** When you exercise regularly, you end up with more muscle tissue than the average bear. Because muscle tissue weighs more than fat tissue, athletes (even weekend warrior types) may end up weighing more than they did before they started exercising to lose weight. But a higher muscle-to-fat ratio is healthier and more important in the long run than actual weight in pounds. Exercise that changes your body's ratio of muscle to fat gives you a leg up in the longevity race. Muscle drives your metabolic rate; therefore, having more muscle means you burn more calories both during any activity you do and when you're sedentary (that means when you're sitting on the couch watching TV). Having more muscle helps you maintain your functionality later in life, which is another way of saying your independence and ability to get around and do the things that you enjoy. As well, active muscles use insulin more efficiently, thereby helping your body use glucose better, and exercise helps keep your cholesterol in check. What more can we say?

✔ **Exercise reduces the amount of fat stored in your body.** People who are fat around the middle as opposed to the hips (in other words an apple shape versus a pear shape) are at higher risk of weight-related illness. Exercise helps reduce abdominal fat and thus lowers your risk of weight-related diseases. Use a tape measure to identify your own body type by comparing your waistline to your hips (around the buttocks). If your waist (abdomen) is bigger, you're an apple. If your hips are bigger, you're a pear.

✔ **Exercise strengthens your bones.** *Osteoporosis* (thinning of the bones that leads to repeated fractures) doesn't happen only to little old ladies. True, on average, a woman's bones thin faster and more dramatically than a man's, but after the mid-30s, everybody — male and female — begins losing bone density. Exercise can slow, halt, or in some cases even reverse the process. In addition, being physically active develops muscles that help support bones. Stronger bones equal less risk of fracture, which, in turn, equals less risk of potentially fatal complications.

✔ **Exercise increases brain power.** You know that aerobic exercise increases the flow of oxygen to the heart, but did you also know that it increases the flow of oxygen to the brain?

When a rush job (or a rush of anxiety) keeps you up all night, a judicious exercise break can keep you bright until dawn. According to Massachusetts Institute of Technology nutrition research scientist Judith J. Wurtman, Ph.D., when you're awake and working during hours that you'd normally be asleep, your internal body rhythms tell your body to cool down, even though your brain is racing along. Simply standing up and stretching, walking around the room, or doing a couple of sit-ups every hour or so speeds up your metabolism, warms up your muscles, increases your ability to stay awake, and, in Dr. Wurtman's words, "prolongs your ability to work smart into the night." Eureka!

The activity doesn't have to be done all at once. You can do it in smaller chunks: ten-minute bits for adults and five-minute bits for children and youth. For tips and guidelines on how to safely include physical activity into your healthy lifestyle, refer to Health Canada's Physical Activity Guide, which can be found at www.phac-aspc.gc.ca/pau-uap/paguide/index.html.

Making Smart Food Choices

Okay. So you have your weight goals firmly in mind, and three, or four, or even seven times a week you manage to *Hup! Two, three, four* at home, or in the gym, or on a walk around the block. The goal of the Food Guide is to put together a diet that supports your new healthy lifestyle. The following will help make your food group choices the best they can be.

Picking the perfect plants

Starting with the Food Guide in 1977, there was more of a push for a diet based on plant foods. Why? Because plant foods

- ✔ Add plenty of bulk and vitamins but few calories to your diet, so you feel full, which may help you to maintain a healthy weight

- ✔ Are usually low in fat and have no cholesterol, which means they reduce your risk of heart disease

- ✔ Are high in fibre, which reduces the risk of heart disease; prevents constipation; reduces the risk of developing hemorrhoids (or at least makes existing ones less painful); moves food quickly through your digestive tract, thus reducing the risk of diverticular disease (inflammation caused by food getting caught in the folds of your intestines and causing tiny out-pouchings of the weakened gut wall); and may lower your risk of some gastrointestinal cancers

- ✔ Are rich in beneficial substances called phytochemicals, which may reduce your risk of heart disease and some forms of cancer (for more, see Chapter 12)

For all these reasons, the Food Guide recommends that fruits and vegetables constitute the largest portion of your diet. Here are some tips for getting the most from your veggies:

✔ **Eat at least one serving of a dark green vegetable and a serving of a dark orange vegetable daily.** Dark green vegetables, like kale, spinach, broccoli, asparagus, arugula, mustard greens, Brussels sprouts, and collards are excellent sources of folate, an important nutrient in the prevention of neural tube defects. And it's believed that folate plays an important role in cardiovascular health (prevention of heart and blood vessel disease, such as heart disease and stroke). Dark green vegetables are also a rich source of lutein, an antioxidant with emerging health-promoting benefits (see Chapter 28 for more details). Orange vegetables such as carrots, sweet potatoes, pumpkin, and winter squash are excellent sources of beta-carotene, something your body can convert to vitamin A.

Some orange-coloured fruits can substitute for vegetables because they also contain an appreciable amount of beta-carotene. These include apricots, papaya, cantaloupe, and mango.

✔ **Avoid vegetables and fruit prepared with added fat, salt, or sugar.** Steamed, raw (wash well), baked, or stir-fried vegetables are much healthier than the deep-fried alternatives.

✔ **Skip the fruit juice; eat the fruit!** Juices can be high in calories and sodium, and low in fibre.

When it comes to choosing your grain products, the Food Guide has a couple of handy tips, too:

✔ **Ensure that at least half of the grain products you eat are whole grain.** This is to help you meet your requirements for magnesium and fibre. Whole grains such as brown rice, oats, quinoa, millet, and bulgar make for cool new additions to your diet. Eating whole-grain products shouldn't be too hard, either; grocery stores are stuffed with whole-grain breads, bagels, pasta, and cereals.

✔ **Avoid high-fat, -sugar, or -salt grain products.** If you want to add spreads such as butter, margarine, or mayonnaise, use small amounts and try to use a low-fat alternative.

To protect your bones, the Food Guide advises washing down your plants with 500 millilitres of lower-fat dairy or fortified alternatives for both their calcium and vitamin D content. For more on vitamin D, mark this page and flip to Chapter 10, for calcium, Chapter 11.

Figuring out fats

As you can plainly see in Chapter 7, dietary fat (the fat in foods) is an essential nutrient. Infants need these fats to thrive, and the same cholesterol that may increase an adult's risk of heart disease is vital to an embryo's healthy development, triggering the action of genes that tell cells to become specialized body structures — arms, legs, backbone, and so forth.

Grown-ups, however, need to control fat intake so they can control calories and reduce the risk of obesity-related illnesses, such as heart disease, diabetes, and some forms of cancer.

Overall, the Food Guide suggests that your adult diet derive no more than 35 percent of its calories from fat and no more than 10 percent of calories from saturated fat, and that it deliver 300 milligrams or less of cholesterol a day. Remember, it's the quality of the fat that's important. For this reason, the new Food Guide recommends getting the equivalent of 30–45 ml (2–3 tablespoons) of unsaturated fat each day. To reach these goals

- Most of your fat calories should come from foods such as fish, nuts, seeds, and vegetable oils that are rich in polyunsaturated and monounsaturated fats. Limit butter, hard (cheap) margarines, lard, and shortening.
- Dairy products, such as milk, yogourt, and cheese, should be low- or no-fat (skim).
- Poultry and meat should be lean (yes, trim off that visible fat).
- With trans fats, less is always better.

To reduce the fat you eat, try low-fat cooking methods such as braising, broiling, poaching, baking, or roasting. These methods require little to no added fat.

Counting on carbs

Carbs are your fastest source of energy, but the trick here is to get your carbs complex (we explain complex versus simple carbs in Chapter 8), which means from plant foods: fruits and vegetables and whole grains. The companion stratagem is to buy and prepare foods with little added sugar.

Puzzling out proteins

When people think protein, they often think of meat: beef, pork, lamb, and chicken.

But the Food Guide category is actually "Meat and Alternatives." The Guide recommends that you eat alternatives such as beans, lentils, and tofu (sometimes called *legumes*) often. Increasing the variety of protein sources is a good idea on two fronts. One, plant sources of protein such as nuts and seeds are chock full of heart-healthy fats and the antioxidant vitamin E. Second, foods such as kidney beans, lentils, and other legumes also provide complex carbohydrates and fibre in addition to an abundance of protein. By having both animal- and plant-based proteins, you get the best of both worlds.

The Guide also advises that you try to eat at least two servings of fish each week — especially cold-water fatty fish, like sardines, herring, mackerel, salmon, and trout. These fish offer healthy omega-3 fats that have been shown to reduce the risk of cardiovascular disease (see Chapter 7 for more).

Limiting salt, balancing potassium

Sodium is a mineral that helps regulate your body's fluid balance, the flow of water into and out of every cell (this process is described in Chapter 13). This balance keeps just enough water inside the cell so that it can perform its daily jobs, but not so much that the cell — packed to bursting — explodes.

Most people have no problems with sodium. They eat a lot one day, a little less the next, and their bodies adjust. Others, however, don't react so evenly. For them, a high-sodium diet appears to increase the risk of high blood pressure. When you already have high blood pressure, you can tell fairly quickly whether lowering the amount of salt in your diet lowers your blood pressure. But no test is available at this point for telling whether someone who doesn't have high blood pressure will develop it by consuming a diet that's high in sodium.

Because limiting sodium intake to a moderate level won't harm anyone, the guidelines advocate avoiding excessive amounts of salt. Doing so helps reduce blood pressure levels for people who are salt sensitive.

What's moderate use? According to Health Canada, you should consume less than 2,400 milligrams (approximately 1 teaspoon) of sodium per day. The easiest way to reach that goal is to choose and prepare foods with very little added salt. At the same time, it pays to consume potassium-rich foods, such as (what else?) fruits, vegetables, whole grains, and even low-fat dairy, because an adequate supply of potassium helps control blood pressure.

By the way, moderating your salt intake has another, unadvertised benefit. It may lower your weight a bit. Why? Because sodium is *hydrophilic* (hydro = water; philic = loving). Sodium attracts and holds water. When you eat less salt, you retain less water, you're less bloated, and you feel thinner.

Don't reduce salt intake drastically without first checking with your doctor. Remember, sodium is an essential nutrient, and Health Canada advocates moderate use, not no use at all.

Where's the sodium?

The foods with the highest amounts of naturally occurring sodium are natural cheeses, sea fish, and shellfish. Some foods are low in sodium but pick up plenty of salt when they're processed. For example, 250 mL (one cup) of cooked fresh green peas has about 2 milligrams (mg) of sodium, but 250 mL (one cup) of canned peas may have 493 mg of sodium. To be fair, many but not all canned and processed vegetables are now available in low-sodium versions, too. The difference is notable: 250 mL (one cup) of low-sodium vegetable cocktail has 140 mg of sodium, more than 500 mg less than the regular version.

You also get added sodium in the salt on snack foods, such as potato chips and peanuts, not to mention the salt you add yourself from the shaker that's on virtually every Canadian table. Not all the sodium you swallow is sodium chloride. Sodium compounds also are used as preservatives, thickeners, and buffers (chemicals that smooth down acidity).

Table 16-1 lists several different kinds of sodium compounds in food. Table 16-2 lists sodium compounds in over-the-counter (OTC) drug products.

Table 16-1	Sodium Compounds in Food
Sodium Compound	*Function*
Monosodium glutamate (MSG)	Flavour enhancer
Sodium benzoate	Keeps food from spoiling
Sodium caseinate	Thickens foods and provides protein
Sodium chloride (table salt)	Flavouring agent
Sodium citrate	Holds carbonation in soft drinks
Sodium hydroxide	Makes peeling the skin off tomatoes and fruits before canning easier
Sodium nitrate/nitrite	Keeps food (cured meats) from spoiling — and gives these foods their distinctive red colour
Sodium phosphates	Mineral supplement
Sodium saccharin	No-calorie sweetener

"The Sodium Content of Your Food," Home and Garden Bulletin, No. 233 (Washington, D.C.: U.S. Department of Agriculture, August 1980); Ruth Winter, A Consumer's Dictionary of Food Additives (New York: Crown, 1978)

Table 16-2	Sodium Compounds in OTC Drug Products
Sodium Compound	*Function*
Sodium ascorbate	A form of vitamin C used in nutritional supplements
Sodium bicarbonate	Antacid
Sodium biphosphate	Laxative
Sodium citrate	Antacid
Sodium fluoride	Mineral used in nutritional supplements and as a decay preventive in tooth powders
Sodium phosphates	Laxative
Sodium saccharin	Sweetener
Sodium salicylate	Analgesic (similar to aspirin)

Handbook of Nonprescription Drugs, 9th ed. (Washington, D.C.: American Pharmaceutical Association, 1990); Physicians' Desk Reference, 48th ed. (Montvale, N.J.: Medical Economics Data Production, 1994)

Moderating alcohol consumption

Telling someone to drink alcohol beverages in moderation sounds like Mom-and-apple-pie advice, right? Right. But — and you've heard this song before — what's *moderation,* anyway? Laypersons (you and me, babe) may define moderate in terms of the effects that alcohol has on the ability to perform simple tasks, such as speaking and thinking clearly or moving in a straight line. Obviously, if the amount of alcohol you drink makes you slur your words or bump into the furniture, that isn't moderation.

The Nutrition Recommendations of the Scientific Review Committee define moderate drinking as no more than 5 percent of total energy from alcohol or two drinks per day (whichever is less) and no alcohol during pregnancy. This works out to roughly one drink per day for women and two for men. Aha, you say, but what's one drink? Good question. Here's the answer, from Health Canada:

- 354 mL (12 ounces) of regular beer (150 calories)

- 142 mL (5 ounces) of wine (100 calories)

- 42 mL (1 ½ ounces) of 80-proof (40 percent alcohol) distilled spirits (100 calories)

Some people shouldn't drink at all, not even in moderation, including people who suffer from alcoholism, people who plan to drive a car or take part in other activities that require attention to detail or real physical skill, and people using medication (prescription drugs or over-the-counter products). For information about who should and should not drink, as well as a list of drugs that interact with alcohol, take a look at Chapter 9.

Clearly, water is the best beverage going, so drink it regularly. You won't consume any calories drinking water, and you'll keep yourself hydrated on hot days and when you're active.

Advice for Different Ages and Stages

Although most of the guidelines in the Food Guide apply to everyone, Health Canada does single out three groups for particular attention. Kids, women of child-bearing age, and adults over the age of 50 all have unique dietary needs that the Food Guide addresses.

Children

Getting kids to eat well — or at all — can be a challenge. They have smaller appetites, and caregivers need to find a balance between that fact and ensuring children get enough to eat, both in terms of calories (energy) and nutrients like vitamins and minerals.

Many caregivers often worry that children won't get enough to eat, but children are actually very good at responding to those cues and signals from their body that tell them when they're hungry and when they're full. Because of their size, preschoolers and young children will tend to graze throughout the day, eating several smaller meals or three meals plus snacks. The amount a child will eat varies from day to day and even within a day based on their activity levels and appetite. If a child eats less at one meal, left on their own they will often naturally eat a little more to make up the difference. Over time, the fluctuations with intake often balance out on their own, and children end up getting enough nutrients.

Don't worry about getting a child to eat a full serving in a single seating; a serving size can be spread out over the day. For example, one serving of milk or alternative can be divided over two meals: 125 mL (½ cup) at breakfast and the other 125 mL (½ cup) with a morning snack or lunch.

For children between the ages of 2 and 5, don't restrict dietary fat or foods higher in fat. Children need those extra calories for growth. Foods such as peanut butter, milk, and cheese or oils such as olive and canola can be an important source of fat calories for growing preschoolers.

Offer a variety of foods from all four food groups and be a good role model to healthy eating — children will pick up healthy habits from their parents and guardians.

Women of child-bearing age

Because of its role in preventing neural tube defects, folic acid is important to women who are either pregnant or could become pregnant, as well as women who are breast-feeding; these women need a multivitamin/mineral with 400 ug (0.4 mg) of folic acid every day. Because many pregnancies are not planned to the month, it is recommended that every woman who could become pregnant should take it. This will ensure that women are meeting the recommendation to get adequate folic acid at least three months prior to conception.

Preconception isn't the only time the need for folic acid is increased — requirements are 600 ug (0.6 mg) per day for women who are pregnant and 500 ug (0.5 mg) during breast-feeding. It's difficult to consistently meet these requirements through food alone, so the Food Guide advises that pregnant women continue to take a multivitamin with folic acid every day.

During pregnancy, a woman's requirements for iron increase as well. This is because the mother's own iron stores in her bone marrow, liver, and spleen will be tapped into to meet the increasing demand. During pregnancy, a woman's total blood volume will increase by 50 percent, thereby increasing the need for iron to make hemoglobin (see Chapter 11 for more). As well, the placenta and fetus need more iron. Consequently, the Food Guide recommends that pregnant women eat plenty of iron-rich foods such as red meats, poultry, fish, and pork, fortified foods like breads and cereals, legumes like lentils and chickpeas, and nuts and seeds. However, getting enough iron from food alone is difficult, if not impossible. Therefore women need to be sure that their multivitamin/mineral contains iron. A health-care professional such as a dietitian, pharmacist, or physician can help you find the multivitamin/mineral that's right for you.

The guide also recommends that pregnant women increase their calorie intake during the last two trimesters. Despite the old saying, "I'm eating for two," the increase in energy requirements is modest: About an extra 350 calories per day in the second trimester and 450 extra calories per day in the third trimester are all that's needed. What does this look like in real food? A bowl with about 165 mL (⅔ cup) of granola and milk or fortified soy beverage, or a sandwich with 30 mL (2 tablespoons) of peanut butter. As a general rule, aim to include two to three extra Food Guide servings each day.

Men and women over 50

The need for vitamin D increases as we get older. Vitamin D is produced when the skin is exposed to UVB radiation from the sun. After the age of 50, however, our skin's capacity to make vitamin D decreases. As well, in Canada, we don't get enough UVB from the sun from October to the end of March to produce vitamin D naturally (this period is even longer in more northern latitudes).

Although some foods such as milk, oily fish like salmon and sardines, and margarine are sources of vitamin D, it's improbable that people over the age of 50 can meet their increased requirement through food alone. Consequently, the Food Guide advises everyone over the age of 50 to take a daily vitamin D supplement of 10 mcg or 400 IU. Most multivitamin/mineral supplements have this much — be sure to check the label.

Okay, Now Relax

Life is not a test. You don't lose points for failing to follow Canada's Food Guide every single day of your life. Nobody's perfect, and the recommendations are meant to be broken — once in a while.

For example, ideally you should hold your daily intake of dietary fat to 20 to 35 percent of your total calories. But you can bet that you'll exceed that amount this Saturday when you stroll by the buffet at your best friend's wedding and see Camembert cheese (70 percent of the calories from fat), sirloin steak (56 percent of the calories from fat), salad with Thousand Island dressing (90 percent of the calories from fat), and whipped cream cake (who can count that high?).

Is this a crisis? Should you stay home? Must you keep your mouth shut tight all night? Are you kidding? Here's the Real Rule: Let the good times roll every once in a while. After the party's over, compensate.

For the rest of the week, go back to your exercise regimen and back to your healthful menu emphasizing lots of the nutritious, delicious, lower-fat foods with plenty of vegetables, fruits, and whole grains that should make up most of your regular diet.

In the end, you're likely to have averaged out to a desirable amount with no fuss and no muss and be right in line with the three main precepts of the Food Guide: balance, moderation, and variety. Remember to take time to enjoy the foods you eat, and remember that eating really is one of life's simplest pleasures. Amen to that.

Chapter 17

Making Wise Food Choices

*T*his chapter features the new Canada's Food Guide and the Nutrition Facts labels — and it tells you how to use them to create a healthful diet.

But consider yourself warned: The following pages are packed with numbers and details, maybe more than you ever wanted to know about your daily bread — and everything else on your plate. Don't let the many, many facts and stats turn you off. The information you find here really is useful for making good food choices. Take a deep breath, keep your highlighter handy, and jump right in.

Playing with Blocks: Basics of the Food Guides

Food guides are building blocks for grown-ups. Instead of letters in the alphabet, these blocks represent food groups that you can put together to create a picture of a healthful diet.

The essential message of all good guides to healthful food choices is that no one food is either good or bad — how much and how often you eat a food is what counts. With that in mind, a food guide delivers three important messages:

- ✔ **Variety:** That the food guide contains several blocks tells you no single food gives you all the nutrients you need.

- ✔ **Moderation:** Having some blocks smaller than others tells you that although every food is valuable, some — such as fats and sweets — are best consumed in small amounts.

- ✔ **Balance:** Blocks of different sizes show that a healthful diet is balanced: the right amount from each food group.

Clearly, the virtue of a food guide is that if you use it you can eat practically everything you like — as long as you follow the recommendations on how much and how frequently (or infrequently).

Canada's food guides from the past

Canada's first food guide, *Canada's Official Food Rules,* was created in 1942 by the Nutrition Division of the federal Department of Pensions and National Health with the help of the Canadian Council on Nutrition. Just before the Food Rules were introduced, the Council developed the first set of Dietary Standards for Canada, which they described as "the amounts of essential nutrients considered adequate to meet the needs of practically all healthy persons." The *Food Rules* were a practical application of the Dietary Standards, and set the model of subsequent food guides: putting the theory of nutritional science into amounts of everyday foods.

Since then, food rules and food guides have been re-created several times over the decades: *Canada's Official Food Rules* (1942) became *Canada's Food Rules* (1944, 1949), then *Canada's Food Guide* (1961, 1977, 1982). *Canada's Food Guide to Healthy Eating* (1992) is now *Eating Well with Canada's Food Guide* (2007). Although the name and look of the guidelines have changed, its core purpose has always been to help Canadians make healthy food choices. The goal of these choices has evolved. The first Food Rules aimed to prevent nutrient deficiencies; more recent guides have aimed to reduce diet-related chronic diseases.

Rainbow revolution: Canada's Food Guide to Healthy Eating

The 1992 version of the guide, *Canada's Food Guide to Healthy Eating,* introduced a new presentation. It did away with the wheel-like sun graphic used in the 1977 and 1982 versions (some of you may remember those guides). The 1992 version established the rainbow concept, made up of four bands. The two outer bands are the largest, and should make up the bulk of your diet. They represent plant foods: grain products, vegetables, and fruits. The two inner bands represent foods derived from animals — milk products, meats, and alternatives. You require these in smaller amounts to round out your diet.

The 1992 guide didn't just abandon circles in favour of rainbows; it presented a whole new approach. In the past, the public was advised to eat the minimum amount of foods from the food groups, and to eat more if you needed more energy. The 1992 version incorporated a wider range of servings from each food group, because different people have different energy needs. The lower end is for people who consume about 1,600 to 1,800 calories a day, and the upper end is for people whose daily dietary intake nears 2,500 calories. The 1992 revision of the food guide was praised for being flexible and simple. It had good visual appeal, and it created widespread awareness — Canadians knew about the new guide.

However, *Canada's Food Guide to Healthy Eating* had some challenges. People were confused about serving sizes and the range of servings. For instance, people would say, "I just can't eat that much bread." They thought they were supposed to eat 12 servings, even though that portion would be more appropriate for a growing teenage boy who was active in high school sports. A sedentary office worker might only need 5 or 6 servings of grain products per day. The guide's images were outdated and didn't reflect the diversity of multicultural foods. So, in 2004, Health Canada set out to revise the guide; they would address critics' concerns but build on the guide's strengths.

The Brand New Canada's Food Guide

Early in 2007, Health Canada unveiled the new food guide, titled *Eating Well with Canada's Food Guide,* along with a new Web site (which you can visit at `www.healthcanada.gc.ca/foodguide`). The new guide made some changes to the rainbow presentation of the previous guide, and also clarified the previous version's serving recommendations, which confused some people.

Revising the rainbow

In the new food rainbow, the largest band is no longer grain products — that honour goes to vegetables and fruits, underscoring a shift towards making these foods the foundation of the diet. Grain products, while nutritious, are a concentrated source of starch and, therefore, calories. Fruits and vegetables are bulkier and take longer to eat (time how long it takes to eat four medium apples versus two cups of cooked macaroni, and you'll see what we're talking about), so it's harder to overeat carbohydrate calories from them.

The milk group has also been changed, to "Milk and Alternatives." This step recognizes fortified soy beverages as an adequate alternative to fluid milk. Fortified soy offers an equal amount of high-quality protein and has a comparable micronutrient profile. Figure 17-1 shows the new food rainbow.

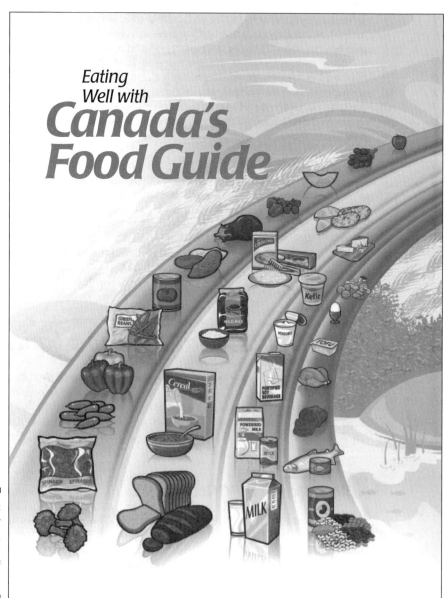

Figure 17-1:
The four food groups, presented in order of importance.

Recognizing the health-promoting benefits of unsaturated fats, the new Food Guide also recommends the addition of a daily source of both polyunsaturated and monounsaturated fats. These fats are found in oils used for cooking (canola, olive, peanut, and soybean), salad dressings, non-hydrogenated margarines, and mayonnaise. Fat isn't a four-letter word!

It's quality that counts — saturated and trans fats should still be limited.

Suggesting servings

The recommended number of servings in the Food Guide represents the average amounts people should try to eat each day. The new Food Guide improves upon the 1992 version by helping to fine-tune the number of servings a person requires, on average, based on sex and age.

Table 17-1 outlines the new Food Guide's recommended servings based on age and sex.

Table 17-1	Recommended Number of Food Guide Servings per Day								
	Children			**Teens**		**Adults**			
Age in Years	**2–3**	**4–8**	**9–13**	**14–18**		**19–50**		**51+**	
Sex	Girls and Boys			Females	Males	Females	Males	Females	Males
Vegetables and Fruit	4	5	6	7	8	7–8	8–10	7	7
Grain Products	3	4	6	6	7	6–7	8	6	7
Milk and Alternatives	2	2	3–4	3–4	3–4	2	2	3	3
Meat and Alternatives	1	1	1–2	2	3	2	3	2	3

Eating Well with Canada's Food Guide (Health Canada, 2007)

How much is a serving? Not to worry. That's spelled out in Figure 17-2.

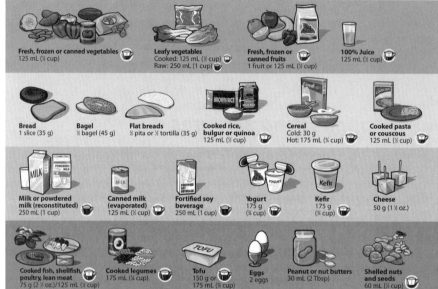

What is One Food Guide Serving?
Look at the examples below.

Figure 17-2:
Standard serving sizes from the new Canada's Food Guide.

The new Food Guide also recommends that women who are pregnant, breast-feeding, or of childbearing age include a daily multivitamin with folic acid and iron. Women older than 50 should take a daily vitamin D supplement providing 10 mcg or 400 IU.

Sizing up the servings

Many people who look at the Food Guide believe that the number of suggested servings is just too much. At first glance, the number may seem like a lot, but when you consider the size of a standard serving, you can see it's a reasonable amount of food — just what your body needs.

Serving sizes are concepts, so the real question is: What does it mean in real food? According to the guide, a 16-year-old female should be eating

- Seven servings of vegetables and fruit
- Six servings of grain products
- Three to four servings of milk and alternatives
- Two servings of meat and alternatives

Table 17-2 provides a sample one-day menu and demonstrates just how those recommendations can be put on the teenager's plate.

Table 17-2:	Sample One-Day Menu for a 16-Year-Old Female				
	Number of Food Guide Servings				
	Vegetables and Fruit	**Grain Products**	**Milk and alternatives**	**Meat and alternatives**	**Added Oils and Fats**
Breakfast					
1 whole-wheat tortilla with 15 mL (1 tbsp) peanut butter		2		½	
1 banana	1				
250 mL (1 cup) skim milk			1		
Snack					
1 apple	1				
Lunch					
Tuna salad sandwich (30 g/1 ounce tuna and mayonnaise) on 2 slices of rye bread	2	½		X	
125 mL (½ cup) orange juice	1				
Baby carrots with dip	1				X

(continued)

Table 17-2: *(continued)*

	Number of Food Guide Servings				
	Vegetables and Fruit	Grain Products	Milk and alternatives	Meat and alternatives	Added Oils and Fats
Dinner					
500 mL (2 cups) spinach salad with 125 mL (½ cup) strawberries and kiwi, 60 mL (¼ cup) almonds, and salad dressing	3			1	X
1 whole-wheat bagel with 50 g (1 ½ ounce) cheese		2	1		
250 mL (1 cup) fortified soy beverage			1		
Total Food Guide Servings for the Day	7	6	3	2	3

Eating Well with Canada's Food Guide: A Resource for Educators and Communicators (Health Canada, 2007)

Building your own Food Guide

Okay, warm up your typing finger(s) and run this one over your keyboard: www.hc-sc.gc.ca/fn-an/food-guide-aliment/myguide-monguide/index_e.html. This takes you to a page of the Food & Nutrition section of Health Canada's Web site, and to a new feature called "My Food Guide."

Click on "Start building my Food Guide" to bring up an interactive tool into which you type your sex and age. From there you can select examples from each food group and choose activities that appeal to you. You'll get a personalized guide that reflects your very own body, tastes, and lifestyle.

Eating Well with Canada's Food Guide: First Nations, Inuit, and Metis

For the first time, we have a Food Guide that includes traditional foods for First Nations, Inuit, and Metis people. This guide aims to incorporate both store-bought and traditional foods, such as bannock (a type of quick bread) and wild game (moose and Artic char). The goal of this unique Food Guide is to show how and where traditional foods fit into a model of healthy eating. In the past, the Food Guide has been modified to meet regional differences in food availability. This is the first nationally tailored Food Guide. To download a copy of the guide, go to www.hc-sc.gc.ca/fn-an/pubs/fnim-pnim/index_e.html.

Understanding the Nutrition Facts Label

Once upon a time, the only reliable consumer information on a food label was the name of the food inside the box. Fortunately, today consumers have a handy tool — nutrition labelling — at their disposal to help them make more informed choices. With 70 percent of Canadians reporting that they use them, nutrition labels have turned out to be an important form of consumer communication. The Food and Drugs Act regulates the labelling of food products in Canada. On January 1, 2003, new labelling guidelines included:

✔ A mini-nutrition guide that shows the food's nutrient content and evaluates its place in a balanced diet

✔ Accurate ingredient listings, with all ingredients listed in order of their weight in the food; for example, the most prominent ingredient in a loaf of bread would be flour

✔ Scientifically reliable, diet-related health claims about the relationship between specific foods and specific chronic health conditions, such as heart disease and cancer

The Nutrition Facts label is required by law for most processed and packaged foods: everything from canned soup to fresh, pasteurized orange juice. For food sold in smaller packages, the Nutrition Facts label may appear on the inside of the package or on an insert. Really small packages — a pack of gum, for example — can omit the nutrition label but must carry a telephone number or address so that an inquisitive consumer (you) can call or write for the information.

The exemptions to the Nutrition Facts label include:

✔ Alcohol beverages

✔ Fresh fruit and vegetables

✔ Raw single-ingredient meat (for example, a steak) and poultry, except for ground meat and ground poultry

✔ Raw single-ingredient fish and seafood

✔ Food containing insignificant amounts of the 13 core nutrients required in the Nutrition Facts table

✔ Food products sold only in the retail establishment where they are prepared or processed

✔ Individual servings of food intended for immediate consumption

Any foods that have been exempted from requiring a Nutrition Facts label will lose their exemption status if their label or advertisements carry a nutrition or health claim (more details later in this chapter), if any vitamins or minerals are added to the food, or if sweeteners are added.

Getting the facts

The star of the Nutrition Facts label is the Nutrition Facts table on the back (or side) of the package. This panel features three important elements: serving size, amounts of nutrients per serving, and Percent Daily Value. (See Figure 17-3.)

Figure 17-3: A typical Nutrition Facts table.

Nutrition Facts
Per 125 mL (87 g)

Amount	% Daily Value*
Calories 80	
Fat 0.5 g	1 %
Saturated Fat 0 g	0 %
+Trans Fat 0 g	
Cholesterol 0 mg	
Sodium 0 mg	0 %
Carbohydrate 18 g	6 %
Fibre 2 g	8 %
Sugars 2 g	
Protein 3 g	

Vitamin A	2 %	Vitamin C	10 %
Calcium	0 %	Iron	0 %

* Percent Daily Values are based on a 2,000 calorie diet. Your daily values may be higher or lower depending on your caloric needs.

Serving size: This varies from package to package. Serving sizes don't always reflect the typical amount that an adult may eat. In some cases, the serving size may be a very small amount.

Calories: The calories contained in a single serving.

% daily values: The percentage of nutrients that one serving contributes to a 2,000-calorie diet. Parents or children may need more or less than 2,000 calories per day.

Nutrient amounts: The nutritional values of the most important, but not all, vitamins and other nutrients in the product.

Serving size

No need to stretch your brain trying to translate gram-servings or ounce-servings into real servings. This label does it for you, listing the servings in comprehensible kitchen terms such as 250 mL (1 cup), or one waffle, or two pieces, or 5 mL (1 tsp). It also tells you how many servings are in the package.

The serving size is exactly the same for all products in a category. In other words, the Nutrition Facts table enables you to compare at a glance the nutrient content for two different brands of yogourt, Cheddar cheese, canned string beans, soft drinks, and so on.

When checking the labels, you may think the suggested serving sizes seem small (especially with so-called low-fat items). Think of these serving sizes as useful guides.

Here's a word to the wise about serving sizes when it comes to prepared foods. The serving sizes in Canada's Food Guide have been standardized. One Food Guide slice of bread is 30 g, but a slice from a food manufacturer can be as much as 45–50 g. This might not seem like much, but five slices of the bigger bread is like eating seven slices of the standardized bread, and a few extra calories here and there can be a recipe for weight gain. Remember that what you buy in the store isn't necessarily what is served up in the Food Guide. Learn to be a savvy label reader.

Amount per serving

The Nutrition Facts table tells you the amount (per serving) for 13 core nutrients:

- ✔ Calories
- ✔ Total fat (in grams and percent Daily Value)
- ✔ Saturated fat and trans fat (in grams and percent Daily Value)
- ✔ Cholesterol (in milligrams)
- ✔ Sodium (in milligrams and percent Daily Value)
- ✔ Total carbohydrate (in grams and percent Daily Value)
- ✔ Dietary fibre (in grams and percent Daily Value)
- ✔ Sugars (in grams — total sugars, the ones occurring naturally in the food *and* the ones added during preparation)
- ✔ Protein (in grams)
- ✔ Vitamin A (percent Daily Value)
- ✔ Calcium (percent Daily Value)
- ✔ Vitamin C (percent Daily Value)
- ✔ Iron (percent Daily Value)

Percent Daily Value

The daily values that were developed for labelling purposes are recommendations for a healthy diet. They refer to the recommended daily intakes for vitamins and minerals as well as reference standards for other nutrients. The Percent Daily Value enables you to judge whether a specific food is high, medium, or low in fat, cholesterol, sodium, carbohydrates, dietary fibre, sugar, protein, vitamin A, vitamin C, calcium, and iron. Some nutrients, like sodium, have a fixed Daily Value, because the amount applies to everyone, regardless of sex, age, and energy intake.

The Percent Daily Value for vitamins and minerals is based on a set of recommendations called the Recommended Nutrient Intakes (RNI), which are similar (but not identical) to the Recommended Dietary Allowances (RDAs) for vitamins and minerals discussed in Chapters 10 and 11.

RNIs are based on allowances set in 1983. Some RNIs now may not apply to all groups of people. For example, the Daily Value for calcium is 1,000 milligrams, but many studies — and two National Institutes of Health Conferences — suggest that postmenopausal women who are not using hormone replacement therapy need to consume 1,500 milligrams of calcium a day to reduce their risk of osteoporosis.

The Percent Daily Values for fats, sodium, and carbohydrates are based on *Reference Standard Values (RSV)*. RSVs are standards for nutrients, such as fat and fibre, known to raise or lower the risk of certain health conditions, such as heart disease and cancer. For example, *Canada's Guidelines for Healthy Eating from 1990* says that no more than 30 percent of your daily calories should come from fat. That means a 2,000-calorie-per-day diet shouldn't have any more than 600 calories from fat. To translate fat calories to grams of fat (the units used in the RSVs), divide the number of calories from fat (600) by 9 (the number of calories in one gram of fat). The answer, 67, is slightly higher than the actual RSV. But it's close enough. For more about the evolving state of dietary recommendations, see Chapter 4. And — dare we say it? — your daily paper. Boy, is nutrition ever a work in progress!

Nutritionists used to use similar calculations to set the RSVs, such as

- ✔ Saturated fat — 10 percent or less of your calories/9 calories per gram
- ✔ Carbohydrates — 60 percent of your calories/4 calories per gram
- ✔ Dietary fibre — at least 25 grams per day
- ✔ Protein — 13 to 15 percent of your calories/4 calories per gram

Having set down this tidy list, we're now compelled to tell you that the %DVs (that's short for Percent Daily Values), as shown on Nutrition Facts labels, are behind the times. New recommendations from both the DRI reports and Canada's Food Guide say

- ✔ Total fat calories should account for 20 to 35 percent of total daily calories.

- ✔ No safe level exists for saturated fats or trans fats, thus no %DV is provided for either one.

  The total amount of saturated fat in the portion is the number of grams of sat fat (saturated fats) plus the number of grams of trans fat. (Who else would tell you these things?)

- ✔ Calories from carbs should account for 45 to 65 percent of daily calories.

- ✔ Women younger than 50 need to consume 25 grams of dietary fibre a day; men younger than 50, 38 grams. After age 51, it's 21 grams for women and 30 grams for men.

- ✔ Calories from protein should account for 10 to 35 percent of total daily calories, an amount much higher than the current RDA for protein.

Will this change the numbers on the Nutrition Facts labels? The sensible answer is, sure it will . . . eventually. Are the current Nutrition Facts labels still useful? Absolutely.

Relying on labels: Health claims

Ever since man (and woman) came out of the caves, people have been making health claims for certain foods. These folk remedies may be comforting, but the evidence to support them is mostly anecdotal: "I had a cold. My mom gave me chicken soup, and here I am, all bright-eyed and bushy-tailed. Of course, it did take a week to get rid of the cold completely. . . ."

On the other hand, nutrient and diet-related health claims approved by Health Canada for inclusion on the new food labels are another matter entirely. If you see a statement suggesting that a particular food or nutrient plays a role in reducing your risk of a specific medical condition, you can be absolutely 100 percent sure that a real relationship exists between the food and the medical condition. You can also be sure that scientific evidence from well-designed studies supports the claim.

In other words, Health Canada–approved, diet-related health claims are medically sound and scientifically specific. Currently there are only five in Canada:

- ✔ A diet adequate in calcium and vitamin D may reduce the risk of osteoporosis.

- ✔ A diet low in saturated fat and trans fat may reduce the risk of heart disease.

- ✔ A diet low in sodium and high in potassium may reduce the risk of high blood pressure.

- ✔ A diet rich in vegetables and fruit may reduce the risk of some types of cancer.

- ✔ A diet with minimal fermentable carbohydrates, found in gum, hard candy, or breath-freshening products, may reduce the risk of dental caries.

Foods with more than 4 grams per serving of saturated fat and/or saturated fat plus trans fat cannot have any health claims at all on their labels.

Figuring out how high is high and how low is low

Today, savvy consumers reach almost automatically for packages labelled "low fat" or "high fibre." But it's a dollars-to-doughnuts sure bet that hardly one shopper in a thousand knows what "low" and "high" actually mean.

Because these are potent terms that promise real health benefits, the new labelling law has created strict, science-based definitions. The following is an abbreviation of the more common nutrient content claims:

- ✔ *High* means that one serving provides 20 percent or more of the Daily Value for a particular nutrient. Other ways to say "high" are "rich in" or "excellent source of," as in "milk is an excellent source of calcium."

- ✔ *Good source* means one serving gives you 10 to 19 percent of the Daily Value for a particular nutrient.

- ✔ *Light* (sometimes written *lite*) is used in connection with calories or fat. It means the product has one-quarter fewer calories or 25 percent less fat as compared to the original version.

  Regarding sodium, the term *lightly salted* means there is 50 percent less sodium than usually is found in a particular type of product.

✔ *Low* means that the food contains an amount of a nutrient that enables you to eat several servings without going over the Daily Value for that nutrient.

- *Low-calorie* means 40 calories or fewer per serving
- *Low-fat* means 3 grams of fat or less
- *Low saturated fat* means 2 grams or less of saturated fat and trans fat combined
- *Low-cholesterol* means 20 milligrams or less

✔ *Reduced saturated fat* means that the amount of saturated fat plus trans fat has been reduced more than 25 percent from what's normal for the given food product.

✔ *Lower in fat* means the food contains at least 25 percent less fat than the regular product.

✔ *Reduced energy* means the food has at least 35 percent fewer calories than the regular product.

✔ *Reduced in saturated fat* means the food has at least 25 percent less saturated fat than the regular product.

✔ *Lower in sugar/reduced sugar* means the product has been reformulated to contain 25 percent less sugar than the regular product.

✔ *Unsweetened/no added sugar* means the food does not contain any added sugars (the food may contain naturally occurring sugars, however).

✔ *Low sodium* means the food has less than 140 mg of salt per serving.

✔ *Free* means an amount that is considered nutritionally insignificant or the amount is "negligible" — not "none."

- *Calorie-free* means fewer than 5 calories per serving.
- *Fat-free* means less than 0.5 grams of fat per serving.
- *Trans fat–free* means less than 0.2 grams trans fat and 0.2 grams saturated fat per serving.
- *Cholesterol-free* means less than 2 milligrams of cholesterol or 2 grams or less of saturated fat per serving
- *Sodium-free* or *salt-free* means less than 5 milligrams of sodium per serving.
- *Sugar-free* means less than 0.5 grams of sugar per serving.

Notice something missing? Right, there's no definition for "low sodium" per serving. On the other hand, a meal plan with less than 1,000 milligrams of sodium per day is considered a low-sodium diet.

Organic — the not-quite-finished evolution of a label term

"*Organic*" (as in organic food) is a highly charged food word. But do you know what it means? Don't be embarrassed to say no. Until recently, neither did most health professionals.

To a chemist, *organic* means a substance that contains carbon, hydrogen, and oxygen. By this chemical standard, all foods — and all human beings — are organic.

Yet some people adopted the word *organic* to describe plant foods grown without pesticides or synthetic chemicals, or to describe the poultry, fish, beef, and lamb from animals raised on a diet with no antibiotics or other medicating chemicals to assure healthy and efficiently producing animals.

But these descriptions were not standards regulated by any federal agency. However, on December 22, 2006, the Minister of Agriculture and Agri-Food and the Minister for the Canadian

Food Inspection Agency (CFIA) announced the final publication of the *Organic Products Regulations*. These regulations will help protect consumers against false and previously unregulated organic claims. Along with the regulations is the introduction of the new Canadian organic logo. The regulation and introduction of the new organic logo will be phased in over the next two years. Only those food products that meet Canadian standards for organic production (which include naturally raised animals and the use of natural fertilizers) and that contain at least 95 percent organic ingredients can bear the new logo. After this two-year period, all foods intended for interprovincial and international trade will be required to bear this logo.

For more information, visit the Canadian Food Inspection Agency's Web site www. inspection.gc.ca/english/fssa/ orgbio/otfgtspbe.shtml.

Listing what's inside

The extra added attraction on the Nutrition Facts label is the complete ingredient listing, in which every single ingredient is listed in order of its weight in the product, heaviest first, lightest last. In addition, the label must spell out the true identity of some classes of ingredients known to cause allergic reactions:

- ✔ Vegetable proteins (*hydrolyzed corn protein* rather than the old-fashioned *hydrolyzed vegetable protein*)
- ✔ Milk products (*non-dairy* products such as coffee whiteners may contain the milk protein caseinate, which comes from milk)
- ✔ Food colourings (FD&C yellow No. 5, a full, formal chemical name instead of *colouring*)

Because it isn't always possible to avoid all potential allergens in food production, manufacturers of food products in which traces of a possible allergen may be present are legally permitted to use precautionary labelling, such as "may contain." This is only permitted in situations when an allergen may inadvertently make its way into a food. If an allergen is most likely to be present, then the use of precautionary labelling is not permitted. Be on alert! Nutrition labelling and ingredient lists are your best weapon to avoiding any problems.

Choosing Foods using the Food Guide and the Nutrition Facts Label

The Food Guide Pyramid helps you to plan balanced meals and snacks. In the kitchen, you can increase the nutritional value by thinking of individual dishes as mini–Food Guides. At snack time, you can use the Food Guide to choose munchies that are a valuable part of your overall daily diet. As a general rule, choose foods from at least three of the four food groups at each main meal and at least two of the four food groups at each snack to ensure you get the nutrients you need every day to stay healthy.

For example, although you know that fruits and veggies are good snacks, that doesn't mean you're stuck with boring carrot sticks or an apple. The Food Guide says "vegetables and fruits," not raw fruits and raw vegetables. Yes, a fresh apple's fine. But so is a baked apple (100 calories), fragrant with cinnamon and decorated with no-fat sour cream (30–45 calories for two tablespoons). Carrot strips are okay. So are vegetarian baked beans — yes, baked beans (140 calories plus 26 grams of carbohydrates, 7 grams of protein, 7 grams of dietary fibre, and 2 grams of fat per 125 mL — ½ cup — serving), which are considered both veggies *and* a member of the high-protein meat/beans group.

As for the Nutrition Facts label, you can use that to eat your cake and have it nutritiously by comparing products to choose the best alternatives.

Here's a good example: You find yourself irresistibly drawn to double dark chocolate ice cream (lots of fat, saturated fat, cholesterol, and a whopping 230 calories per 125 mL — ½ cup — serving). But then, just as your hand is opening the freezer door, ready to reach for the ice cream, suddenly . . . out of the corner of your eye, you see the Nutrition Facts table on the label of the no-fat but equally irresistible chocolate sorbet. It says, "No fat, no saturated fat, no cholesterol, and only 90 to 130 calories per serving." When you put the labels side by side, do you need to ask which one comes out the winner?

Balancing Diagrams and Stats

At the beginning of this chapter, you were warned: Keeping track of all the facts may be difficult. But by now you can pretty much boil them all down to one nutritional Golden Rule, exemplified by the Food Guide and the Nutrition Facts label: *Keep things in proportion.*

Come to think of it, that's not a bad philosophy for life.

Chapter 18

Eating Smart When Eating Out

In This Chapter

▶ Navigating a restaurant menu

▶ Ordering without overdoing

▶ Finding nutritious fast-food favourites

*E*ating out is in. You don't have to cook, and somebody else washes the dishes. The challenge is to avoid letting luxury lull you into ceding responsibility for your food choices to some chef whose heart belongs to butter. This chapter lays out strategies for making your excellent adventure nutritionally sound. You find out how to edit a menu in a *white-tablecloth* restaurant (the food professional's description of an upscale eatery) to balance gustatory pleasure with common-sense nutrition. And you figure out how to juggle fast food so that it fits into a healthful diet. No cooking, no dishes, no guilt. Who could ask for anything more?

Interpreting a Restaurant Menu

Restaurants are businesses, and that means they respond to consumer demand. What consumers have demanded for years are rich foods and big portions, which means that the restaurant concept of a portion or of a healthy alternative is seriously out of whack with what the nutrition experts recommend. Does that mean you should stop eating out? Heck, no! But it does mean you need to use caution when navigating a menu.

Pinpointing portions

Restaurants don't make friends by serving up teensy little portions. In fact, tiny servings probably sank *nouvelle cuisine*, the 1980s fad that put one string bean, three garden peas, half an artichoke heart, and one sliced cherry tomato on a lettuce leaf and called it the salad course.

Reality dictates that the portions on restaurant plates rarely come within hailing distance of the official serving sizes issued by Health Canada. To protect yourself from humongous servings, you need to store real-life versions of the recommended portions in your memory banks. To do that, use a 250mL (8-ounce) measuring cup and a kitchen scale to run through some basic practice drills at home:

- ✔ Broil a small steak or roast a chicken breast. Use a kitchen scale to weigh an 85g (3-ounce) portion. Does the steak look like a deck of cards? How about a small calculator? Maybe it's closer to the size of a computer mouse (this is a little bigger at 114 g or 4 ounces — still close enough). That's one serving.

- ✔ Boil some rice. After the rice is done, fill the measuring cup to the halfway mark. Take out the rice and roll it into a tennis ball or a billiard ball. Alternatively, it's about the size of a standard light bulb or a small fist. Whatever. That's one serving.

- ✔ Shred some greens. You want only enough to fit into a cupped hand. Or fill the measuring cup to the 250mL (8-ounce) mark. Turn the greens out onto a salad plate. That's one serving.

- ✔ Open one can of beets or fruit cocktail. Fill the measuring cup to the halfway mark. Spoon the beets or fruit onto a plate. Again, the food should be about the size of a standard light bulb or a small fist. That's one serving.

- ✔ Open a can of soda. Pour it into the measuring cup, right up to the 250mL (8-ounce) mark. Pour that into a glass. Add some ice. It's probably more than you get in an upscale restaurant, less than you get at the burger barn. No matter: It's still one standardized Canada Food Guide serving.

Now that you have a picture of a serving in your mind, you can slice away the extra from your restaurant plate — and take it home for lunch or dinner the next day. That's what *doggie bags* are for.

Checking out the Eat Smart! program

In an attempt to make healthy eating easier, the Government of Ontario has created the Eat Smart! program. Eat Smart! is designed to both award and designate restaurants and cafeterias that make dining out a healthier experience. Restaurants and cafeterias that offer a smoke-free environment and healthy food choices are given the Eat Smart! designation as awarded by the local Public Health Unit, the Canadian Cancer Society, and the Heart and Stroke Foundation of Canada. When you eat away from home, all you have to do is look for the Eat Smart! symbol.

Being an Eat Smart! restaurant or cafeteria doesn't mean that everything on the menu is considered healthy, but it does mean healthier choices are available. You still need to be prudent when you make choices. Recognizing that healthy eating is more than just offering more vegetables, fruits, and lower-fat options, the program also ensures that the establishment has demonstrated a consistent food safety record and at least one full-time person certified in food safety and handling is on staff.

The Eat Smart! Web site (`eatsmart.web.ca/en/index.php`) enables you to search for participating restaurants before heading out. From the home page, click on the link "Find an Eat Smart! Restaurant." Don't live in Ontario? No problem. You can also search for Eat Smart! restaurants on `www.foodinc.ca`, an online directory for restaurants across Canada. To date there are more than 50,000 restaurant listings, so finding something in your neck of the woods should be easy.

Making Smart Menu Choices

From a nutritional point of view, restaurant dining has three basic pitfalls:

- Serving sizes are too big.
- Garnishes and side dishes are too rich.
- Meals have too many courses.

Not to worry. Exercise a little care and caution, and you can order from any menu, secure in the knowledge that pleasing your palate doesn't mean tossing away all nutritional common sense. A few strategies can make any restaurant experience a joy.

Starting simple

Set the nutritional tone of dinner right off the bat with your choice of appetizer. You have two possible alternatives. The first is opting for a really rich, high-calorie dense food such as pâté de foie gras (literally: fat liver paste) and then coasting downward, calorie-fat-and-cholesterol-wise, for the rest of the meal. A second alternative is choosing a tasty but low-calorie, low-fat appetizer such as clear soup, a salad with lemon juice dressing, or shellfish such as shrimp cocktail (10 to 30 calories a shrimp) with no-fat (ketchup/horseradish) sauce. This choice allows you more food later.

Elevating appetizers to entrees

For smaller portion sizes or to skip the calorie-laden sides that come with most entrees, order an appetizer as your main course. A perfect example of this would be an appetizer consisting of a bowl of steamed mussels in their shells in a low-oil, fresh-tomato sauce with one piece of crusty French bread underneath to sop it up with. Add a glass of cold, dry, white wine and one more piece of bread, and this appetizer becomes a meal in itself — with a lot fewer calories and less fat than most any entree on the menu. Less expensive, too.

Skipping the fat on the bread

Don't butter your bread. Don't oil it, either. Many chic and trendy restaurants now serve up a dish of flavoured olive oil in place of butter. True, the olive oil has less saturated fat than butter, and it has no cholesterol, but the calorie count is exactly the same. All fats and oils (butter, margarine, vegetable oils) give you about 100 calories a tablespoon. *Note:* You may get even more calories from the oil if you do a lot of dipping.

Consumer alert: Don't assume that your bread is low-fat just because you didn't butter it. Many different types of breads come already buttered (or oiled). One example is foccacia, the thick squares of savoury Italian bread. Others are popovers and muffins.

To test the fat content of your bread, pick up a piece or put it on your napkin. If your hand feels greasy or the bread leaves an oily spot on your napkin, you have your answer.

Going naked: Undressed veggies

Victorians boiled vegetables into a yucky muck — no colour, no texture, no taste. Then came 20th-century butter, cheese, and cream sauces, often burnished under the broiler to a browned crust. Now, smart restaurant cooks rely on herbs and spices, reduced (boiled down and thickened) fat-free bouillons, unusual salad combinations, and imaginative treatments such as purées and kabobs to make their vegetables tasty but trim. The result? Food heaven and nutrition joy. The vegetable flavours come through, and the calories stay very, very, very low.

You don't have to settle for that boring steamed stuff or for veggies so raw they have no taste. The difference between raw cauliflower and cauliflower that's been steamed for 15 or 20 minutes and dusted with dill is so vast that people who insist on passing out the stuff cold should be charged with vegetable abuse.

To reap the low-calorie rewards, avoid veggie dishes labelled

- ✔ Au beurre (with butter)
- ✔ Au gratin (with cheese sauce)
- ✔ Batter-dipped (eggs, oil, fried)
- ✔ Breaded (breadcrumbs, oil, fried)
- ✔ Fritters (fried)
- ✔ Fritto (fried)
- ✔ Hollandaise (sauce with butter and egg yolks)
- ✔ Tempura (battered and fried)

Minimizing the main dish

I won't insult you by telling you to avoid fried foods.

If you're reading this book, you already know that the best choice is something broiled, baked, or roasted — without added fat, and with the drippings siphoned off. But I can't avoid noting that you can lower the fat content of any main dish simply by wielding a mean knife and fork to cut away the vestiges of visible fat on your chop or steak or poultry.

Another approach is to order a main course meat dish without the "main" part. That is, order your meat, fish, or poultry as a small-serving appetizer, and then ask your waiter for a veggie entree. Or opt for all the nifty little extras that usually accompany the meat course, ordering the veggie side dishes à la carte instead of as a veggie entree.

Demand tiny boiled onions. Baby peas with mint. Pickled beets and red cabbage. Sugared carrots. Sautéed spinach. Darling little boiled or baked potatoes with a crust of paprika or cumin. The more, the merrier. The result may not be entirely fat free, but it almost certainly has fewer calories, less fat, more dietary fibre, and a wider variety of vitamins than plain meat or poultry.

Sidelining sauces

Dining out is a treat, so treat yourself — within reason. You can have your béarnaise (egg yolks, butter), béchamel (butter, flour, heavy cream), brown sauce (beef drippings, flour), and hollandaise (butter, egg yolks), as long as you have them in reasonable amounts.

Ask the waiter to bring the sauce on the side, take one tablespoonful (about a soup spoonful), and hand the rest back to the waiter. When ordering from an Italian menu, the general rule is to avoid the olive-oil-based sauces and choose the tomato-based red sauce. (If the chef where you're eating fattens up the tomato sauce with olive oil, forget this rule.) Many restaurants now make their red sauces skinny — all tomato, little or no oil.

Satisfying your sweet tooth

After a heavy meal, your body often craves something sweet. Lower your calories, fat, and so on by splitting a dessert with your dinner partner. Or opt for rich but fat-free sweetened coffees: espresso, Greek, and Turkish brews seem most satisfying. Hate coffee? Have a diet cola.

Discovering the Healthful Side of Fast Food

Fast food can be good food. By choosing carefully, you can enjoy burgers and still meet recommended daily dietary allowances for all important vitamins and minerals. A fast-food burger on a bun, plus a salad and a small, low-fat milk shake, a 250mL (8-ounce) container of milk, a small cola, or plain old water may not sound like great nutrition, but the version served up in fast-food restaurants can actually be relatively low in fat and relatively high in valuable nutrients.

Choosing wisely at the drive-through

The greatest problem with fast food is *very* big servings. More food means more calories — and more you. Several people recently have filed lawsuits charging that fast-food restaurants made them overeat, which, in turn, made them overweight. At least one such suit was tossed out of court, but that doesn't mean another won't be filed down the road. So the question of the day becomes, does a smart cookie like you check your brains at the door when you enter a fast-food restaurant — or do you have the intelligence to choose wisely regardless of where you plunk yourself down for a meal?

Eating smart is a skill you can exercise in any location. For example, Table 18-1 compares the nutrient values of three basic McDonald's meals. All three meals derive about 30 percent of their calories from fat (although all three dish up about one-third the percent Daily Value for artery-clogging saturated fat). They're relatively low in cholesterol and provide plenty of vitamin A, vitamin C, and bone-building calcium. And the servings are reasonable:

- The burger is the basic, small, no-frills hamburger.
- The salad is a Caesar salad (no chicken) with one packet of Newman's Own low-fat Italian dressing.
- The parfait is the Fruit 'n Yogurt without granola.
- The milk is a 250mL (8-ounce) container of low-fat (1 percent) milk.
- The cola is a 500mL (16-ounce) cup (small).

The initials DV stand for Daily Value, a nutritional guideline suggesting how much of each nutrient you need each day on a 2,000-calorie diet. For the complete skinny on the DV and how it's used on food labels, check out Chapter 17.

Stop! Before you bite into that burger, look at the following chart, but remember that it's only a guide. Menus and ingredients may change, so check the nutrition brochure at your local burger haven, and do it every single time you eat there. You never know when something new will pop up on your plate.

Table 18-1	Nutritious Fast-Food Meals? Yes!		
Nutrient (% Daily Value)	*Burger, Salad, Milk (490 Calories)*	*Burger, Salad, Parfait (520 Calories)*	*Burger, Salad, Small Cola (540 Calories)*
Calories from fat	33%	30%	26%
Saturated fat	30.5%	34%	29%
Cholesterol	16%	15%	13%
Dietary fibre	31%	31%	31%
Vitamin A	132%	155%	122%
Vitamin C	60%	67%	56%
Calcium	65%	45%	35%

McDonald's Corporation, as of November 21, 2005

Trans fat: The Boooo! factor

Once upon a time, fast-food restaurants — indeed, most restaurants — fried up their foods in butter, which is loaded with the saturated fat and cholesterol that gum up your arteries and increase your risk of heart disease. Then, prodded by the Food Police, restaurants switched to vegetable fats, which are lower in saturated fat and have no cholesterol. Hooray? Well, not exactly. Instead of using heart-healthy vegetable oils, fast-food restaurants sometimes use solid vegetable shortenings, and there's a crucial

difference. The shortenings are solid in part because they contain partially hydrogenated vegetable oils. Chapter 7 explains the chemistry of *hydrogenation* (adding hydrogen atoms to fats).

Partially hydrogenated vegetable oils are high in trans fatty acids, a form of fat that may clog your arteries as badly as saturated fats and cholesterol do. With trans fats in the mix, an order of fries may have as much artery-hostile fat as a 4-ounce burger. Boooo!

Finding fast-food ingredient guides

Fast-food restaurants now make nutrition information available. McDonald's even puts its numbers on the food wrapper. If your local eatery doesn't have brochures on hand or post nutrition info on the wall, don't be shy: Write, call, or click for a copy. *Note:* Companies that don't give you a mailing address usually have a "write us" e-mail form on their Web sites.

Arby's of Canada Inc.
7045 Edward's Blvd.
Mississauga ON, L5S 1X2
Phone 800-263-7040
Web site www.arbys.com (Click on "Nutrition.")

Burger King Restaurants of Canada Inc.
700 – 401 The West Mall
Toronto, ON M9C 5J4
Phone 416-626-6696
Web site www.burgerking.ca (Click on "Nutrition.")

Tim Hortons
874 Sinclair Rd.
Oakville, ON L6K 2Y1
Phone 905-845-6511
Web site www.timhortons.com (Select "Nutrition" under "In our Store.")

KFC Canada (Kentucky Fried Chicken)
101 Exchange Ave.
Vaughan, ON L4K 5R6
Phone 866-664-5696
Web site www.kfc.ca (Click on "Nutritional Information.")

McDonald's Restaurants of Canada Limited
McDonald's Place
Toronto, ON M3C 3L4
Phone 416-446-3443
Web site www.mcdonalds.ca (Click on "Nutrition" under "Our Food.")

Pizza Hut
101 Exchange Ave.
Vaughan, ON L4K 5R6
Phone 866-664-5696
Web site www.pizzahut.ca (Click on "Nutrition Facts" under "Menu.")

Subway
325 Bic Dr.
Milford, CT 06460
Phone 800-888-4848 or 203-877-4281
Web site www.subway.ca (Click on "Nutrition.")

Note: there isn't one corporate address for Subway Canada but rather regional development offices. You can find the local contact closest to you by clicking on "Franchise Opportunities" on the home page.

Wendy's Restaurants of Canada
Consumer Relations
240 Wyecroft Rd.
Oakville, ON L6K 2G7
Phone 905-849-7685
Web site www.wendys.com (Click on "Country and Language" and then "Food" and "Nutrition.")

Fingers too fatigued to troll through the separate sites? Check out www. nutritiondata.com. Slide your mouse to the right side of the page and run it down the list of fast-food restaurants. Choose one. Click. Choose your dish. Click. Up comes the most complete nutrition analysis known to man. Or woman. Yay NutritionData.com!

Part IV
Food Processing

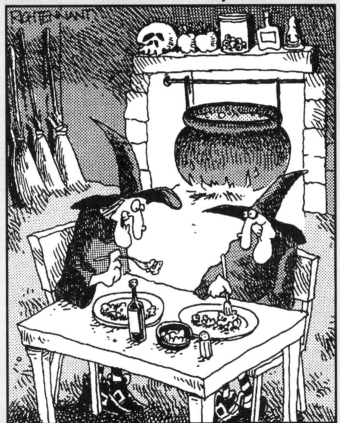

"I substitute tofu for eye of newt in all my recipes now. It has twice the protein and doesn't wriggle around the cauldron."

In this part . . .

Have you ever wondered why canned green beans aren't as green as fresh ones? Or why an originally translucent egg white turns white when you cook it? Or why frozen carrots are mushy when you defrost them? Or — modern technology at its most mysterious — why exposing food to radiation keeps it fresh longer? Wonder no more. Just shift your eyes to the right to find out what happens when you cook, freeze, dry, or zap food.

Chapter 19

What Is Food Processing?

S ay "processed food," and most people think "cheese spread." They're right, of course. Cheese spread is, in fact, a processed food. But so are baked potatoes, canned tuna, frozen peas, skim milk, pasteurized orange juice, and scrambled eggs. In broad terms, food processing is any technique that alters the natural state of food — everything from cooking to freezing to pickling to drying, and more and more and more.

In this chapter, you can read all about how each form of processing changes food from a living thing (animal or vegetable) into an integral component of your healthful diet — and at the same time

✔ Lengthens shelf life

✔ Reduces the risk of food-borne illnesses

✔ Maintains or improves a food's texture or flavour

✔ Upgrades the nutritional value of foods

What a set of bonuses!

Preserving Food: Five Methods of Processing

Where food is concerned, the term *natural* doesn't necessarily translate as "safe" or "good to eat." Food spoils (naturally) when microbes living (naturally) on the surface of meat, a carrot, a peach, and so on reproduce (naturally) to a population level that overwhelms the food.

Sometimes you can see, feel, or smell when this is happening. You can see mould growing on cheese, feel how meat or chicken turns slippery, and smell when the milk turns sour. The mould on cheese, slippery slickness on the surface of the meat or chicken, and odour of the milk are caused by exploding populations of micro-organisms. Don't even argue with them; just throw out the food.

All food processing is designed to prevent what happens to the chicken (or the cheese or the milk). It aims to preserve food and extend its *shelf life* (the period of time when it's nutritious and safe to consume) by stemming the natural tide of biological destruction. (But wait! Not all microbes are bad guys. We use "good" ones to ferment milk to yogourt or cheese and to produce wines and beers.)

Reducing or limiting the growth of food's natural microbe population not only lengthens its shelf life but also lowers the risk of food-borne illnesses. Increased food safety is a natural consequence of most processing that keeps foods usable longer. This section discusses how food processing works.

For simplicity's sake, here's a list of the methods used to extend the shelf life of food. (These methods are discussed in even more detail in Chapter 20, Chapter 21, and Chapter 22.)

- Temperature methods
  - Cooking
  - Canning
  - Refrigeration
  - Freezing
- Air control
  - Canning
  - Vacuum packaging
- Moisture control
  - Dehydration
  - Freeze-drying (which combines methods of controlling temperature, air, and moisture)
- Chemical methods
  - Acidification
  - Mould inhibition
  - Salting (dry salt or brine)
- Irradiation
- High-pressure processing

Tantalizing tidbit of food nomenclature

Central American Indians dried meat to produce *chaqui,* a name carried north by Spanish explorers who used it to describe the dried meats of the Southwestern Indians, which eventually became — you saw this coming, right? — jerky.

Temperature control

Exposing food to high heat for a sufficiently long time reduces the natural population of bacterial spoilers and kills microbes that otherwise may make you sick. For example, pasteurization — heating milk or other liquids such as fruit juice to between 63 and 68°C (between 145 and 154.4°F) for 30 minutes — kills nearly all disease-causing and most other bacteria, as does high-temperature, short-time pasteurization (72°C or 161°F for 15 seconds).

Chilling also protects food. It works by slowing the rate of microbial reproduction. For example:

✔ Milk refrigerated at 10°C (50°F) or colder may stay fresh for almost a week because the cold prevents organisms that survived pasteurization from reproducing.

✔ Fresh chicken frozen to 32°C (0°F) or colder may remain safe for up to 12 months (whole) or 9 months (cut up).

Removing the water

Like all living things, the microbes on food need water to survive. Dehydrate the food, and the bugs won't reproduce, which means the food stays edible longer. That's the rationale behind raisins, prunes, and *pemmican,* a dried mix of meat, fat, and berries adapted from East Coast Native Americans and served to 18th- and 19th-century sailors of every national stripe. Dehydration (loss of water) occurs when food is

✔ Exposed to air and sunlight

✔ Heated for several hours in a very low oven (120°C or 250°F) or smoked (the smokehouse acts as a very low oven)

Controlling the air flow

Just as microbes need water, most also need air. Reducing the air supply almost always reduces the bacterial population. The exception is anaerobes (micro-organisms that can live without air), such as *botulinum* organisms, which thrive in the absence of air. Go figure!

Foods are protected from air by vacuum packaging. A *vacuum* — from *vacuus,* the Latin word for "empty" — is a space with virtually no air. The food is put in a container — a plastic bag or glass jar — then the air is vacuumed out of the container and the container is immediately sealed. When you open a vacuum-packed container, you hear a sudden little pop as the vacuum is broken.

If there's no popping sound, the seal has already been broken, allowing air in, and that means the food inside may be spoiled or may have been tampered with. Do not taste-test: Throw out the entire package, food and all.

Chemical warfare

About two dozen chemicals are used as *food additives* or *food preservatives* to prevent spoilage. (If the mere mention of chemicals or food additives makes the hair on the back of your neck rise, chill out with Chapter 22.) Here are the most common chemical preservatives:

- ✔ **Acidifiers:** Most microbes don't thrive in highly acidic settings, so a chemical that makes a food more acidic prevents spoilage. Wine and vinegar are acidifying chemicals, and so are *citric acid,* the natural preservative in citrus fruits, and *lactic acid,* the natural acid in yogourt.

- ✔ **Mould inhibitors:** Sodium benzoate, sodium propionate, and calcium propionate slow (but do not entirely stop) the growth of mould on bread. Sodium benzoate also is used to prevent the growth of moulds in cheese, margarine, and syrups.

- ✔ **Bacteria busters:** Salt is *hydrophilic* (hydro = water; phil = loving). When you cover fresh meat with salt, the salt draws water up and out of the meat — and up and out of the cells of bacteria living on the meat. Presto: The bacteria die; the meat dries. And you get to eat corned beef (which gets its name from the fact that large grains of salt were once called "corns").

Irradiation

Irradiation is a technique that exposes food to electron beams or to *gamma radiation,* a high-energy light stronger than the X-rays your doctor uses to make a picture of your insides. *Gamma rays* are ionizing radiation, the kind that kills living cells. As a result, irradiation prolongs the shelf life of food by

- ✔ Killing microbes and insects on plants (wheat, wheat powder, spices, dry vegetable seasonings)
- ✔ Preventing potatoes and onions from producing new sprouts at the eyes
- ✔ Slowing the rate at which some fruits ripen
- ✔ Killing disease-causing organisms such as *Trichinella, Salmonella, E. coli,* and *Listeria* (the organism responsible for a recent outbreak of food poisoning from packaged meats and cold cuts) on meat and poultry

And, no, irradiating food *does not make* the food radioactive. But you already knew that, right?

Making Food Better and Better for You

Some food processing really does make your food taste better; a well-broiled steak beats a raw one anytime. Processing also allows you to sample a wide variety of seasonal foods (mostly fruits and vegetables) all year long, and it enables food producers to improve the nutritional status of many basic foods, such as grains and milk, by enriching or altering them to meet the needs of modern consumers.

Intensifying flavour and aroma

One advantage of food processing is that it enables you to enjoy things never seen in nature, such as the ever-popular — and ever-criticized — cheese spread. A more mundane benefit of food processing is that it intensifies aroma and flavour, almost always for the better. Here's how:

- ✔ **Drying concentrates flavour.** A prune has a different, darker, more intensely sweet flavour than a fresh plum. On the other hand, dried food can be hard and tough to chew (think beef jerky).

✓ **Heating heightens aroma by quickening the movement of aroma molecules.** In fact, your first tantalizing hint of dinner usually is the scent of cooking food. Chilling has the opposite effect: It slows the movement of the molecules. To sense the difference, sniff a plate of cold roast beef versus hot roast beef straight from the oven. Or sniff two glasses of vodka, one warm, one icy from the freezer. One comes up scent-free; the other has the olfactory allure of pure gasoline. Guess which is which. Or you can pass up the guessing and try for yourself. Nothing like first-hand experience!

✓ **Warming foods intensifies flavours.** This development is sometimes beneficial (warm roast beef is somehow more savoury than cold roast beef), sometimes not (warm milk is definitely not as popular as the icy-cold version).

✓ **Changing the temperature also changes texture.** Heating softens some foods (butternut squash is a good example) and solidifies others (think eggs). Chilling keeps the fats in pâté firm so the stuff doesn't melt down into a puddle on the plate. Ditto for the gelatin that keeps dessert moulds and dinner aspics standing upright.

Adding nutrients

The addition of vitamins and minerals to basic foods has helped eliminate many once-common nutritional deficiency diseases. The practice is so common that you take the following for granted:

✓ Breads, cereals, and grains are given extra B vitamins to replace the vitamins lost when whole grains are stripped of their nutrient-rich covering to make white flour or white rice or degermed cornmeal. Adding the vitamins reduces the risk of the B vitamin–deficiency diseases beriberi and pellagra.

✓ Breads, cereals, and grains also are given iron to replace what's lost in milling and to make it easier for North American women to reach the RDA (Recommended Dietary Allowance) for this important mineral.

✓ All milk sold in Canada has added vitamin D to reduce the risk of the bone-deforming vitamin D–deficiency diseases rickets (among children) and osteomalacia (among adults).

✓ Added fat-free milk proteins turn *skim milk* — milk from which the fat has been removed — into a creamier liquid with more calcium and protein but less fat and cholesterol than whole milk.

Combining benefits

Adding genes from one food (such as corn) to another food (such as tomatoes) may make the second food taste better and stay fresh longer. You can
bet your bottom flapjack that this is one hot topic, so for more about genetic
engineering at the dinner table, check out Chapter 22.

Faking It: Alternative Foods

In addition to its many other benefits, food processing offers you some
totally fake but widely appreciated substitute sweeteners. Actually, these
may be just the tip of the iceberg, so to speak. Two years ago, the Brits
sprang Quorn (a meat substitute), food made from fungi (yes, fungi), on an
unsuspecting U.S. public (it didn't make it to Canada). Quorn seems to have
slipped back into the nutritional netherworld, but as processing becomes
more adventurous, who knows what strange and wonderful dishes lie just
beyond the entrance to the Nutritional Twilight Zone? Dum-de-dum-dum . . .

Alternative foods: Substitute sweeteners

Here's a scientific tidbit. Most substitute sweeteners were discovered by
accident in laboratories where researchers touched a paper or a pencil,
then stuck their fingers in their mouths to discover, "Eureka! It's sweet." As
Harold McGee wrote in the first edition of his wonderful *On Food and Cooking*
(Collier Books, 1988), "These stories make one wonder about the standards
of laboratory hygiene."

Because substitute sweeteners are not absorbed by your body and don't provide any nutrients, scientists call them by their proper name: *non-nutritive
sweeteners.* The best-known (listed in order of their discovery and/or Health
Canada approval) are:

- **Saccharin (Hermesetas):** This synthetic sweetener was discovered by
  accident (the fingers-in-the-mouth syndrome) at Johns Hopkins in 1879.
  Saccharin was banned in 1977, after it was linked to bladder cancer in
  rats; however, diabetics who have used saccharin for years in other
  countries where its use is allowed show no excess levels of bladder
  cancer. Health Canada is currently revisiting the ban to decide whether
  to allow its use. Saccharin is available in tablet form in Canada from
  pharmacists under the brand name Hermesetas and cannot be added to
  packaged foods or beverages. Avoid this sweetener during pregnancy.
  Note: Most people think saccharin is very sweet, but if you hate broccoli,
  you're likely to think saccharin's bitter. Check out Chapter 15 to see why.

✔ **Cyclamates (Sucaryl, Sugar Twin, Sweet'n Low):** These surfaced (on somebody's finger, of course) in 1937 at the University of Illinois. They were tied to cancer in laboratory animals and banned (1969) in the U.S. but not in Canada and many other countries. Never has any evidence of ill effects in human beings been attributed to cyclamates, which are available for use as a tabletop sweetener in Canada in packets, tablets, liquid, and granulated form, but not allowed in packaged foods and beverages Avoid this sweetener during pregnancy. Cyclamates cannot be used in cooking or baking; they are affected by heat.

✔ **Aspartame (Equal, NutraSweet, Sugar Twin):** Another accidental discovery (1965), *aspartame* is a combination of two amino acids, aspartic acid and phenylalanine. The problem with aspartame is that during digestion, it breaks down into its constituent ingredients. The same thing happens when aspartame is exposed to heat. That's trouble for people born with a *phenylketonuria (PKU),* a metabolic defect characterized by a lack of the enzyme needed to digest phenylalanine. The excess amino acid can pile up in brain and nerve tissue, leading to mental retardation in young children. Aspartame is available in packets, tablets, or granulated form. It can be added to prepared foods such as drinks, yogourt, cereals, low-calorie desserts, chewing gum, and many other packaged foods. It is not heat stable, so it cannot be used in cooking or baking. It is considered safe for pregnant women.

✔ **Sucralose (Splenda):** *Sucralose,* which was discovered in 1976, is a no-calorie sweetener made from sugar. But your body doesn't recognize it as a carbohydrate or a sugar, so it zips through your intestinal tract unchanged. More than 100 scientific studies conducted during a 20-year period attest to its safety, and Health Canada has approved its use in a variety of foods, including baked goods, candies, substitute dairy products, and frozen desserts. What sets sucralose apart from the other sweeteners is that it is heat stable and can be substituted for sugar in cooking and baking.

✔ **Acesulfame-K (Sunett):** The *K* is the chemical symbol for potassium, and this artificial sweetener, with a chemical structure similar to saccharin, is found in baked goods, chewing gum, and other food products, but it's not available for purchase as a single ingredient. It is considered safe for pregnant women.

✔ **Neotame:** This free-flowing, water-soluble sweetener is derived from amino acids (the building blocks of protein, the nutrient that stars in Chapter 6). It is estimated to be 7,000 to 13,000 times sweeter than sucrose (regular table sugar). In December 2006, Health Canada received an application to amend the *Food and Drug Regulations* to permit the use of Neotame. At this time it is still under review. To date, more than 113 animal and human studies worldwide have shown absolutely no adverse effects.

✔ **Tagatose (Naturlose, Shugr):** A white powder made from lactose, the sugar in milk. This product is still under review for use in Canada. In other countries that have approved it, it's used in cereal, soft drinks, frozen desserts, candy, chewing gum, and cake frosting. Although tagatose may cause gastric upset (gas, bloating, nausea, and diarrhea), it can also serve as an aid to digestion.

✔ **Sugar Alcohols (sorbitol, mannitol, maltitol, xylitol, lactitol, isomalt, polydextrose):** Sugar alcohols are neither sugars nor alcohols. Small amounts are naturally found in fruits and vegetables, or sugar alcohols can be manufactured. They are often used in products labelled "sugar free" or "no added sugar." They can't be bought as table sweeteners but are used by food manufacturers in candy, frozen desserts, and ice cream products. Sugar alcohols aren't "true" artificial sweeteners — they do provide small amounts of calories, which may affect blood glucose (sugar) levels, because they are only partially absorbed by your body. But they do have fewer calories than sugar. Large amounts (more than 10 grams per day) can cause diarrhea, cramps, gas, and bloating. Sugar alcohols are safe for pregnant women.

Table 19-1 compares the calorie content and sweetening power of sugar versus the substitute sweeteners. For comparison, sugar has 4 calories per gram.

Table 19-1	Comparing Substitute Sweeteners to Sugar	
Sweetener	*Calories Per Gram*	*Sweetness Relative to Sugar**
Sugar (sucrose)	4	
Saccharin	0	200–700 times sweeter than sugar
Cyclamates	0	30–60 times sweeter than sugar
Aspartame	4**	160–200 times sweeter than sugar
Sucralose	0	600 times sweeter than sugar
Acesulfame-K	0	150–200 times sweeter than sugar
Neotame	0	7,000–13,000 times sweeter than sugar
Tagatose	1.5**	Similar to sugar
Sorbitol	2.6	50–70% as sweet as sugar

(continued)

Table 19-1 *(continued)*

Sweetener	Calories Per Gram	Sweetness Relative to Sugar*
Mannitol	1.6	50–70% as sweet as sugar
Maltitol	3	90% as sweet as sugar
Xylitol	3	As sweet as sugar
Lactitol	2	30–40% as sweet as sugar
Isomalt	2	45–65% as sweet as sugar
Polydextrose	1	0***

* The range of sweetness reflects estimates from several sources.
** Aspartame has 4 calories per gram and tagatose 1.5, but you need so little to get a sweet flavour that you can count the calorie content as 0.
*** Polydextrose is not sweet but slightly tart in taste.

A Last Word: Follow That Bird

You can sum up the essence of food processing by following the trail of one chicken from the farm to your table. (Vegetarians are excused from this section.)

A chicken's first brush with processing comes right after slaughtering. It's plucked, packed in ice to slow the natural bacterial decomposition, and shipped off to the food processor or the supermarket. In the food factory, your chicken may be boiled and canned whole, or boiled and cut up and canned in small portions like tuna fish, or boiled into chicken soup to be canned or dehydrated into bouillon cubes, or cooked with veggies and canned as chicken à la king, or fried and frozen in whole pieces, or roasted, sliced, and frozen into a chicken dinner, or . . . you get the picture (and if you don't, check out Figure 19-1).

When you buy a fresh (raw) chicken instead of a cooked one, you perform similar rituals in your own kitchen. First, the chicken goes to the refrigerator (or freezer), then to the stove for thorough cooking to make sure that no stray bacteria contaminate your dinner table (or you), and then back to the fridge for the leftovers. In the end, the chicken's been processed. And you have eaten. That's the point of this story.

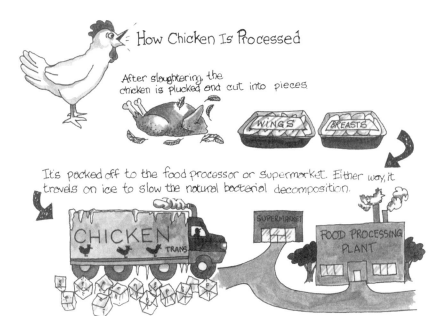

How Chicken Is Processed

After slaughtering, the chicken is plucked and cut into pieces

It's packed off to the food processor or supermarket. Either way, it travels on ice to slow the natural bacterial decomposition.

In the food factory, your chicken may be boiled and canned whole, or boiled and canned in small portions, or boiled into chicken soup, or dehydrated into bouillon cubes, or fried or frozen into whole pieces, or ... you get the picture....

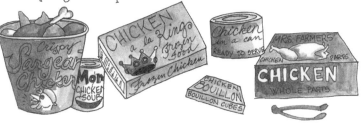

Figure 19-1:
From the farm to your table: chicken processing.

Chapter 20

Cooking and Nutrition

*Y*ou can bet that the first cooked dinner was an accident involving some poor wandering animal and a bolt of lightning that — zap! — charred the beast into medium sirloin. Then a caveman attracted by the aroma tore off a sizzled hunk and forthwith offered up the first restaurant rating: "Yum."

After that, it was but a hop, a skip, and a jump, anthropologically speaking, to gas ranges, electric broilers, and microwave ovens. This chapter explains how these handy technologies affect the safety, nutritional value, appearance, flavour, and aroma of the foods that you heat.

For more (much, much more) detail on what and how to cook, check out *Cooking Basics For Dummies,* 3rd edition (written by Brian Miller, Marie Rama, Eve Adamson, and Wolfgang Puck), a compilation of the kind of no-nonsense, easy-to-follow instructions that you've come to expect from the big books with the yellow-and-black covers. If cutting fat and calories is your pleasure (or necessity), choose *Lowfat Cooking For Dummies,* by Lynn Fisher and W. Virgil Brown. Wiley publishes both books.

What's Cooking?

Ever since humankind discovered fire and how to control cooking — rather than having to wait for a passing thunderbolt — the human race has generally relied on three simple ways of heating food:

> ✔ **An open flame:** You hold the food directly over — or under — the flame or put the food on a griddle on top of the flame. The electric heating coil is a 20th-century variation on the open flame.

✔ **Hot air:** You put the food in a closed box (an oven) and heat the air in the oven to create high-temperature dry heat.

✔ **Hot liquid:** You submerge the food in hot liquid or suspend the food over the liquid so that it cooks in the steam escaping from the surface.

Cooking food in a wrapper such as aluminum foil combines two methods: open fire (the grill) or hot air (the oven) plus the steam from the food's own juices (hot liquid).

Here are the basic methods used to cook food with heat generated by fire or an electric coil:

Open Flame	*Hot Air*	*Hot Liquid*
Broiling	Baking	Boiling
Grilling	Roasting	Deep-frying
Toasting		Poaching
		Simmering
		Steaming
		Stewing

Cooking with electromagnetic waves

A gas or electric stove generates thermal energy (heat) that warms and cooks food. A microwave oven generates electromagnetic energy (microwaves) produced by a device called a magnetron (see Figure 20-1).

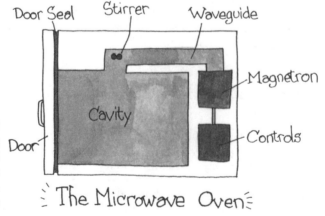

Figure 20-1: Your typical microwave oven.

TECHNICAL STUFF

How hot is boiling water?

Water is a molecule (H2O) composed of three atoms: two hydrogen and one oxygen. When water is exposed to energy (heat), some of the water molecules *vapourize* (or separate into their gaseous components). These vapours collect in tiny pockets at the bottom of the vessel (pot) in which the water's contained. Continued heating energizes the vapours, and they begin to push up against the water.

To break through the water's surface, the vapours must acquire enough energy to equal the force (pressure) of the atmosphere (air) pushing down on the water. The temperature at which this happens is called the *boiling point.*

At sea level (elevation: 0 metres), the atmosphere is heavier (has more oxygen) than at higher elevations. That's why you breathe more easily in Charlottetown, PEI (elevation: sea level), than in Banff, Alberta (elevation: 1,463 metres, or 4,800 feet).

The heavier air at sea level exerts more pressure against the surface of the water in your pot, so making the water boil takes more energy (higher heat).

At sea level, the boiling point of water is 100 degrees on the Celsius — C — scale (212 degrees on the Fahrenheit — F _ scale). As a general rule, the boiling point of water drops about half a degree Celsius (one degree Fahrenheit) for every 152.4-metre (500-foot) increase in altitude above sea level. In other words, at an altitude 152.4 metres (500 feet) above sea level, the boiling point for water is 99.4 degrees Celsius (211 degrees Fahrenheit); at 305 metres (1,000 feet), it's 98.9 degrees Celsius (210 degrees Fahrenheit).

The following chart shows the approximate boiling points for water in specific Canadian cities at specific altitudes.

Altitude	Place	Boiling Point °C	Boiling Point °F
Sea level	Charlottetown, PEI	100	212
75 m (246 feet)	Toronto, ON	99.45	211.5
577 m (1,893 feet)	Regina, SK	94.8	208
1,097 m (3,600 feet)	Kimberley, BC	96.3	205
1,534 m (5,033 feet)	Lake Louise, AB	92.2	198

Note: How fast the water is boiling does not affect the temperature; a slow boil (few bubbles) is as hot as a fast one (lots of bubbles).

Microwaves transmit energy that excites water molecules in food. The water molecules leap about like hyperactive 3-year-olds, producing friction, which then produces the heat that cooks the food. The dish holding food in a microwave oven generally stays cool because it has so few water molecules.

Cooking away contaminants

Many micro-organisms that live naturally in food are harmless or even beneficial. For example:

- *Lactobacilli* (lacto = milk; bacilli = rod-shaped bacteria) are used to digest sugars in milk and convert the milk to yogourt.

- Nontoxic moulds convert milk to blue cheese. The blue ribbons in the cheese are safe, edible mould.

Some organisms, however, carry the risk of food poisoning. For example:

- *Clostridium botulinum (C. botulinum),* a bad bug that thrives in the absence of air (as in low-acid canned food), produces the potentially fatal toxin that causes botulism.

- *Campylobacter jejuni (C. jejuni),* which flourishes in raw meat and poultry and unpasteurized milk, has been linked to Guillain-Barré syndrome, a paralytic illness that sometimes follows flu infection.

  Are you surprised to find out that, every year, an estimated 11 to 13 million Canadians experience diarrhea and other more serious symptoms of food-borne illness after eating food contaminated with such an organism? Health Canada estimates that food-borne illnesses cost Canadian health services, industry, and society as a whole between 12 and 15 billion dollars annually.

Although simply heating food to the temperatures shown in Table 20-2 is not a guaranteed protection against food-borne illness, cooking food thoroughly and keeping it hot (or chilling it quickly) after it has been cooked destroys many dangerous bugs or slows the rate at which they reproduce, thus reducing the risk. Table 20-1 lists some common *pathogens* (disease-causing organisms) linked to food-borne illnesses and notes the foods likely to harbour them; Table 20-2 shows the recommended safe cooking temperatures for various foods. Use a food thermometer to make sure you reach the recommended temps. Because some things are more complicated than they seem, read the directions that come with the thermometer to be sure you're doing it right. Really.

Although pathogens (disease-causing organisms) in food are equal-opportunity bad guys — anyone who eats food carrying them may get sick — they are most dangerous for the very young, the very old, and those whose immune systems have been weakened by illness or medication.

Converting between Fahrenheit and Celsius

Pssst! Here's how to convert temperatures from Fahrenheit (F) to Celsius (C) and back again:

1. Degrees Celcius = $\dfrac{(\text{degrees F} - 32)}{9} \times 5$

For example, to convert the Fahrenheit boiling point of water (212 degrees F) to the Celsius boiling point of water (100 degrees C):

$$\frac{(212 - 32) \times 5}{9} = 100$$

2. Degrees Fahrenheit = $\dfrac{(\text{degrees C}) \times 9}{5} + 32$

For example, to convert the Celsius boiling point of water (100 degrees C) to the Fahrenheit boiling point of water (212 degrees F):

$$\frac{(100 \times 9)}{5} + 32 = 212$$

Table 20-1	Disease-Causing Organisms in Food
The Bug	**Where You Find It**
Campylobacter jejuni	Raw meat and poultry, unpasteur-ized milk
Clostridium botulinum	Poorly processed canned low-acid foods or vacuum-packed smoked fish
Clostridium perfringens	Foods made from poultry or meat
E. coli	Raw beef
Listeria monocytogenes	Raw meat and seafood, raw milk, some raw cheeses
Salmonella bacteria	Poultry, meat, eggs, dried foods, dairy products
Staphylococcus aureus	Custards, egg, chicken, and tuna salads

Canadian Food Inspection Agency

Table 20-2	How Hot Is Safe?
This Food . . .	*Is Done (Generally Safe to Eat) When Cooked to This Internal Temperature*
Eggs and Egg Dishes	
Eggs	Cook until yolk and white are firm
Egg dishes	71°C (160°F)
Ground Meat and Meat Mixtures*	
Turkey, chicken	74°C (165°F)
Veal, beef, lamb, pork	74°C (165°F)
Fresh Beef*	
Medium rare	63°C (145°F)
Medium	71°C (160°F)
Well-done	77°C (170°F)
Fresh Pork	
Medium	71°C (160°F)
Well-done	77°C (170°F)
Poultry	
Chicken, whole	82°C (180°F)
Turkey, whole	82°C (180°F)
Poultry breasts, roasts	77°C (170°F)
Poultry thighs, wings	Cook until juices run clear
Stuffing (cooked in bird)**	74°C (165°F) on thermometer inserted into the centre of the stuffing**
Duck and goose	82°C (180°F)
Ham	
Fresh (raw)	71°C (160°F)
Precooked (to reheat)	60°C (140°F)

* Undercooked hamburger is a major source of the potentially lethal organism E. coli 0157:H7. To be safe, the internal temperature of the meat must read 74°C (165°F).
** After the bird is cooked, the stuffing should be removed immediately and stored separately in the refrigerator.
Canadian Partnership for Consumer Food Safety Education www.canfightbac.org

Two hours — and you're out!

Micro-organisms thrive on food at temperatures between 4 and 60 degrees Celsius or 40 and 140 degrees Fahrenheit (the cooking temperature that inactivates many — though not all — bad guys).

For maximum safety, follow Health Canada's Two-Hour Rule: After cooking the food to the proper temperature, never allow it to sit at temperatures between 4 and 60 degrees Celsius (40 and 140 degrees Fahrenheit) for more than two hours.

More questions about food safety? Call or click:

✔ Canadian Partnership for Consumer Food Safety Education
Phone 519-651-2466
Web site www.canfightbac.org

✔ Canadian Food Inspection Agency
Web site www.inspection.gc.ca

✔ Health Canada
Web site www.hc-sc.gc.ca

✔ Food Safety Network at the University of Guelph
Phone 866-503-7638
Web site (English) www.foodsafety network.ca/en/

Making Changes: How Cooking Affects Food

Cooking foods changes the way they feel, look, taste, and smell. In fact, the appetizing texture of food, its rich colour, intense flavour, and fragrant aroma all are products of, yes, that's right: cooking.

Cook me tender: Changing texture

Exposure to heat alters the structures of proteins, fats, and carbohydrates, so it changes food's *texture* (the way food particles are linked to make the food feel hard or soft). In other words, cooking can turn crisp carrots mushy and soft steak to shoe leather.

Protein

Proteins are made of very long molecules that sometimes fold over into accordion-like structures (see Chapter 6 for details about proteins). Although heating food doesn't lower its protein value, it does

✔ Break protein molecules into smaller fragments

✔ Cause protein molecules to unfold and form new bonds to other protein molecules

✔ Make proteins clump together

Need an example? Consider the egg. When you cook one, the long protein molecules in the white unfold, form new connections to other protein molecules, and link up in a network that tightens, then squeezes out moisture so the egg white hardens and turns opaque. The same unfold-link-squeeze reaction turns translucent poultry firm and white and makes gelatin set. The longer you heat proteins, the stronger the network becomes, and the tougher, or more solid, the food will be.

To see this work, scramble two eggs — one beaten and cooked plain and one beaten with milk and then cooked. Adding liquid (milk) makes squeezing out all the moisture more difficult for the protein network. So the egg with the added milk cooks up softer than the plain egg.

Fat

Heat melts fat, which can run off food, lowering the calorie count. In addition, cooking breaks down connective tissue — the supporting framework of the body, which includes some adipose (fatty) tissue — thus making the food softer and more pliable. You can see this most clearly when cooking fish. The fish flakes when it's done because its connective tissue has been destroyed.

When meat and poultry are stored after cooking, their fats continue to change, this time by picking up oxygen from the air. Oxidized fats have a slightly rancid taste more politely known as *warmed-over flavour.* You can slow — but not entirely prevent — this reaction by cooking and storing meat, fish, and poultry under a blanket of food rich in *antioxidants,* chemicals that prevent other chemicals from reacting with oxygen. Vitamin C is a natural antioxidant, so gravies and marinades made with tomatoes, citrus fruits, tart cherries, or blueberries slow the natural oxidation of fats in cooked or stored foods.

Carbohydrates

Cooking has different effects on simple carbohydrates and complex ones (if you're confused about carbohydrates, see Chapter 8). When heated

✔ Simple sugars — such as sucrose or the sugars on the surface of meat and poultry — caramelize, or melt and turn brown. (Think of crème caramel.)

✔ Starch, a complex carbohydrate, becomes more absorbent, which is why pasta expands and softens in boiling water.

✔ Some dietary fibres (plant cell walls, such as gums, pectins, hemicellulose) dissolve, so vegetables and fruits soften when cooked.

Grains: Split personality performers

In cooking, grains, such as corn, exhibit split personalities — part protein, part complex carbohydrates. When you boil an ear of corn, the protein molecules inside the kernels do the break-unfold-network dance (the molecules break their links, the protein unfolds, and the molecules form new links). At the same time, carbohydrate starch granules begin absorbing moisture and then soften.

The trick to boiling perfect corn is controlling this process, removing the corn from the water when starch granules have absorbed enough moisture to soften the kernels but before the protein network has tightened.

That's why cookbooks advise a short stay in the pot. But if you're a person who likes corn chewy, just let it boil away, 15 minutes, 30 minutes — you be the judge.

The last two reactions — absorption and dissolved cell walls — can improve the nutritional value of foods by making the nutrients inside previously fibre-stiffened cells more available to your body.

A less-beneficial effect of heat on carbs surfaced early in 2002 when Swedish researchers set off a nutritional hoo-ha with the announcement that exposing starchy carbohydrate foods — such as potatoes and bread — to the high heat of baking or frying produces *acrylamides,* a family of chemicals known to cause cancer in rats. Then things got worse when scientists at the City of Hope Cancer Research Center (Los Angeles) said that acrylamides could trigger cell changes that lead to cancer in human beings. But a 2003 analysis of data from a study of 987 cancer patients and 538 healthy "controls" conducted by researchers at Harvard School of Public Health and the Departments of Oncology-Pathology and Medical Epidemiology at Karolinska Institute in Stockholm shows no evidence of an increased risk of bowel, bladder, or kidney cancer among fans of fries and toast. And in June 2004, an expert panel at the National Toxicology Program of the National Institute of Environmental Health Sciences said the level of acrylamides in a normal Canadian diet — even one that includes baked and fried carbs — is too low to be carcinogenic. Fries on toast, anyone?

At a follow-up U.N.–sponsored meeting in Geneva, a group of really important international food scientists confirmed the Stockholm discovery of acrylamide in carbs but couldn't agree on what to do about it other than to call for another study, which showed up pretty quickly. By the end of the year, kitchen scientists agreed that moderate amounts of fries are safe. Nutritious, too. The most healthful potato, it's true, is one that hasn't been fried, but even when crisped to a fare-thee-well, 28 g (1 ounce) of potato chips nevertheless may still deliver up to 12 percent of the RDA for vitamin C, up to 7 percent of the RDA for folate, up to 4 percent of the RDA for iron, and more than a gram of dietary fibre. In other words, as one part of a varied diet, the chip may still be okay to dip. The problem is: Are you sure you can have just one? Or two? Or . . .

Enhancing flavour and aroma

Heat degrades (breaks apart) flavour and aroma chemicals. As a result, most cooked food has a more intense flavour and aroma than raw food.

A good example is the mustard oils that give cruciferous vegetables, such as cabbage and cauliflower, their distinctive (some may say offensive) odours. The longer you cook these vegetables, the worse they smell. On the other hand, heat destroys *diallyl disulfide,* which is the chemical that gives raw garlic its bite and bark. So cooked garlic tastes and smells milder than the raw version.

Altering the palette: Food colour

Carotenoids — the natural red and yellow pigments that make carrots and sweet potatoes orange and tomatoes red — are practically impervious to heat and the acidity or alkalinity of cooking liquids. No matter how you cook them or how long, carotenoids stay bright and sunny.

Cheeseburgers for your health: A hot story

When you heat fats, their molecules break apart into chemicals known as *free radicals,* molecule fragments that may hook up together to form potentially carcinogenic (cancer-causing) compounds. These compounds are produced in higher numbers at higher heats; the usual safe cutoff is around 260°C (500°F) — right before "broil" on the oven dial. Burned fat or smoking oil, for example, has more nasties than plain melted fat or oil that is warm but not smoking.

As a result, many nutritionists warn against eating the crisp, crinkly, absolutely yummy browned top layer of foods, especially burned meats, which in 1998 were tentatively linked to a higher risk of breast cancer in women. Of course, the theory has yet to be proven, and as is true with so much in modern nutrition, the story may be more complicated than it seems at first glance.

Why? Because in 1996, Martha Belury, of Purdue University, discovered that cheeseburgers — yes, cheeseburgers ... grilled, fried, broiled, whatever — are rich in CLA (short for conjugated linoleic acid), a form of an essential fatty acid (a topic discussed in Chapter 7).

In Belury's lab, CLA slowed or reversed skin, breast, and stomach cancers in mice at the three stages of tumour development: early, when the cell is first damaged; midway in the process, when precancerous cells multiply to form tumours; and late, when tumours begin to enlarge and spread to other organs.

Whether this benefit happens in people nobody knows, but it sure reminds me of the Woody Allen movie *Sleeper,* in which the hero wakes up at some point in the future to discover that corned beef sandwiches are health food. Hey, you can't make this stuff up!

Red to blue and back again

The following experiment lets you see colours change right before your very eyes. Gather

✔ 1 small can sliced beets

✔ 1 saucepan

✔ 3 small glass bowls

✔ 1 cup water

✔ 1 teaspoon baking soda

✔ 3 tablespoons white vinegar

Line up the glass bowls on your kitchen counter. Open the can. Remove six slices of beets. Put two slices in the first glass bowl and four slices in the saucepan. Put the rest of the beets from the can in a small container and refrigerate for dinner. No sense wasting good beets!

Mix the baking soda into the water and add this alkaline solution to the saucepan. Heat for 4 minutes; don't heat too high — the solution foams. Turn off the heat. Remove the beets from the pan. Put two slices each in the second and third glass bowls.

Ignore the second bowl. Add the vinegar (an acid) to the third bowl. Wait two minutes. Now look: The beets in the first bowl (straight from the can) should still be bright red. Alkaline compounds darken colours, so the beets in the second bowl, straight from the baking soda bath, should be almost navy blue. Acids reverse the reaction, so the beets in the third bowl, with added vinegar, should be heading back to bright red. Not yet? Add another tablespoon of vinegar.

Ain't chemistry grand?

You can't say the same for the other pigments in food: The other pigments that make food naturally red, green, or white react — usually for the worse — to heat, acids (such as wine, vinegar, or tomato juice), and basic (alkaline) chemicals (such as mineral water or baking soda and water). Here's a brief rundown on the colour changes that you can expect when you cook food:

✔ Red beets and cabbage get their colours from pigments called *anthocyanins*. Acids make these pigments redder. Alkaline solutions fade anthocyanins from red to bluish purple.

✔ Potatoes, cauliflower, rice, and white onions are white because they contain pigments called *anthoxanthins*. When anthoxanthins are exposed to alkaline chemicals (mineralized water or baking soda), they turn yellow or brownish. Acids prevent this reaction. Boil cauliflower florets in tomato juice, rinse off the juice, and you'll see — white cauliflower!

✔ Green veggies are coloured by *chlorophyll*, a pigment that reacts with acids in cooking water (or in the vegetable itself) to form *pheophytin*, a brown pigment. The only way to short-circuit this reaction is to protect the vegetables from acids. Old-time cooks added alkaline baking soda to the cooking water, but that increases the loss of certain vitamins (see "Protecting the Nutrients in Cooked Foods" later in this chapter) and softens the vegetables. Fast cooking at high heat or cooking in lots of water (which dilutes acids) lessens these colour changes.

✔ The natural red colour of fresh meat comes from *myoglobin* in the muscle tissue and *hemoglobin* in blood. When meat is heated, the pigment molecules are *denatured,* or broken into fragments. They lose oxygen and turn brown or — after long cooking — the really unappetizing grey characteristic of steam-table meats. This inevitable change is more noticeable in beef than in pork or veal because beef starts out naturally redder.

Choosing Cookware: How Pots and Pans Affect Food

A pot is a pot is a pot, right? No way! In fact, your choice of pots can affect the nutrient value of food by

✔ Adding nutrients to the food

✔ Slowing the natural loss of nutrients during cooking

✔ Actively increasing the loss of nutrients during cooking

In addition, some pots make the food's natural flavours and aromas more intense, which, in turn, can make the food more — or less — appetizing. Read on to find out how your pot can change your food. And vice versa.

Aluminum

Aluminum is lightweight and conducts heat well. That's good. But the metal

✔ Makes some aroma chemicals smellier (particularly those in the cruciferous vegetables — cabbage, broccoli, Brussels sprouts, and so on)

✔ Flakes off, turning white foods (such as cauliflower or potatoes) yellow or brownish

Early speculation aside, aluminum flaking is not hazardous to your health: Cooking with aluminum pots does not increase your risk for developing Alzheimer's disease. True, cooking salty or acidic foods (wine, tomatoes) in aluminum pots increases the flaking, but even then, the amount of aluminum you get from the pot is less than you get naturally every day from food and water.

Copper

Copper pots heat steadily and evenly. To take advantage of this property, many aluminum or stainless steel pots are made with a layer of copper sandwiched into the bottom. But naked copper is a potentially poisonous metal. That's why copper pots are lined with tin or stainless steel. Whenever you cook with copper, periodically check the lining of the pot. If it's damaged — meaning that you can see the orange copper peeking through the silvery lining — have the pot relined or throw it out.

Ceramics

The chief virtue of plain terra cotta (the orange clay that looks like red bricks) is its *porosity,* a fancy way of saying that terra cotta roasting and baking pans allow excess steam to escape while holding in just enough moisture to make bread so moist and chicken such tender pickings.

Decorated — or glazed — ceramic vessels are another matter. For one thing, the glaze makes the pot much less porous, so that meat or poultry cooked in a covered painted ceramic pan steams instead of roasts. The practical result: a soggy surface rather than a crisp one.

More important, some pigments used to paint or glaze the pots contain lead. To seal the decoration and prevent lead from leaching into food, the painted pots are *fired* (baked in an oven). If the pots are fired in an oven that isn't hot enough or if they aren't fired for a long enough time, lead will leach from ceramics when in contact with acidic foods, such as fruit juices or foods marinated in wine or vinegar.

Ceramics made in Canada, the United States, Japan, and Great Britain generally are considered safe, but for maximum protection, hedge your bets. Unless the pot comes with a tag or brochure that specifically says it's acid-safe, don't use it for cooking or storing foods. And always wash decorated ceramics by hand; repeated passes through the dishwasher can wear down the surface.

Copper and egg whites: A chemical team

When you whip an egg white, its proteins unfold, form new bonds, and create a network that holds air in. That's why the runny white turns into stable foam.

You can certainly whip egg whites successfully in a glass or ceramic bowl — chilled, and absolutely free of any fat, including egg yolk, which would prevent the proteins from linking tightly. But the best choice is copper: the ions (particles) flaking off the surface bind with and stabilize the foam. (Aluminum ions stabilize but darken the whites.)

But wait. Isn't copper toxic? (See Chapter 11.) Yes, but the amount you get in an occasional batch of whites is so small it's insignificant, safetywise.

Enamel ware

Enamelled pots are made of metal covered with *porcelain,* a fine translucent china. Enamel ware heats more slowly and less evenly than plain metal. A good-quality enamelled surface resists discolouration and does not react with food. But the enamel can chip, and it's easily marked or scratched by cooking utensils other than wood or hard plastic. If the surface chips and you can see the metal underneath, discard the pot lest metals flake into your food.

Glass

Glass is a neutral material that does not react with food. Two cautions with glass:

- ✔ Do not use a glass-and-metal pot in the microwave oven. The metal blocks microwaves. More important, it can cause *arcing* — a sudden electrical flare that may damage the oven and scare you out of your wits.

- ✔ Remember that glass breaks — sometimes all over the floor. Are you a person who often drops things? Pass on the glass.

Iron

Like aluminum, iron pots are a good news/bad news item. Iron conducts heat well and stays hot significantly longer than other pots. It's easy to clean. It lasts forever, and it releases iron ions into food, which may improve the nutritional value of dinner.

In 1985, nutrition researchers at Texas Tech University in Lubbock set out to measure the iron content of foods cooked in iron pots. Among their discoveries: Beef stew (0.7 milligrams of iron per 100 grams/3.5 ounces, raw) can end up with as much as 3.4 milligrams of iron per 100 grams after cooking slightly longer than an hour in an iron pot.

Alas! There's a downside. The iron that flakes off the pot may be a form of the mineral that your body can't absorb. Also, more iron is not necessarily better. It encourages oxidation (bad for your body) and can contribute to excess iron storage in people who have *hemochromatosis,* a condition that leads to iron buildup that may damage internal organs.

By the way, did I mention that pumping iron is not a bad way to describe the experience of cooking with iron pots? They're really, really heavy.

Nonstick

Nonstick surfaces are made of plastic (polytetrafluoroethylene to be exact; PTFE for short) plus perfluorooctanoic acid (PFOA), a synthetic chemical used to make nonstick coating — chemicals that make the surface, well, hard. As long as the surface is unscratched and intact, the nonstick surface does not react with food.

Nonstick pots are a dieter's delight. They enable you to cook without added fat, but using them may also lighten your wallet. They scratch easily. Unless you stick scrupulously to wooden or plastic spoons, your pot can end up looking like chickens have been stomping on the surface.

Note: Scratched nonstick pots and pans are not a health hazard. If you swallow tiny pieces of the nonstick coating, they pass through your body undigested.

Health Canada has determined that nonstick coatings are safe for use at temperatures less than 350°C (662°F). However, when nonstick surfaces get very hot, they may

- ✔ Separate from the metal to which they're bound (the sides and bottom of the pot)

- ✔ Emit odourless fumes

  If your kitchen is not properly ventilated, this may cause *polymer fume fever* — flulike symptoms with no known long-term effect. To prevent this, keep the stove flame moderate and the windows open.

Many manufacturers in the U.S. are planning to phase out the use of PFOA entirely by the year 2015.

Stainless steel

Stainless steel is an alloy, a substance composed of two or more metals. Its virtues are hardness and durability; its drawback is poor heat conduction. In addition, the alloy includes nickel, a metal to which many people are sensitive. Finally, stainless steel isn't *really* stainless. When exposed to high heat, stainless steel develops a characteristic multi-hued "rainbow" discolouration. Starchy foods, such as pasta and potatoes, may darken the pot. Undissolved salt can pit the surface. Sorry about that!

If your stainless steel pot is scratched deeply enough to expose the inner layer under the shiny surface, the metals in the alloy may flake into your food. So toss the pot.

Plastic and paper

Plastic melts and paper burns, so you obviously can't use plastic or paper containers in a stove with an open flame (gas) or heat source (electric). But can you use them in the microwave? You bet! As long as you pick a proper plastic.

When plastic dishes or plastic wrap are heated in a microwave oven, they may emit potentially carcinogenic compounds that can migrate into your food. To reduce your exposure to these compounds, choose only plastic containers labelled "for microwave oven use." Thin plastic storage bags, margarine tubs, and whipped topping bowls are convenient, but way, way off-limits.

The Food and Drugs Act and Regulations of Health Canada control the safety of all materials used for packaging foods. The Act aims to ensure that food is packaged in materials that are safe and that won't leach chemicals into the food. The limitation of the Act is that it places this responsibility on the man-ufacturer of any packaged food.

The Canadian Plastics Industry Association offers the following guidelines on their Web site (www.cpia.ca):

✔ **Only cook or reheat foods in containers intended for microwave use.** These containers are designed to withstand the high temperatures pos-sible when the foods you're heating contain fat or sugar.

✔ **Remove food from store wrap before thawing or reheating in a microwave oven unless the manufacturer indicates that it's meant for microwave use.** Some plastic trays, wraps, or containers can melt or warp when the food gets hot, which could cause spills and burns.

✔ **Understand that most cold-food packages — such as margarine tubs, cottage cheese containers, and foam meat trays — aren't intended for microwave use.**

✔ **Place plastic wraps over bowls or dishes during rewarming to help keep moisture in and provide even cooking.** Wrap that touches the food could get overly hot and possibly melt.

✔ **Be sure to carefully follow the manufacturer's directions when microwaving.**

Because Health Canada requires microwave-safe plastics to meet strict safety standards, repeated studies show no ill effects from their minimal leakage. On the other hand, if even very small exposure makes you edgy, you can switch to glass or ceramic dishes that are made specifically to be used in microwave ovens. Splatter-proof the dish with wax paper, parchment paper, or white paper towels labelled safe for microwave use.

Protecting the Nutrients in Cooked Foods

Myth: All raw foods are more nutritious than cooked ones.

Fact: Some foods (such as meat, poultry, and eggs) are positively dangerous when consumed raw (or undercooked). Other foods are less nutritious raw because they contain substances that destroy or disarm other nutrients. For example, raw dried beans contain enzyme inhibitors that interfere with the work of enzymes that enable your body to digest protein. Heating disarms the enzyme inhibitor.

But there's no denying that some nutrients are lost when foods are cooked. Simple strategies such as steaming food rather than boiling, or broiling rather than frying, can significantly reduce the loss of nutrients when you're cooking food.

Maintaining minerals

Virtually all minerals are unaffected by heat. Cooked or raw, food has the same amount of calcium, phosphorus, magnesium, iron, zinc, iodine, selenium, copper, manganese, chromium, and sodium. The single exception to this rule is potassium, which — although not affected by heat or air — escapes from foods into the cooking liquid.

Those volatile vitamins

With the exception of vitamin K and the B vitamin niacin, which are very stable in food, many vitamins are sensitive and are easily destroyed when exposed to heat, air, water, or fats (cooking oils). Table 20-3 shows which nutrients are sensitive to these influences.

Table 20-3	What Takes Nutrients Out of Food?			
Nutrient	*Heat*	*Air*	*Water*	*Fat*
Vitamin A	X			X
Vitamin D				X
Vitamin E	X	X		X
Vitamin C	X	X	X	
Thiamin	X		X	

(continued)

Table 20-3 (continued)

Nutrient	Heat	Air	Water	Fat
Riboflavin			X	
Vitamin B6	X	X	X	
Folate	X	X		
Vitamin B12	X		X	
Biotin			X	
Pantothenic acid	X			
Potassium			X	

To avoid specific types of vitamin loss, keep in mind the following tips:

- **Vitamins A, E, and D:** To reduce the loss of fat-soluble vitamins A and E, cook with very little oil. For example, bake or broil vitamin A–rich liver oil free instead of frying. Ditto for vitamin D–rich fish.

- **B vitamins:** Strategies that conserve protein in meat and poultry during cooking also work to conserve the B vitamins that leak out into cooking liquid or drippings: Use the cooking liquid in soup or sauce. *Caution:* Do not shorten cooking times or use lower temperatures to lessen the loss of heat-sensitive vitamin B12 from meat, fish, or poultry. These foods and their drippings must be thoroughly cooked to ensure that they're safe to eat.

  Do not rinse grains (rice) before cooking unless the package advises you to do so (some rice does need to be rinsed). Washing rice once may take away as much as 25 percent of the thiamin (vitamin B1). Toast or bake cakes and breads only until the crust is light brown to preserve heat-sensitive Bs.

- **Vitamin C:** To reduce the loss of water-soluble, oxygen-sensitive vitamin C, cook fruits and vegetables in the least possible amount of water. For example, when you cook 1 cup of cabbage in 4 cups of water, the leaves lose as much as 90 percent of their vitamin C. Reverse the ratio — one cup water to 4 cups cabbage — and you hold on to more than 50 percent of the vitamin C.

  Serve cooked vegetables quickly: After 24 hours in the fridge, vegetables lose one-fourth of their vitamin C; after two days, nearly half.

  Root vegetables (carrots, potatoes, sweet potatoes) baked or boiled whole, in their skins, retain about 65 percent of their vitamin C.

Chapter 21

What Happens When Food Is Frozen, Canned, Dried, or Zapped

. . . .

In This Chapter

▶ Freezing food safely

▶ Creating canned food

▶ Explaining the ancient art of drying food

▶ Using radiation to protect food

. . . .

Cold air, hot air, no air, and radioactive rays all can be used to make food safer for longer periods of time by reducing or eliminating damage from exposure to air or organisms (microbes) that live on food.

The methods described in this chapter all have one important thing in common: Used correctly, each process can dramatically lengthen a food's shelf life. The downside? Nothing's perfect, so you still have to monitor your food to make sure that the preservation treatment has, well, preserved it. The following pages tell you how.

Cold Comfort: Chilling and Freezing

Keeping food cold, sometimes very cold, slows or suspends the activity of microbes bent on digesting your food before you do.

Unlike heat, which actually kills many of the microbes (see Chapter 20), chilling food (or freezing it) may not kill all the microbes, but the cold will reduce the microbial population to some degree, depending on the microflora present, and will sideline the microbes for a while. For example, *mould spores* (hibernating mould organisms) snuggle inside frozen food to sleep quietly like so many comfy bears inside a wintry cave. When spring comes, the bears bounce back to life; thaw the food, and the mould does the same.

How long things stay safe in the refrigerator or freezer varies from food to food and to some extent on the packaging (better packaging, longer freezing time). Table 21-1 provides a handy guide to the limits of safe cool storage. These ranges depend on foods being fresh to start out and on the refrigerator/freezer maintaining a constant temperature. Whenever these conditions aren't met, food may spoil more quickly. Use your common sense: If food seems in any way questionable, *throw it out without tasting.* Or as the catchy saying goes: When in doubt, throw it out.

Table 21-1   How Long Foods Generally Stay Safe in Cold Storage

Food	Refrigerator (4°C or 40°F)	Freezer (–18°C or 0°F)
Eggs		
Fresh, in shell	See best before date (about 3 weeks)	Don't freeze
Raw yolks, whites	2–4 days	4 months
Hard cooked	5–7 days	Don't freeze well
Liquid pasteurized eggs or egg substitutes, opened	3 days	Don't freeze well
Liquid pasteurized eggs or egg substitutes, unopened	See best before date (about 2 weeks)	1 year
Mayonnaise, Commercial		
Unopened jar	See best before date	Don't freeze
Open jar	2 months	Don't freeze
TV Dinners, Frozen Casseroles		
As originally packed, until ready to serve	Don't refrigerate: Keep frozen	3–4 months
Deli and Vacuum-Packed Products		
Prestuffed pork and lamb chops, chicken breasts stuffed with dressing	1 day	Don't freeze well
Store-cooked convenience meals	1–2 days	Don't freeze well
Soups and Stews		
Vegetable or meat-added	3–4 days	4 months

Food	Refrigerator (4°C or 40°F)	Freezer (–18°C or 0°F)
Ground Meats and Stew Meats		
Hamburger and stew meats	1–2 days	2–3 months
Ground turkey, veal, pork, lamb, and mixtures of these meats	1–2 days	2–3 months
Hot Dogs** and Lunch Meats*		
Hot dogs, opened	3–5 days	In freezer wrap, 1–2 months
Hot dogs, unopened	2 weeks	In freezer wrap, 1–2 months
Lunch meats, opened	3–5 days	In freezer wrap, 1–2 months
Lunch meats, unopened	2 weeks	In freezer wrap, 1–2 months
Bacon and Sausage		
Bacon*	7 days	1–2 months
Sausage, raw — pork, beef, turkey	1–2 days	2–3 months
Smoked breakfast links, patties	7 days	1–2 months
Hard sausage — pepperoni, jerky sticks	2–3 weeks	1–2 months
Ham, Corned Beef		
Corned beef in pouch with pickling juices*	5–7 days	Drained and wrapped, 1 month
Ham, canned, label says to keep refrigerated	6–9 months	Don't freeze
Ham, fully cooked — whole	7 days	1–2 months
Ham, fully cooked — half	3–5 days	1–2 months
Ham, fully cooked — slices	3–4 days	1–2 months

(continued)

Table 21-1 *(continued)*

Food	Refrigerator (4°C or 40°F)	Freezer (−18°C or 0°F)
Fresh Meat		
Steaks — beef	2–3 days	6–9 months
Chops — pork	2–3 days	6–9 months
Chops — lamb	2–3 days	6–9 months
Roast — beef	2–4 days	6–9 months
Roast — lamb	2–4 days	6–9 months
Roast — pork, veal	2–4 days	4–5 months
Cooked Meat, Leftovers		
Meat, meat dishes	2–3 days	2–3 months
Gravy, broth	1–2 days	2–3 months
Variety meats — tongue, brain, kidneys, liver, heart, chitterlings	1–2 days	3–4 months
Fish & Shellfish		
Fish, raw (cleaned)	1–2 days	
Fat species (salmon, mackerel, trout, herring)	1–2 days	2 months
Lean species (cod, haddock, pike)	1–2 days	6 months
Fish, cooked	3–4 days	Doesn't freeze well
Crabs, clams, lobsters, mussels (live)	12–24 hours	Don't freeze
Oysters (live)	1 week	Don't freeze
Scallops, shrimps (fresh)	1–2 days	2–4 months
Shellfish (cooked)	1–2 days	2–4 months
Salmon, smoked	1–2 days	Don't freeze
Kippered cod, whiting, smoked	6–7 days	Don't freeze
Fresh Poultry		
Chicken or turkey, whole	1–2 days	1 year
Pieces	1–2 days	6 months
Giblets	1–2 days	3–4 months

Food	Refrigerator (4°C or 40°F)	Freezer (–18°C or 0°F)
Cooked Poultry, Leftover		
Chicken, fried	2–3 days	1–3 months
Casseroles	2–3 days	1–3 months
Pieces, plain	2–3 days	1–3 months
Pieces, with broth or gravy	1–2 days	6 months
Chicken, nuggets, patties	1–2 days	1–3 months

*Follow date on package.
**Caution: Even when food is in date and has been properly refrigerated, always boil or broil hot dogs to an internal temperature of 74°C (165°F).
Sources: www.eggs.ca; Health Link Alberta, www.healthlinkalberta.ca; "Food Storage in the Home," (www.homefamily.net); Food Safety and Inspection Service, "A Quick Consumer's Guide to Safe Food Handling," Home and Garden Bulletin, No. 248 (U.S. Department of Agriculture, August 1995)

How freezing affects the texture of food

When food freezes, the water inside each cell forms tiny crystals that can tear cell walls. When the food is thawed, the liquid inside the cell leaks out, leaving thawed food dryer than fresh food.

Beef that has been frozen, for example, is noticeably drier than fresh beef. Dry cheeses, such as Cheddar, turn crumbly. Bread dries, too. You can reduce the loss of moisture by thawing the food in its freezer wrap so that it has a chance to reabsorb the lost moisture, which is still in the package.

What's that brown spot on my burger?

Freezer burn is a dry brownish spot left when moisture evaporates from the surface of frozen food. Because freezer burn changes the composition of fats on the surface of foods such as meat and poultry, it may cause some change in flavour, as well.

To prevent freezer burn, wrap food securely in freezer paper or aluminum foil and seal in a plastic bag. The more air you keep out, the fewer brown spots will develop.

You can't restore the crispness of cooked vegetables that get their crunch from stiff, high-fibre cell walls. After ice crystals puncture the walls, the vegetable (carrots are a good example) turns mushy. The solution? Remove carrots and other crunchies, such as cabbage, before freezing the stew.

Refreezing frozen food

The official word from the Food Safety Network (a collaboration of the Food Safety Network at Kansas State University and the University of Guelph in Ontario) is that you can refreeze frozen food — as long as the food still has ice crystals or feels refrigerator-cold to the touch.

Although some people may feel safer just throwing out any partially thawed food, the experts at the universities know their stuff. Be sure to follow general food safety guidelines, and be sure that foods are cooked to the recommended internal temperatures (see Chapter 20 for more details).

Canning Food: Keeping Out Contaminants

Food is canned by heating what goes into the container, then sealing the container to keep out air and microbes, then heating the sealed can or jar. Like cooked food, canned food is subject to changes in appearance and nutritional content. Heating food often changes its colour and texture (see Chapter 20). It also destroys some vitamin C. But canning effectively destroys a variety of pathogens, and it deactivates enzymes that could otherwise harm the food.

A modern variation on canning is the sealed plastic or aluminum bag known as the *retort pouch*. Food sealed in the pouch is heated, but for a shorter period than that required for canning. As a result, the pouch method does a better job of preserving flavour, appearance, and heat-sensitive vitamin C.

The sealed can or pouch also protects food from deterioration caused by light or air, so the seal must remain intact. When the seal is broken, air seeps into the can or pouch, spoiling the food.

A more serious hazard associated with canned food is *botulism,* a potentially fatal form of food poisoning caused by the failure to heat the food to high-enough temperatures or for a long-enough time to kill all *Clostridium botulinum* (or *C. botulinum*) bacteria. Canning is based on temperatures and times necessary to destroy *C. bot* spores. *C. botulinum* is an *anaerobic* (an = without; aerobic = air) organism that thrives in the absence of oxygen, a condition nicely fulfilled by a sealed can. *Botulinum* spores not destroyed by high heat during the canning process may produce a toxin that can kill by paralyzing your heart muscles and the muscles that enable you to breathe.

The essence of canned food

The technique of canning food in glass containers was discovered (depending on your source) in either 1809 or 1810 by Nicholas Appert, a Frenchman who noted that if he sealed food in a container while it was heating, the food stayed edible longer — much longer — than fresh food. According to Harold McGee, author of *On Food and Cooking: The Science and Lore of the Kitchen* (Simon & Schuster), a wonderful guide to food technology, a tin of 114-year-old canned meat once was eaten without making anyone sick. Of course, nobody cried, "Oh, wow, this is good," either.

According to Joseph Nathan Kane's *Famous First Facts* (H.W. Wilson Company), the first foods canned in tin — salmon, oysters, and lobsters — were introduced in 1819 by New Yorkers Ezra Daggett and Thomas Kensett. Four years later, Daggett and Kensett took out a patent to "preserve animal substances in tin." New York inventor J. Osterhoudt patented the first can with a key opener on October 2, 1866. (For the most part, keys have been replaced by pull tabs.) The first beer in cans (from the Gottfried Krueger Brewing Company of Newark, New Jersey) went on sale on January 24, 1935, in Richmond, Virginia. Pop!

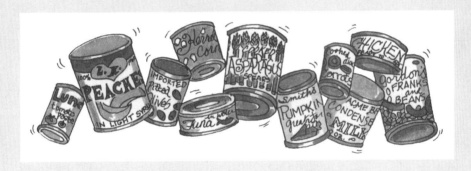

To avoid potentially hazardous canned food, do not buy, store, or use any can that is

✔ Swollen, which indicates that bacteria are growing inside and producing gas

✔ Damaged, rusted, or deeply dented along the seam, because a break in the can permits air to enter and may promote the growth of organisms (other than *botulinum*)

Consumer alert: Never, never, *never* taste any food from a swollen or damaged can "just to see if it's all right." ***Remember:*** When in doubt, throw it out.

Drying Food: No Life without Water

Drying protects food by removing the moisture that bacteria, yeasts, and moulds need to live. Drying is an ancient technique, used to produce the famous dates of the desert and the dried meat of the North American plains.

Drying food the low-tech way means putting it out in the sun and waiting for it to dry on its own. Drying food the high-tech, modern way means putting food out on racks and employing fans to quick-dry the food at a low temperature under vacuum pressure.

Another form of drying is spray drying. *Spray drying* is a technique used to dry liquids, such as milk, by blowing the liquids (in very small droplets) into a heated chamber where the droplets dry into a powder that can be reconstituted (made back into a liquid) by adding water. Instant coffee is a spray-dried product. So are instant teas and all the various instant fruit beverages.

How drying affects food's nutritional value

As always, exposure to heat and/or air (oxygen) reduces a food's vitamin C content, so dried foods have less vitamin C than fresh foods.

One good example is the plum versus the prune (a dried plum):

- One fresh, medium-size plum, weighing 66 grams (a bit more than 2 ounces) without the pit, has 6 milligrams of vitamin C, 7 to 8 percent of the Recommended Dietary Allowance for a healthy adult.

- An equivalent amount of uncooked dried (low-moisture) prunes (66 grams) has only 1.3 milligrams of vitamin C.

But wait! Before you leap to the conclusion that fresh is always more nutritious than dried, feed these facts into your memory banks: Dried fruit has less water than fresh fruit. That means its weight reflects more solid fruit. Although drying destroys some vitamin C, removing water concentrates what's left, along with other nutrients, jamming more calories, dietary fibre, and/or air-resistant vitamins and minerals into a smaller space.

As a result, dried food often has surprisingly more nutritional bounce to the ounce than fresh food. Once again, consider the plum and the prune:

- A medium-size, pit-free plum weighing 66 grams — slightly more than 2 ounces — provides 35 calories, 0.1 milligram of iron, and 670 IU (67 RE) of vitamin A. (What's IU? What's RE? Check out Chapter 4.)

✔ In 66 grams (almost 2 ounces) of uncooked, low-moisture prunes, there are about 193 calories, 2 milligrams of iron, and 952 IU (72 RE) of vitamin A. In other words, if you're trying to lose weight, you need to be aware that although dried fruit is low in fat and rich in nutrients, it's also high in calories.

When dried fruit may be hazardous to your health

Many fruits contain an enzyme (polyphenoloxidase) that darkens the fruit flesh when the fruit is exposed to air. To prevent the darkening, the fruits are treated with sulphur compounds known as sulphites. The sulphites — sulphur dioxide, sodium bisulphite, sodium metabisulphite — can cause potentially serious allergic reactions in sensitive individuals. For more about sulphites, see Chapter 22.

Irradiating What We Eat: A Hot Topic

Irradiation is a technique that exposes food to electron beams or gamma radiation, a high-energy light stronger than the X-rays your doctor uses to make a picture of your insides. Gamma rays are ionizing radiation, the kind of radiation that kills living cells. Ionizing radiation can sterilize food or at least prolong its shelf life by

✔ Killing microbes and insects on plants (wheat, wheat powder, spices, dry vegetable seasonings)

✔ Killing disease-causing organisms on pork *(Trichinella),* poultry *(Salmonella),* and ground beef (pathogenic *E. coli)*

✔ Preventing potatoes and onions from sprouting during storage

✔ Slowing the rate at which some fruits ripen

Irradiation does not change the way food looks or tastes. It does not change food texture. It does not make food radioactive. It does, however, alter the structure of some chemicals in foods, breaking molecules apart to form new substances called *radiolytic products* (radio = radiation; lytic = break).

About 90 percent of all compounds identified as radiolytic products (RP) also are found in raw, heated, and/or stored foods that have not been deliberately exposed to ionizing radiation. A few compounds, called *unique radiolytic products* (URPs), are found only in irradiated foods.

Are irradiated foods harmful?

Many scientific organizations, including the 27,000-member Institute of Food Technologists and an international Expert Committee on the Wholesomeness of Irradiated Foods (which includes representatives from the United Nations, the International Atomic Energy Agency, and the World Health Organization), believe that irradiation is a safe and important weapon in the fight against food poisoning caused by microbial and parasitic contamination.

Health Canada has been approving various uses of food irradiation since 1960. In addition, irradiation is approved for more than 40 food products in more than 37 countries around the world. Fifty-one percent of Canadians surveyed in 2000 said they approved of the use of irradiation for the prevention of food-borne illness; 42 percent disagreed and stated they wouldn't buy irradiated food because they thought it was unsafe.. Before a food can be listed in the *Food and Drug Regulations* as safe to irradiate, it must be accepted through an application process to evaluate the effects of irradiation on the proposed food's nutritional content and food safety.

Some consumers, however, remain leery of irradiation, fearful that it may expose them to radiation (it can't; no radioactive residues are present in irradiated food) or that URPs (unique radiolytic products) — compounds produced only when foods are irradiated — may eventually turn out to be harmful. For now, irradiated food seems safe, but it's fair to point out that the story of irradiating foods is still unfolding, a situation that makes many people uneasy.

Around the world, all irradiated packaged food is identified with an international symbol. Just in case that isn't enough to get the message across, the package must also carry the words "treated by irradiation" or "treated with irradiation." If the food isn't packaged, then there needs to be a visible sign with this information displayed near the food itself. The only exception is commercially produced food that contains some irradiated ingredients such as spices. If the total amount of that ingredient is less than 10 percent of the finished product, it is exempt from being labeled as such, If the irradiated ingredient makes up more than 10 percent, then the product must state that the ingredient in the ingredient list has been irradiated. The symbol and/or wording isn't required, for example, on the packaging for a frozen pizza that's seasoned with irradiated oregano if the amount of oregano is less than 10 percent of the whole pizza.

You can get answers online to the most commonly asked questions about food irradiation at the Canadian Food Inspection Agency Web site, www.inspection.gc.ca/english/fssa/concen/tipcon/irrade.shtml, as well as Health Canada's site, www.hc-sc.gc.ca/fn-an/securit/irridation/index_e.html. Another good reference is the Web site maintained by the Centers for Disease Control and Prevention in the U.S. (CDC): www.cdc.gov/ncidod/dbmd/diseaseinfo/foodirradiation.htm.

Table 21-2 tells you when certain irradiated foods were deemed safe in Canada.

Table 21-2	Foods Approved for Irradiation in Canada
Food	*Approval date*
Potatoes	November 9, 1960
Onions	March 25, 1965
Wheat, wheat flour	February 25,1969
Spices	October 3, 1984
Vegetables seasonings (dried)	October 3, 1984
Herbs	October 3, 1984

Health Canada, Canadian Food Inspection Agency

Ground beef, mangoes poultry, shrimp, and prawns are currently under review to be approved for irradiation by Health Canada.

Is that food still good to eat? Understanding the dates on food labels

The following terms can help you decide when to check whether your food's still good:

✔ **Sell-by:** The last date on which the food can be offered for sale. If stored properly, most perishable foods such as milk, cheese, and packaged meats are safe for a few days past the sell-by date.

✔ **Best if used by or Use by:** Refers to the food's flavour and quality, not its safety; the manufacturer's recommendation of the last date on which the food is likely to taste best.

✔ **Expires or Do not use after:** The last date on which a product either provides the highest nutritional value or works best (for instance, the last date on which yeast or baking powder is likely to make your bread or cake rise).

Chapter 22

Better Eating through Chemistry

In This Chapter

▶ Understanding food additives

▶ Considering additives that cause health problems

▶ Creating new foods with biotechnology

*I*f the title of this chapter turns you off, you're not alone. More people than you can shake a stick — heck, a whole oak tree — at think that when you're talking food, natural's good and chemical's bad. Period. But it ain't necessarily so.

This chapter is about the natural *and* synthetic ingredients and the technological processes that help make food more nutritious; enhance its appearance, flavour, and texture; and keep it fresh on the shelf longer. More to the point, this chapter explains that without these products and processes, human beings would still have to gather (or kill) dinner fresh each day and serve it up fast before it spoils.

And, yes, this chapter talks about new and unusual processes, such as genetic engineering (which we discuss in the section "Looking Beyond Additives: Foods Nature Never Made" at the end of this chapter). Try it. You may like it.

Exploring the Nature (And Science) of Food Additives

What are food additives? Here's a really simple definition: *Food additives* are substances added to food. But not everything that's added to food is considered a food additive. Food additives are regulated under the *Food and Drug Regulations* and don't include such things as vitamins, minerals, amino acids (building blocks of protein), veterinary drugs like growth hormones, or flavour enhancers such as spices and herbs or sugar and salt. The list of common food additives includes

- ✔ Antioxidants
- ✔ Colouring agents
- ✔ Gelling agents
- ✔ Some flavours and flavour enhancers (such as artificial and natural flavourings)
- ✔ Preservatives

Food additives may be natural or synthetic. For example, vitamin C is a natural preservative. Butylated hydroxyanisole (BHA) and butylated hydroxytoluene (BHT) are synthetic preservatives. Many people think natural additives are safer than synthetic ingredients, probably because "synthetic" seems synonymous with "chemical," a sort of scary word. Besides, synthetic additives often have names no one can pronounce, much less translate, which makes them even more forbidding.

In fact, every single thing in the world is made of chemicals: your body, the air you breathe, the paper on which this book is printed, and the glasses through which you read it, not to mention every single bite of food you eat and every mouthful of beverage you drink.

To ensure your safety, the natural *and* synthetic food additives used in Canada must meet Canadian regulatory standards. Health Canada has created a list of all approved food additives and their approved uses, referred to as the "Food Additive Dictionary." This is found in Division 16 of the *Food and Drug Regulations* and is available on Health Canada's Web site (`www.hc-sc.gc.ca/index_e.html`).

All additives in the Food Additive Dictionary

- ✔ Are approved by Health Canada, meaning that it is satisfied the additive is safe and effective
- ✔ Must be used only in specifically limited amounts
- ✔ Must be used to satisfy a specific need in food products, such as protection against moulds
- ✔ Must be effective, meaning that they must actually maintain freshness and safety
- ✔ Must be listed accurately on the label

Adding nutrients

Some nutrients also are useful preservatives. For example, vitamin C is an antioxidant that slows food spoilage and prevents destructive chemical reactions. Manufacturers must add a form of vitamin C *(isoascorbic acid)* to bacon to prevent the formation of potentially cancer-causing compounds.

Another example of a nutrient that can be added to food for reasons other than enhancing your health is riboflavin, which is also known as vitamin B2. This vitamin is often added because it gives food a distinctive yellow colour. Some nutrients, such as ferrous sulphate (a form of iron), are added to food as a nutrient for organisms, such as yeast, that are used in food production. Yeasts make breads rise, and they need iron to thrive; the iron added to bread is for them, not you!

Adding colours and flavours

Colours, flavouring agents, and flavour enhancers make food look and taste better. Like other food additives, these three may be either natural or synthetic.

Colours

Colouring agents make food look better. An example of a natural colouring agent is *beta carotene,* the natural yellow pigment in many fruits and vegetables. Beta carotene is used to make margarine (which is naturally white) look like creamy yellow butter. Other natural colouring agents are *annatto,* a yellow-to-pink pigment from a tropical tree; *chlorophyll,* the green pigment in green plants; *carmine,* a reddish extract of *cochineal* (a pigment from crushed beetles); *saffron,* a yellow herb; and *turmeric,* a yellow spice.

An example of a synthetic colouring agent is FD&C Blue No. 1, a bright blue pigment made from coal tar and used in soft drinks, gelatin, hair dyes, and face powders, among other things. And, yes, as scientists have discovered more about the effects of coal-tar dyes, including the fact that some are carcinogenic, many of these colouring agents have been banned from use in food but are still allowed in cosmetics.

To avoid these dyes entirely, read the label and choose foods made with only natural colours.

Alphabet soup: Understanding artificial colours

When you read the label on a food, drug, or cosmetic product containing artificial colours, you may see the letters *F, D,* and *C* — as in FD&C Yellow No. 5. The *F* stands for food. The *D* stands for drugs. The *C* stands for cosmetics. An additive whose name includes all three letters can be used in food, drugs, and cosmetics. An additive without the *F* is restricted to use in drugs and cosmetics or is for external use only (translation: You don't take the products by mouth). For example, D&C Green No. 6 is a blue-green colouring agent used in hair oils and pomades. FD&C Blue No. 2 is a bright blue colouring agent used in hair rinses, as well as mint jellies, candies, and cereals.

Flavours and flavour enhancers

Every cook worth his or her spice cabinet knows about natural flavour ingredients, especially the most basic natural ones: salt, sugar, vinegar, wine, and fruit juices.

Artificial flavouring agents reproduce natural flavours. For example, a teaspoon of fresh lemon juice in the batter lends cheesecake a certain *je ne sais quoi* (French for "I don't know what" — a little something special), but artificial lemon flavouring works just as well. You can sweeten your morning coffee with natural sugar or with the artificial sweetener saccharin. (For more about substitute sweeteners, see Chapter 19.)

Flavour enhancers are a slightly different kettle of fish. They intensify a food's natural flavour instead of adding a new one. The best-known flavour enhancer is *monosodium glutamate (MSG),* which is widely used in Asian foods. MSG may trigger headaches and other symptoms in people sensitive to the seasoning.

Adding preservatives

Food spoilage is a totally natural phenomenon. Milk sours. Bread sprouts mould. Meat and poultry rot. Vegetables lose moisture and wilt. Fats turn rancid. The first three kinds of spoilage are caused by *microbes* (bacteria, mould, and yeasts). The last two happen when food is exposed to *oxygen* (air).

All preservative techniques — cooking, chilling, canning, freezing, drying — prevent spoilage either by slowing the growth of the organisms that live on food or by protecting the food from the effects of oxygen. Chemical preservatives do essentially the same thing:

✔ *Antimicrobials* are natural or synthetic preservatives that protect food by slowing the growth of bacteria, moulds, and yeasts.

✔ *Antioxidants* are natural or synthetic preservatives that protect food by preventing food molecules from combining with oxygen (air).

Table 22-1 is a representative list of some common preservative chemicals and the foods in which they're found.

Table 22-1	Preservatives in Food
Preservative	*Found in . . .*
Ascorbic acid	Sausages, luncheon meats, flour
Benzoic acid	Beverages (soft drinks), ice cream, baked goods
BHA (butylated hydroxyanisole)	Potato chips and other foods
BHT (butylated hydroxytoluene)	Potato chips and other foods
Calcium propionate	Breads, processed cheese
Guar gum	Yogourt, sour cream, cream cheese
Sodium ascorbate	Luncheon meats and other foods
Xylitol	Chewing gum, protein and energy bars

Food Additive Dictionary, Health Canada, 2007

Naming some other additives in food

Food chemists use various types of natural and chemical additives to improve the texture of food, to keep it smooth, or to prevent mixtures from separating:

✔ *Emulsifiers,* such as lecithin and polysorbate, keep liquid-plus-solids such as chocolate pudding from separating into, well, liquid and solids. They can also keep two unfriendly liquids, such as oil and water, from divorcing so that your salad dressing stays smooth.

✔ *Stabilizers,* such as the alginates (alginic acid) derived from seaweed, make foods such as ice cream feel smoother, richer, or creamier in your mouth.

✔ *Thickeners* are natural gums and starches, such as apple pectin or cornstarch, that add body to foods.

✔ *Texturizers,* such as calcium chloride, keep foods such as canned apples, tomatoes, or potatoes from turning mushy.

Although many of these additives are derived from foods, their real benefit is aesthetic (the food looks and tastes better), not nutritional.

Determining the Safety of Food Additives

The safety of any chemical approved for use as a food additive is based on whether it is

- Toxic
- Carcinogenic
- Allergenic

Defining toxins

A *toxin* is a poison. Some chemicals, such as cyanide, are toxic (poisonous) in very, very small doses. Others, such as sodium ascorbate (a form of vitamin C), are nontoxic even in very large doses. All chemicals listed in the Food Additive Dictionary are considered nontoxic in the amounts that are permitted in food. By the way, did you realize that both examples — cyanide and vitamin C — are *natural* chemicals?

Explaining carcinogens

A *carcinogen* is a substance that causes cancer. In 1958, New York Congressman James Delaney proposed, and Congress enacted into law, an amendment to the Food, Drug, and Cosmetic Act that banned from food any synthetic chemical known to cause cancer (in animals or human beings) when ingested in any amount. (Canada doesn't have any similar legislation.)

Since then, the only exception to the Delaney clause has been saccharin, which was exempted in 1970. Although ingesting very large amounts of the artificial sweetener is known to cause bladder cancer in animals, no similar link can be found to human cancers. In addition, saccharin can be helpful for those who are trying to control the total amount of carbohydrate in their diets, most notably people with diabetes. ***Note:*** In 1977, Congress required all products containing saccharin to carry a warning statement: *Use of this product may be hazardous to your health. This product contains saccharin, which has been determined to cause cancer in laboratory animals.* This requirement was lifted in 2000; the warning is no more. In Canada, saccharin is still banned from being added to foods, but it can be purchased at pharmacies to be used as a tabletop sweetener. Health Canada is in the process of reviewing the current ban on saccharin as a food additive, which has been in place since 1977.

The nitrate/nitrite conundrum

Some preservatives are double-edged — good and not-so-good at the same time. For example, nitrates and nitrites are effective preservatives that prevent the growth of disease-bearing organisms in cured meat. But when they reach your stomach, nitrates and nitrites react with natural ammonia compounds called *amines* to form *nitrosamines,* substances known to cause cancer in animals fed amounts of nitrosamines much higher than found in any human food. But humans aren't animals, and it's unclear whether the nitrates and nitrites that we're exposed to increase our risk for stomach cancer. Evidence supports both sides of the argument.

What's interesting is that we're exposed to many sources of nitrates and nitrites every day. These include air, water, and food (both naturally occurring and those nitrates that are added to foods), so avoiding foods with added nitrates and nitrites won't keep you from having to cope with nitrosamines. Beets, celery, eggplant, lettuce, radishes, spinach, and turnip greens all contain naturally occurring nitrates and nitrites. When the nitrates and nitrates in these vegetables shake hands in your stomach, they make — you got it! — nitrosamines.

Some evidence suggests that vitamin C helps reduce the carcinogenic effect of nitrosamines. Studies that looked specifically at nitrates and nitrites have found that higher intakes of fruits and vegetables, both good sources of vitamin C, are associated with lower rates of stomach cancer. Although the jury is still out, here's yet another reason to eat more fruits and vegetables at each meal!

As of this writing, the Delaney clause is still in effect in the U.S., even though many scientists, including cancer specialists, consider it to be outmoded because it imposes an impossible standard — zero risk — and applies only to synthetic chemicals. The Delaney clause does not apply to natural chemicals, even those known to cause cancer, such as aflatoxins, poisons produced by moulds that grow on peanuts.

Listing allergens

Allergens are substances that trigger allergic reactions. Some foods, such as peanuts, contain natural allergens that can provoke fatal allergic reactions.

The best-known example of an allergenic food additive is sulphites, preservatives that

- ✔ Keep light-coloured fruits and vegetables (apples, potatoes) from browning when exposed to air

- ✔ Prevent shellfish (shrimp and lobster) from developing black spots

- ✔ Reduce the growth of bacteria in fermenting wine and beer

✔ Bleach food starches

   ✔ Make dough easier to handle

Here is a list of foods that may contain sulphites (also see Figure 22-1):

✔ Beer	✔ Molasses
✔ Cakes, cookies, pies	✔ Potatoes (dehydrated, precut, peeled fresh)
✔ Cider (hard)	
✔ Condiments	✔ Shrimp
✔ Dried fruit	✔ Soup mixes
✔ Fruit juices	✔ Tea
✔ Jams and jellies	✔ Vegetables (canned)
✔ Gravy	✔ Vegetable juices
✔ Maraschino cherries	✔ Wine

Sulphites — One of the nine most common food products causing severe adverse reactions, Health Canada, 2007

Sulphites are safe for most people, but not for all. In fact, the Food and Drug Administration (FDA) in the U.S. estimates that 1 out of every 100 people is sensitive to these chemicals; among people with asthma, the number rises to 5 out of every 100. For people sensitive to sulphites, even infinitesimally small amounts may trigger a serious allergic reaction, and asthmatics may develop breathing problems by simply inhaling fumes from sulphite-treated foods.

The Canadian Food Inspection Agency recommends that anyone who has a sensitivity to sulphites try to avoid them as much as possible. They recommend avoiding any food or any product that has sulphites or sulphite derivatives. The best way to determine if a food contains sulphites is to read its ingredient list. Look for names such as sodium bisulphate, potassium bisulphate, or metasulphite or sulphur dioxide. If you're unclear about whether a food contains sulphites, or if a food doesn't have an ingredient list, avoid it. For a list of the many names of sulphites and the common food sources, check out the Canadian Food Inspection Agency Web site (www.inspection.gc.ca/english/fssa/labeti/allerg/sulphe.shtml).

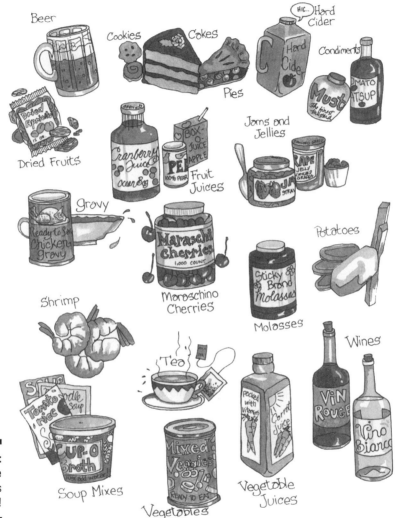

Figure 22-1:
Where the
sulphites
may be!

Looking Beyond Additives:
Foods Nature Never Made

Genetically engineered foods, also known as bioengineered foods or genetically modified foods (GM), are foods with extra genes added artificially through special laboratory processes. Like preservatives, flavour enhancers, and other chemical boosters used in food, the genes — which may come from plants, animals, or micro-organisms such as bacteria — are used to make foods

- ✔ More nutritious
- ✔ Better tasting
- ✔ More resistant to disease and insects

Genetic engineering may also help plants and animals grow faster and larger, thus increasing the food supply. And it may enable us to produce foods with medicines bred right into the food itself. (Check out Chapter 26.)

The Big Question is: Are genetically engineered foods safe? Boy, oh boy, can you get a fight going over that one! The best answer may be that only time will tell. As you can imagine, many ordinary people don't want to wait to find out. For them, genetically engineered foods are simply unacceptable, characterized dismissively as "Frankenfoods" (as in Dr. Frankenstein's monster).

To permit consumers to make a clear choice — "Yes, I'll take that biotech food" or "No, I won't" — the European Union requires food labels to specifically state the presence of any genetically altered ingredients.

In Canada, both Health Canada and the Canadian Food Inspection Agency (CFIA) are responsible for food labelling with respect to GM foods. Health Canada develops policy and sets the standards, and the CFIA enforces them. When it comes to labelling GM foods, Health Canada requires wording that alerts consumers to any potential allergen that may be present, be it naturally occurring or derived from a GM food (such as corn genes in tomatoes). In general, both GM and traditional foods are treated the same with respect to labelling, provided the GM food is proven to be safe: All ingredients in the food product must be listed in the ingredient list in descending order based on the amount of the ingredient present.

So, if a food contains tomatoes that have a modified gene to maintain its flavour, the ingredient list won't distinguish between that tomato and a traditional tomato. If, however, a product contains an ingredient specifically chosen to change the properties of that food, then that ingredient must be listed on the ingredient list in a common name. The best example is a variety of soybean oil designed to have a higher concentration of oleic acid (a heart-healthy monounsaturated fat). An oil using this type of soybean will list "high oleic acid soybean oil" as its ingredient; an oil made with a traditional soybean will simply read "soybean oil."

Whether the wording on the label matters to most consumers or whether most consumers are willing to accept genetically altered foods seems to depend on whom you ask. The International Food Information Council (IFIC), a trade group for the food industry, accepts the current label wording rules. The Center for Science in the Public Interest (CSPI), a Washington-based consumer advocacy group that also has an active presence in Canada, wants to see the words "genetically altered" on all foods that have been, well, genetically altered.

Naturally, each organization has conducted a survey to bolster its point of view. For example, IFIC's survey says that nearly two-thirds (61 percent) of Americans expect food technology to serve up better-quality, better-tasting food. CSPI's competing survey says, "Not so fast." The difference lies in the questions. The IFIC's survey questions emphasize the benefits of biotech; CSPI's survey questions lean more heavily on the drawbacks. Here are a couple of comparable questions from the CSPI and IFIC surveys:

1. **Question**

   CSPI Version: Should food labels tell you if a food has been genetically altered in any way? 70 percent (Yes)

   IFIC Version: Would you say you support or oppose FDA's [current labelling] policy? 59 percent (Support)

2. **Question**

   CSPI Version: Would you buy food labelled "genetically engineered"? 43 percent (Yes)

   IFIC Version: Would you buy a food if it had been modified by biotechnology to taste better or fresher? Or stay fresher? 54 percent (Yes)

In other words, despite a slight wariness about exploring new nutritional ground, Americans seem intrigued by the promise of food innovations and are willing to give the whole idea a try. As well, according to a 1999 Environics poll, 80 percent of Canadians want clear and understandable labelling with respect to GM foods. After that, the proof of the — genetically engineered — pudding is in the eating.

To read the CSPI survey, click on www.cspinet.org, choose Reports, and scroll down to "National Opinion Poll on Labeling of Genetically Engineered Foods." To read the IFIC survey, visit this URL: http://www.ific.org/research/upload/IFIC-Survey-Americans-Acceptance-of-Food-Biotechnology-Matches-Growers-Increased-Adoption-of-Biotech-Crops.pdf.

Part V
Food and Medicine

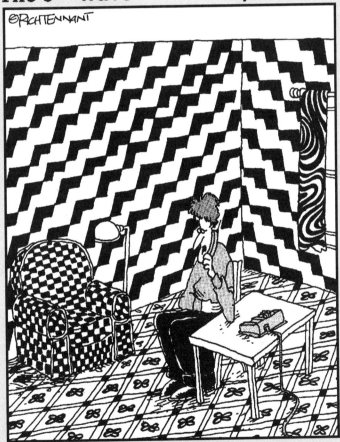

"Doctor, I'm feeling nauseous and disoriented. Do you think I'm having a reaction to something I ate?"

In this part . . .

How come a civilization (yours) that has antibiotics, analgesics, and decongestants still serves up chicken soup for a cold, coffee for a headache, and chocolate for a broken heart? Because they work!

Food and medicine are natural partners. Sometimes they fight (the technical term is *food/drug interactions*), but more often — as you find out in this part — they go hand in hand on the road to keeping your body in tip-top shape.

Chapter 23

When Food Gives You Hives

A ccording to Anaphylaxis Canada, at least 2 percent of Canadians, or about 600,000 people, have true food allergies (also known as food hypersensitivity); this number includes more children than adults because many childhood allergies seem to fade with age.

So, you may ask, if allergies are likely to disappear, why do I need a whole chapter about them? Good question, for which there are two good answers. First, food allergies that don't disappear can trigger reactions ranging from the trivial (a stuffy nose the day after you eat the food) to the truly dangerous (immediate respiratory failure). Second, a person with food allergies is likely to be allergic to other things, such as dust, pollen, or the family cat. Forewarned (about food allergies) is forearmed (against the rest), right? Right.

Finding Out More about Food Allergies

Your immune system is designed to protect your body from harmful invaders, such as bacteria. Sometimes, however, the system responds to substances normally considered harmless. The substance that provokes the attack is called an *allergen;* the substances that attack the allergen are called *antibodies.*

When you have a food allergy, your body releases antibodies to attack specific proteins in food. When this happens, some of the physical reactions include

✔ Hives

✔ Itching

✔ Swelling of the face, tongue, lips, eyelids, hands, and feet

NUTRITION SPEAK

Allergy lingo

So you think you have allergies. Now you need to know the lingo of allergies. These words and definitions (an allergy glossary, if you will) can help you understand what's going on with allergies:

allergen: Any substance that sets off an allergic reaction (see "antigen" in this sidebar)

anaphylaxis: A potentially life-threatening allergic reaction involving many body systems that creates a cascade of adverse effects beginning with sudden, severe itching and moving on to tissue swelling in the air passages, which can lead to breathing difficulties, falling blood pressure, unconsciousness, and death

antibody: A protein in your blood that reacts to an antigen by trying to render it harmless

antigen: A substance that stimulates a response from the immune system; an allergen is a specific type of antigen

basophil: A white blood cell that carries immunoglobulin E and releases histamine

ELISA: Short for *enzyme-linked immunosorbent assay,* a test used to determine the presence of antibodies in your blood, including antibodies to specific allergens

histamine: The substance released by the immune system (specifically by basophils and mast cells) that produces the symptoms of an allergic reaction such as itching and swelling

IgE: An abbreviation for *immunoglobulin E,* the antibody that reacts to allergens

intolerance: A nonallergic adverse reaction to food

mast cell: A cell in body tissue that releases histamine

RAST: An abbreviation for *radioallergosorbent test,* a blood test used to determine whether you're allergic to certain foods

urticaria: The medical name for hives

American Academy of Allergy & Immunology, International Food Information Council Foundation, "Understanding Food Allergy" (April 1995)

✔ Rashes

✔ Headaches, migraines

✔ Nausea, vomiting

✔ Diarrhea, sometimes bloody

✔ Sneezing, coughing

✔ Asthma

✔ Breathing difficulties caused by *tightening* (swelling) of tissues in the throat

✔ Loss of consciousness (from anaphylactic shock)

If you're sensitive to a specific food, you may not have to eat the food to have the reaction. For example, people sensitive to peanuts may break out in hives just from touching a peanut or peanut butter; they could suffer a fatal reaction from tasting chocolate touched by factory machinery that previously touched peanuts. People sensitive to seafood — fin fish and shellfish — have been known to develop breathing problems after inhaling the vapours or steam produced by cooking the fish.

Understanding how an allergic reaction occurs

When you eat a food containing a protein to which you're sensitive, your immune system releases antibodies that hitch a ride on white blood cells called *basophils.* The basophils circulate through your entire body, giving the antibodies the chance to hop off and bind to immune system cells called *mast cells.*

Basophils and mast cells produce, store, and release *histamine,* a natural body chemical that causes the symptoms — itching, swelling, hives — associated with allergic reactions. Yes, that's why some allergy pills are called anti-histamines. When the antibodies carried by the basophils and mast cells come in contact with food allergens, boom! You have an allergic reaction.

Investigating two kinds of allergic reactions

Your body may react to an allergen in one of two ways — immediately or later:

- ✔ Immediate reactions are more dangerous because they involve a fast swelling of tissue, sometimes within seconds after contact with the offending food.

- ✔ Delayed reactions, which may occur as long as 24 to 48 hours after you've been exposed to the offending food, are usually much milder, perhaps a slight cough or nasal congestion caused by swollen tissues.

Most allergic reactions to food are unpleasant but essentially mild. However, it is possible to die from a severe reaction to a food allergy.

Call 911 immediately if you — or a friend or relative — show any signs of an allergic reaction — including an allergic reaction to food — that affects breathing.

It's all in the family: Inheriting food allergies

A tendency toward allergies (although not the particular allergy itself) is inherited. If one of your parents has a food allergy, your risk of having the same problem is two times higher than if neither of your parents were allergic to foods. If both your mother and your father have food allergies, your risk is four times higher.

Considering Foods Most Likely to Cause Allergic Reactions

Here's something to chew on: According to Anaphylaxis Canada, more than 90 percent of all allergic reactions to foods are caused by just eight foods (see Figure 23-1):

- Milk
- Eggs
- Peanuts
- Tree nuts (almonds, Brazil nuts, cashews, hazelnuts [filberts], macadamia nuts, pecans, pine nuts, pistachios, walnuts)
- Soy-based foods (miso, soy milk, tempeh, tofu)
- Wheat
- Fish
- Shellfish

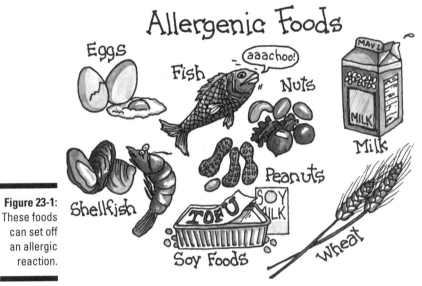

Figure 23-1:
These foods
can set off
an allergic
reaction.

Testing, Testing: Identifying Food Allergies

To identify the culprit causing your food allergy, your doctor may suggest an *elimination diet*. This regimen removes from your diet foods known to cause allergic reactions in many people. Then, one at a time, the foods are added back. If you react to one, bingo! That's a clue to what triggers your immune response.

To be absolutely certain, your doctor may challenge your immune system by introducing foods in a form (maybe a capsule) that neither you nor he can identify as a specific food. Doing so rules out any possibility that your reaction has been triggered by emotional stimuli — that is, seeing, tasting, or smelling the food.

Two more-sophisticated tests — *ELISA* (enzyme-linked immunosorbent assay) and *RAST* (radioallergosorbent test) — can identify antibodies to specific allergens in your blood. But these two tests are rarely required.

Elimination diets

Because different people are sensitive to different foods, more than one elimination diet exists. The three listed here eliminate broad groups of foods known to cause allergic reactions in many people. Your doctor will pick the one that seems most useful for you.

Diet No. 1: No beef, pork, poultry, milk, rye, or corn

Diet No. 2: No beef, lamb, rice, or milk

Diet No. 3: No lamb, poultry, rye, rice, corn, or milk

The Merck Manual, 16th ed. (Rahway, N.J.: Merck Research Laboratories, 1992)

Coping with Food Allergies

After you know that you're allergic to a food, the best way to avoid an allergic reaction is to avoid the food. Unfortunately, that task may be harder than it sounds because the offending ingredient may be hidden — peanuts in the chili or caviar (fish eggs) in the dip.

Sometimes the hidden ingredient is hidden in plain sight on a food label that uses chemical code names for allergens. Example? How about "whey" or "casein" or "lactoglobulin" for "milk." Currently in Canada the *Food and Drug Regulations* require most packaged foods to have a food label with the ingredients listed in descending order based on the amount of those ingredients in the food. There are, however, some ingredients that are exempt from this legislation, which makes it difficult for those with food allergies to distinguish between a food product that is safe and one that is not. An amendment to the regulation is currently under review; the amendment would improve the labelling of high-priority allergens such as wheat (sometimes called gluten) and peanuts, for example.

In the meantime, the Canadian Food Inspection Agency is actively sending advisories to remind food manufacturers, importers, distributors, and retailers that the labelling of common food allergens is their responsibility. Failure to declare a priority allergen could result in punitive measures, for example, a product recall.

If you have a potentially life-threatening allergy to food (or another allergen, such as wasp venom), your doctor may suggest that you carry a syringe filled with *epinephrine,* a drug that counteracts the reactions. You may also want to wear a tag that identifies you as a person with a serious allergic problem. One company that provides these tags is MedicAlert Canada, located in Toronto (visit the Web site at www.medicalert.ca).

The food industry takes food allergies so seriously that the Canadian Restaurant and Foodservices Association (CRFA) has produced a booklet that includes an overview of the history and nature of food allergies and those foods most responsible for allergic reactions. You can order a hard copy of the booklet from the CRFA Web site, `www.cfra.ca`, and you can view the content online as well.

Recognizing Other Bodily Reactions to Food

Allergic reactions aren't the only way your body registers a protest against certain foods.

Food intolerance is a term used to describe reactions that are common, natural, and definitely not allergic, which means that these reactions do not involve production of antibodies by the immune system. Some common food intolerance reactions are

- ✔ **A metabolic food reaction:** This response is an inability to digest certain foods, such as fat or lactose (the naturally occurring sugar in milk). Metabolic food reactions can produce gas, diarrhea, or other signs of gastric revolt, and are an inherited trait.

- ✔ **A physical reaction to a specific chemical:** Your body may react to things such as the laxative substance in prunes or monosodium glutamate (MSG), the flavour enhancer commonly found in Asian food. Although some people are more sensitive than others to these chemicals, their reaction is a physical one that doesn't involve the immune system.

- ✔ **A bodily response to psychological triggers:** When you're very fearful or very anxious or very excited, your body moves into hyperdrive, secreting hormones that pump up your heartbeat and respiration, speed the passage of food through your gut, and cause you to empty your bowels and bladder. The entire process, called the *fight-or-flight response,* prepares your body to defend itself by either fighting or running. On a more prosaic level, a strong reaction to your food may cause diarrhea. It isn't an allergy; it's your hormones.

- ✔ **A change in mood and/or behaviour.** Some foods, such as coffee, contain chemicals, such as caffeine, that have a real effect on mood and behaviour, but that's the subject of Chapter 24. Turn the page, and it's yours.

Getting help with food allergies

There are some great resources on the topic of food allergies and food safety. For more information, write, call, or e-mail the following groups:

Anaphylaxis Canada
2005 Sheppard Avenue East, Suite 800
Toronto, Ontario M2J 5B4
Phone 416-785-5666 or 866-785-5660
Fax 416-785-0458
E-mail info@anaphylaxis.ca
Web site www.anaphylaxis.org

Canadian Celiac Association
190 Britannia Rd. E., Unit 11
Mississauga, Ontario L4Z 1W6
Phone 905-507-6208 or 800-363-7296
Fax 905-507-4673
E-mail celiac@web.net
Web site www.celiac.ca

Canadian Food Inspection Agency
59 Camelot Drive
Nepean, Ontario K1A 0Y9
Phone 613-225-2342
Fax 613-228-6608
Web site www.cfia-acia.agr.ca

Canadian MedicAlert Foundation
2005 Sheppard Avenue East, Suite 800
Toronto, Ontario M2J 5B4
Phone 416-696-0267 or 800-668-1507
Fax 416-696-0156 or 800-392-8422
E-mail general@medicalert.ca
Web site www.medicalert.ca

Canadian Restaurant and Foodservices Association
316 Bloor Street West
Toronto, Ontario M5S 1W5
Phone 416-923-8416 or 800-387-5649
Fax 416-923-1450
E-mail info@crfa.ca
Web site www.crfa.ca

Health Canada
Chief
Chemical Health Hazard Assessment Division
Bureau Chemical Safety, Food Directorate
Sir Frederick Banting Building
Postal Locator: 2201B1
Ottawa, Ontario K1A 0L2
Phone 613-957-1700
Fax 613-990-1543
E-mail john_salminen@hc-sc.gc.ca
Web site www.hc-sc.gc.ca/food-aliment

Chapter 24

Food and Mood

· ·

· ·

*D*raw the curtains. Turn down the lights. Come a little closer. We're going to talk about something nutritionists never seem to write about: Food can make you feel good. And we don't mean the simple, warm, good feelings that follow a fine meal. We mean the pick-me-up-when-I'm-low, calm-me-down-when-I'm-hyper kind of good you usually associate with serious mood-altering drugs.

Why do most nutrition books ignore this subject? Who knows? But this book gives you a bunch of information that you may otherwise never see.

So here's a chapter on mood and food. The chapter names some of the common, naturally occurring, mood-alerting chemicals in food; explains how these chemicals work; and presents some simple strategies for increasing their effectiveness. Sit back, open a box of chocolates, pour a glass of wine, brew up the espresso — and enjoy.

How Chemicals Alter Mood

A *mood* is a feeling, an internal emotional state that can affect how you see the world. For example, if your team wins the World Series, your happiness may last for days, making you feel so mellow that you simply shrug off minor annoyances such as finding a ticket on your windshield because your parking metre expired while you were having lunch. On the other hand, if you feel sad because the project you spent six months setting up didn't work out, your disappointment can linger long enough to make your work seem temporarily unrewarding or your favourite television show unfunny.

Most of the time, after shifting one way or the other, your mood swings back to centre fairly soon. You come down from your high or recover from your disappointment, and life resumes its normal pace — some good stuff here, some bad news there, but all in all, a relatively level field.

Occasionally, however, your mood may go haywire. Your happiness over your team's victory escalates to the point where you find yourself rushing from store to store buying things you can't afford, or your sadness over your failure at work deepens into a gloom that steals joy from everything else. This unpleasant state of affairs — a mood out of control — is called a *mood disorder.*

About one in every four human beings (women more often than men) experiences some form of mood disturbance during his or her lifetime. Eight or nine out of every 100 people experience a *clinical mood disorder,* a mood disorder serious enough to be diagnosed as a disease.

The two most common moods are happiness and sadness. The two most common mood disorders are *clinical depression,* an elongated period of overly intense sadness, and *clinical mania,* an elongated period of overly intense elation. Clinical depression alone is called a *unipolar (one-part) disorder;* clinical depression plus clinical mania is a *bipolar (two-part) disorder.*

Today, scientists have identified naturally occurring brain chemicals that affect mood and play a role in mood disorders. Your body makes a group of substances called *neurotransmitters,* which are chemicals that enable brain cells to send messages back and forth. Three important neurotransmitters are

- Dopamine *(DOE-pa-meen)*
- Norepinephrine *(NOR-e-pe-NEF-rin)*
- Serotonin *(ser-a-TOE-nin)*

Dopamine and *norepinephrine* are chemicals that make you feel alert and energized. *Serotonin* is a chemical that can make you feel smooth and mellow.

Some forms of clinical depression and mania appear to be malfunctions of the body's ability to handle these chemicals. Drugs known as antidepressants adjust mood by making neurotransmitters more available to your brain or enabling your brain to use them more efficiently. Medications used to treat mood disorders include

- **Tricyclic antidepressants:** These drugs are named for their chemical structure: three ring–shaped groups of atoms (tri = three; cyclic = ring). They relieve symptoms by increasing the availability of serotonin. One well-known tricyclic is amitriptyline (Elavil).

✔ **Selective serotonin reuptake inhibitors (SSRIs):** These medicines slow your body's reabsorption of serotonin so that more of that chemical is available to your brain. SSRIs are reported to have fewer side effects than the tricyclics. Two well-known SSRIs are fluoxetine (Prozac) and paroxetine (Paxil).

✔ **Monoamine oxidase inhibitors (MAO inhibitors):** These drugs slow your body's natural destruction of dopamine and other neurotransmitters so that they remain available for your brain. Phenelzine (Nardil) and tranylcypromine (Parnate) are MAO inhibitors.

✔ **Lithium:** This drug's precise actions remain unknown, but it may increase the availability of serotonin and lower the availability of norepinephrine.

✔ **A number of chemicals unrelated to each other or to other groups of antidepressants:** Some are known to regulate the availability of serotonin; others work in ways that have not yet been identified. This group includes bupropion (Wellbutrin, Zyban) and sertraline (Zoloft).

How Food Affects Mood

Good morning! Time to wake up, roll out of bed, and sleepwalk into the kitchen for a cup of coffee.

Good afternoon! Time for a moderate glass of whiskey or wine to soothe away the tensions of the day.

Good grief! Your lover has left. Time for chocolate, lots of chocolate, to soothe the pain.

Good night! Time for milk and cookies to ease your way to Dreamland.

For centuries, millions of people have used these foods in these situations, secure in the knowledge that each food will work its mood magic. Today, modern science knows why. Having discovered that your emotions are linked to your production or use of certain brain chemicals, nutrition scientists have been able to identify the natural chemicals in food that change the way you feel by

✔ Influencing the production of neurotransmitters

✔ Hooking onto brain cells and changing the way the cells behave

✔ Opening pathways to brain cells so that other mood-altering chemicals can come on board

The following sections describe chemicals in food most commonly known to affect mood.

Alcohol

Alcohol is the most widely used natural relaxant. Contrary to common belief, alcohol is a depressant, not a mood elevator. If you feel loosey-goosey and exuberant after one drink, the reason isn't that the alcohol is speeding up your brain; it's that alcohol relaxes your *controls,* the brain signals that normally tell you not to put a lampshade on your head or take off your clothes in public.

For more about alcohol's effects on virtually every body organ and system, turn to Chapter 9. Here in this chapter, it's enough to say that many people find that, taken with food and in moderation — defined as one drink a day for a woman and two for a man — alcohol can comfortably change one's mood from tense to mellow.

Anandamide

Anandamide is a *cannabinoid,* a chemical that hooks up to the same brain receptors that catch similar ingredients in marijuana smoke. Your brain produces some anandamide naturally, but you also get very small amounts of the chemical from (what else?) chocolate. In addition, chocolate contains two chemicals similar to anandamide that slow the breakdown of the anandamide produced in your brain, thus intensifying its effects. Maybe that's why eating chocolate makes you feel very mildly mellow. Not mellow enough to get you hauled off to the hoosegow (jail) or to bring in the Feds to confiscate your candy; just enough to wipe away the tears of lost love. (Don't worry; you'd need to eat at least 25 pounds of chocolate at one time to get any marijuana-like effect.)

Caffeine

Caffeine is a mild stimulant that

- ✔ Raises your blood pressure
- ✔ Speeds up your heartbeat
- ✔ Makes you burn calories faster
- ✔ Makes you urinate more frequently
- ✔ Causes your intestinal tract to move food more quickly through your body

As well, caffeine is a mood elevator. Although it increases the level of serotonin, the calming neurotransmitter, it also hooks up at specific receptors (sites on the surface of brain cells) normally reserved for another naturally occurring tranquilizer, adenosine *(a-DEN-o-seen)*. When caffeine latches on in place of adenosine, brain cells become more reactive to stimulants such as noise and light, making you talk faster and think faster. Lately, athletes who take coffee before an event have reported that it also improves performance in some endurance events.

However, how people react to caffeine is a highly individual affair. Some can drink seven cups of regular ("with caffeine") coffee and still stay calm all day and sleep like a baby at night. Others tend to hop about on decaf. Perhaps those who stay calm have enough brain receptors to accommodate both adenosine and caffeine, or perhaps they're more sensitive to the adenosine that manages to hook up to brain cells.

A more plausible explanation probably lies in the speed at which you can *metabolize* (break down and get rid of) caffeine. A study in the *Journal of the American Medical Association* in 2006 found that some people are "fast" metabolizers and others are "slow" metabolizers of caffeine. Study co-author Ahmed El-Sohemy, of the University of Toronto, explains that a gene (cytochrome P450 1A2) determines the rate at which a person can clear caffeine from his or her body. The study found that those individuals under the age of 50 that had the "slow" version of the gene were up to four times as likely to experience a nonfatal heart attack if they drank two or more cups of coffee per day compared to those without the "slow" gene.

This study highlights the role of genes and their influence on nutrition — an emerging field of research called *nutrigenomics* and *nutrigenetics* (the study of how genes influence a person's response to different nutritional factors, and how, in turn, nutrition can modulate or affect those genes). Who knows, maybe one day we'll have different diet therapies based on an individual's genes.

In the meantime, it's best to follow Health Canada's guidelines on caffeine consumption, and limit it to 400 milligrams per day — which is about four small coffees.

Either way, caffeine's bouncy effects may last anywhere from one to seven hours. Some people can count on missing a night's sleep when they have real (as opposed to decaffeinated) coffee after 5 p.m. Espresso at dinner? Some of us will still be awake when the birds get up the next morning. Table 24-1 lists some common food sources of caffeine.

Table 24-1	Foods That Give You Caffeine
Food	*Amount of Caffeine (mg)*
150 mL (5 ounces)	
Coffee, regular, drip	80–150
Coffee, regular, instant	40–108
Coffee, decaffeinated	1–6

(continued)

Table 24-1 *(continued)*	
Food	*Amount of Caffeine (mg)*
Tea	20–110
Tea, instant	25–60
Cocoa	2–50
355 mL (12 ounces)	
Soft drinks	30–72
250 mL (8 ounces)	
Chocolate milk	2–7
28 g (1 ounce)	
Milk chocolate	1–15
Semisweet chocolate	5–35
Bitter (baker's) chocolate	26

George M. Briggs and Doris Howes Callaway, Nutrition and Physical Fitness, 11th ed. (New York: Holt, Rinehart and Winston, 1984); Current Medical Diagnosis and Treatment, 36th ed. (Stamford, CT: Appleton and Lange, 1997)

Tryptophan and glucose

Tryptophan is one of the *amino acids,* a group of chemicals commonly called the building blocks of protein (see Chapter 6). Glucose, the end product of carbohydrate metabolism, is the sugar that circulates in your blood, the basic fuel on which your body runs (see Chapter 8). Milk and cookies, a classic calming combo, owe their power to the tryptophan-glucose team.

Start with the fact that neurotransmitters dopamine, norepinephrine, and serotonin are made from the amino acids tyrosine and tryptophan, which are found in protein foods (like milk). *Tyrosine* is the most important ingredient in dopamine and norepinephrine, the alertness neurotransmitters. *Tryptophan* is the most important ingredient in serotonin, the calming neurotransmitter.

All amino acids ride into your brain like little trains on tiny chemical railroads. But Mother Nature — clearly a party animal! — has arranged the switches so that your brain makes way for the bouncy tyrosine train first and the soothing tryptophan train last. That's why a high-protein meal heightens your alertness.

To move the tryptophan train up the track, you need glucose, and that means you need carbohydrate foods (like those cookies). When you eat carbs, your pancreas releases *insulin,* a hormone that enables you to metabolize the carbs and produce glucose. The insulin also keeps tyrosine and other amino acids circulating in your blood so the tryptophan trains can travel on plenty of open tracks to the brain. With more tryptophan coming in, your brain can increase its production of soothing serotonin. That's why a meal of starchy pasta (starch is composed of chains of glucose molecules, as explained in Chapter 8) makes you calm, cool, and kind of groovy.

The effects of simple sugars such as sucrose (table sugar) are more complicated. If you eat simple sugars on an empty stomach, the sugars are absorbed rapidly, triggering an equally rapid increase in the secretion of insulin, a hormone needed to digest carbohydrates. The result is a rapid decrease in the amount of sugar circulating in your blood, a condition known as *hypoglycemia* (hypo = low; glycemia = sugar in the blood) that can make you feel temporarily jumpy rather than calm. However, when eaten on a full stomach — dessert after a full meal — simple sugars are absorbed more slowly and may exert the calming effect usually linked to complex carbohydrates (starchy foods).

So some foods, such as meat, fish, and poultry, make you more alert. Others, such as pasta, bread, potatoes, or rice and other grains, calm you down. The effect of the food depends on its ability to alter the amount of serotonin available to your brain (see Figure 24-1).

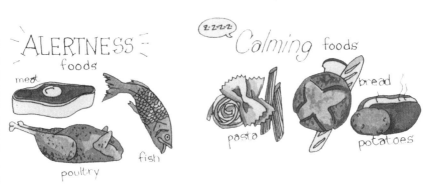

Figure 24-1: Some foods may calm you, and some foods may make you more alert.

Phenylethylamine (PEA)

Phenylethylamine — sometimes abbreviated PEA — is a natural chemical that your body releases when you're in love, making you feel, well, good all over. A big splash occurred in the late 1980s when researchers discovered that chocolate, the food of lovers, is a fine source of PEA.

In fact, many people think that PEA has a lot to do with chocolate's reputation as the food of love and consolation. Of course, to be fair about it, chocolate also contains the mood-elevator caffeine, the muscle stimulant theobromine, and the cannabinoid anandamide (see the discussion on anandamide earlier in this chapter). What is there to say other than, "Hey, can you please pass that box of chocolates down to this end of the table?"

Using Food to Manage Mood

No food will change your personality or alter the course of a mood disorder. But some may add a little lift or a small moment of calm to your day, increase your effectiveness at certain tasks, make you more alert, or give you a neat little push over the finish line.

The watchword is balance:

✔ One cup of coffee in the a.m. is a pleasant push into alertness. Seven cups of coffee a day can make your hands shake, and caffeine may not be the best way to manage a busy lifestyle.

✔ One alcohol drink is generally a safe way to relax. Three may be a disaster.

✔ A grilled chicken breast (white meat, no skin) for breakfast — yes, breakfast — on a day when you have to be on your toes before lunch can help make you sharp as a tack.

✔ Got an important lunch meeting? Order starches without fats or oils: pasta with fresh tomatoes and basil, no oil, no cheese; rice with veggies; rice with fruit. Your aim is to get the calming carbs without the high fat that slows thinking and makes you feel sleepy.

In this, as in other aspects of a healthy life, the point is to make sure that you use the tool (in this case, food), not the other way around.

Caution! Medicine at work

Some of the mood-altering chemicals in food interact with medicines. As you may have guessed, the two most notable examples are caffeine and alcohol.

✔ Caffeine makes painkillers such as aspirin and acetaminophen more effective. On the other hand, many over-the-counter (OTC) painkillers and cold medicines already contain caffeine. If you take the pill with a cup of java, you may increase your caffeine intake past the jitters stage.

✔ Alcohol is a no-no with most medicines because it increases the sedative or depressant effects of some drugs, such as antihistamines and painkillers, and alters the rate at which you absorb or excrete others.

When you fill a prescription, always ask your pharmacist about food and drug interactions (you can read more about this in Chapter 25). When you're choosing OTC products, read the labels very carefully.

Chapter 25

Food and Drug Interactions

. . . .

. . . .

*F*oods nourish your body. Medicines cure (or relieve) what ails you. You'd think the two would work together in perfect harmony to protect your body. Sometimes they do. Occasionally, however, foods and drugs square off like boxers slugging it out in the ring. The drug keeps your body from absorbing or using the nutrients in food, or the food (or nutrient) prevents you from getting the benefits of certain medicines.

The medical phrase for this sad state of affairs is *adverse interaction.* This chapter describes several adverse interactions and lays out some simple strategies that enable you to short-circuit them.

Explaining How Some Foods and Drugs Interact

When you eat, food moves from your mouth to your stomach to your small intestine, where the nutrients that keep you strong and healthy are absorbed into your bloodstream and distributed throughout your body. Take medicine by mouth, and it follows pretty much the same path from your mouth to your stomach, where it's dissolved and passed along to the small intestine for absorption. Nothing is unusual about that.

The problem, however, arises when a food or drug brings the process to a screeching halt by behaving in a way that stops your body from using either the drug or the food or both (see Figure 25-1). Many possibilities exist:

> ✔ Some drugs or foods change the natural acidity of your digestive tract so that you absorb nutrients less efficiently. For example, your body

absorbs iron best when your stomach is acidic. Taking antacids (such as Tums, which contains calcium carbonate) reduces stomach acidity — and iron absorption.

✔ Some drugs or foods change the rate at which food moves through your digestive tract, which means that you absorb more (or less) of a particular nutrient or drug. For example, eating prunes (a laxative food) or taking a laxative drug speeds things up so that foods (and drugs) move more quickly through your body, giving you less time to absorb medicine or nutrients.

✔ Some drugs and nutrients *bond* (link up with each other) to form insoluble compounds that your body can't break apart. As a result, you get less of the drug and less of the nutrient. The best-known example: Calcium (in dairy foods) bonds to the antibiotic tetracycline so that both zip right out of your body.

✔ Some drugs and nutrients have similar chemical structures. Taking them at the same time fools your body into absorbing or using the nutrient rather than the drug. One good example is warfarin (a drug that keeps blood from clotting) and vitamin K (a nutrient that makes blood clot). Eating lots of vitamin K–rich leafy greens counteracts the intended effect of the warfarin.

✔ Some foods contain chemicals that either lessen or intensify the natural side effects of certain drugs. For example, the caffeine in coffee, tea, and cola drinks reduces the sedative effects of antihistamines and some antidepressant drugs, but increases the nervousness, insomnia, and shakiness common with some diet pills and cold medications containing caffeine or a *decongestant* (an ingredient that temporarily clears a stuffy nose).

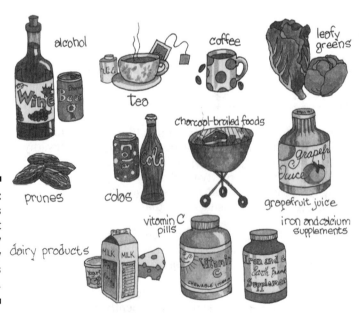

Figure 25-1:
Some foods may affect the way your body interacts with drugs.

alcohol

coffee

leafy greens

tea

charcoal-broiled foods

prunes

colas

grapefruit juice

vitamin C pills

iron and calcium supplements

dairy products

Duking It Out: Drugs versus Nutrients versus Foods

Sometimes the combinations of interacting foods and drugs are positively astounding. Or, as the next paragraph suggests, breathtaking.

Here's a prime example. Everyone knows that people with asthma may find it hard to take a deep breath around the barbecue. The culprit's the smoke, right? Yes. And no. True: Breathing in smoke irritates air passages. But the kicker is that eating charcoal-broiled food speeds the body's elimination of theophylline, a widely used asthma drug, and reduces the drug's ability to protect against wheezing. Take the drug, eat the food, and end up wheezing. Yipes.

Another potential troublemaker is fruit juice. Acidic beverages (colas as well as fruit juice) can send the antibiotics erythromycin, ampicillin, and penicillin down for the count.

Grapefruit juice is another acidic actor. In the mid-1990s, researchers tracking the effects of alcohol beverages on the blood-pressure drug felodipine (Plendil) tripped across the *Grapefruit Effect,* a dramatic reduction in your ability to metabolize and eliminate certain drugs. Grapefruit juice contains substances that suppress the effectiveness of Cytochrome P450 3A4, an intestinal enzyme required to convert many drugs to water-soluble substances you can flush out of your body; without the enzyme, you can't get rid of the drug. The result may be a dramatic rise in the amount of medication in your body, leading to unpleasant side effects. The list of drugs that interact with grapefruit juice has now expanded beyond felodipine to include a second blood-pressure med, nifedipine (Adalat, Procardia), plus — among others — the cholesterol-lowering drugs lovastatin (Mevacor), pravastatin (Pravachol), and simvastatin (Zocor); the antihistamine loratadine (Claritin); the immunosuppressant drug cyclosporine; and saquinavir (Invirase), a protease (enzyme) inhibitor used to treat HIV. Ask your doctor or pharmacist whether you should avoid grapefruit or grapefruit juice when starting any new medication.

Water pills, more properly known as *diuretics,* make you urinate more often and more copiously, thus increasing your elimination of the mineral potassium. To make up what you lose, experts suggest adding potatoes, bananas, oranges, spinach, corn, tomatoes, and other high-potassium foods to your diet. Consuming less sodium (salt) while you're using water pills makes the water pills more effective and decreases your loss of potassium.

Oral contraceptives seem to reduce the ability to absorb B vitamins, including folate. Taking lots of aspirin or other NSAIDs (nonsteroidal anti-inflammatory drugs) such as ibuprofen can trigger a painless, slow, but steady loss of small amounts of blood from the lining of your stomach; this loss may lead to iron-deficiency anemia.

Persistent use of antacids made with aluminum compounds may lead to loss of the bone-building mineral phosphorus, which binds to aluminum and rides right out of the body. Laxatives increase the loss of calcium and other minerals in feces.

The antiulcer drugs cimetidine (Tagamet) and ranitidine (Zantac) can make you positively giddy. These drugs reduce stomach acidity, which means the body absorbs alcohol more efficiently. According to experts at the Mayo Clinic, taking ulcer medication with alcohol leads to twice the wallop, like drinking one beer and feeling the effects of two.

The point? Read the label and check with your doctor or pharmacist for any potential food and drug interactions whenever you take medication.

Finally, consider nutritional supplements. The vitamins and minerals in nutritional supplements are simply food reduced to its basic nutrients, so interactions between drugs and supplements aren't a surprise. Table 25-1 lists some common interactions between drugs, vitamins, and minerals. (For more information on supplements, see Chapter 5.)

Table 25-1	Battling Nutrients and Medications
You Absorb Less	*When You Take*
Vitamin A	Aluminum antacids Bisacodyl (laxative) Mineral oil (laxative) Neomycin (antibiotic)
Vitamin D	Bisacodyl (laxative) Mineral oil (laxative) Neomycin (antibiotic)
Vitamin K	Bisacodyl (laxative) Mineral oil (laxative) Neomycin (antibiotic)
Vitamin C	Aspirin Barbiturates (sleeping pills) Cortisone and related steroid drugs
Thiamin	Antacids (calcium) Aspirin Cortisone and related steroid drugs
Riboflavin	Birth control pills

You Absorb Less	When You Take
Folate	Aspirin Penicillin Phenobarbital, primidone (antiseizure drugs) Sulfa drugs
Vitamin B12	Neomycin (antibiotic)
Calcium	Cortisone and related steroid drugs Diuretics (water pills) Magnesium antacids Neomycin (antibiotic) Phosphorus laxatives Tetracycline (antibiotic)
Phosphorus	Aluminum antacids
Magnesium	Diuretics (water pills) Tetracycline (antibiotic)
Iron	Aspirin and other nonsteroidal anti-inflammatory drugs Calcium antacids Calcium supplements (with meals) Neomycin (antibiotic) Penicillin (antibiotic) Tetracycline (antibiotic)
Zinc	Diuretics (water pills)

Health Canada — Drug Product Database, 2007

Avoiding Adverse Food and Drug Interactions

When you pick up an over-the-counter drug or get a new prescription, *read the label.* Repeat: Read. The. Label. Warnings and interactions often are right there on the package. If they're not, ask your doctor or pharmacist whether you need to avoid any specific foods while you're taking the drug. Go on, now — ask.

Or you can plunk down a few bucks for your very own copy of *Understanding Prescription Drugs For Canadians For Dummies* (Wiley, 2007). The book is affordable, readable, reliable, and fun. Go for it.

Using Food to Improve a Drug's Performance

Not every food and drug interaction is an adverse one. Sometimes a drug works better or is less likely to cause side effects when you take it on a full stomach. For example, aspirin is less likely to upset your stomach if you take the painkiller with food, and eating stimulates the release of stomach juices that improve your ability to absorb griseofulvin, an antifungus drug.

Table 25-2 lists some drugs that may work better when your stomach is full.

Table 25-2	Drugs That Work Better on a Full Stomach
Purpose	*Drug*
Analgesics (painkillers)	Acetaminophen Aspirin Codeine Ibuprofen Indomethacin Mefenamic acid Metronidazole Naproxen/naproxen sodium
Antibiotics, Antivirals, Antifungals	Biaxin Isoniazid Pyrimethamine
Antidiabetic Agents	Glimepiride Glialazide Glyburide Tolbutamide
Cholesterol-Lowering Agents	Cholestyramine Colestipol Lovastatin
Gastric Medications	Cimetidine Ranitidine

Health Canada — Drug Product Database, 2007

Don't guess about drugs and food. Every time you take a pill, read the package label or check with your doctor or pharmacist to find out whether taking the medicine with food improves or reduces its ability to make you better. Or thumb through your brand-new copy of *Understanding Prescription Drugs For Canadians For Dummies* (Wiley, 2007).

With this medicine, who can eat?

Interactions aren't the only drug reactions that keep you from getting nutrients from food. Some drugs have side effects that also reduce the value of food. For example, a drug may

✔ Sharply reduce your appetite so that you simply don't eat much. The best-known example may be the amphetamine and amphetamine-like drugs such as fenfluramine used (surprise!) as diet pills.

✔ Make food taste or smell bad or steal away your senses of taste or smell so that eating isn't pleasurable. One example is the antidepressant drug amitriptyline (Elavil), which can leave a peculiar taste in your mouth.

✔ Cause nausea, vomiting, or diarrhea so that you either can't eat or do not retain nutrients from the food you do eat. Examples include the antibiotic erythromycin and many drugs used to treat cancer.

✔ Irritate the lining of your gut so that even if you do eat, your body has a hard time absorbing nutrients from food. One example is cyclophosphamide, an antitumour medication.

The moderately good news is that new medications appear to make some drugs (including anticancer drugs) less likely to cause nausea and vomiting. The best news is that many drugs are less likely to upset your stomach or irritate your gut if you take them with food (see Table 25-2). For example, taking aspirin and other non-prescription painkillers such as ibuprofen with food or a full glass of water may reduce their natural tendency to irritate the lining of your stomach.

Chapter 26

Using Food as Medicine

A healthful diet gives you the nutrients you need to keep your body in top-flight condition. In addition, evidence suggests that eating well may prevent or minimize the risk of a long list of serious medical conditions, including heart disease, high blood pressure, and cancer.

This chapter describes what nutritionists know right now about how to use food to prevent, alleviate, or cure what ails you — with a couple of hints about what's to come in the evolving world of medical nutrition.

Defining Food as Medicine

Start with a definition. A food that acts like a medicine is one that increases or reduces your risk of a specific medical condition or cures or alleviates the effects of a medical condition. For example:

✔ Eating foods with lots of lutein (the yellow pigment you can see in foods like corn, which is also in spinach, kale, broccoli, and collard greens, where the pigment is masked by chlorophyll) — along with vitamin C, vitamin E, and zinc — protects your vision by reducing the risk of age-related degeneration of the macula, the organ at the back of your eye that enables you to perceive light.

✔ Eating foods such as wheat bran that are high in insoluble dietary fibre (the kind of fibre that doesn't dissolve in your gut) moves food more quickly through your intestinal tract and produces soft, bulky stool that reduces your risk of constipation.

✔ Eating foods such as beans that are high in soluble dietary fibre (fibre that dissolves in your intestinal tract) seems to help your body mop up the cholesterol circulating in your bloodstream, preventing it from sticking to the walls of your arteries. This reduces your risk of heart disease.

✔ Eating sufficient amounts of calcium-rich foods ensures the growth of strong bones early in life and protects bone density later.

✔ Eating very spicy foods, such as chili, causes the membrane lining your nose and throat to weep a watery fluid that makes blowing your nose or coughing up mucus easier when you have a cold.

✔ Eating (or drinking) foods (or beverages) with mood-altering substances such as caffeine, alcohol, and phenylethylamine (PEA) may lend a lift when you're feeling down, or help you chill when you're tense.

The joy of food-as-medicine is that it's cheaper and much more pleasant than managing illness with drugs. Given the choice, who wouldn't opt to control cholesterol levels with oats or chili (all those yummy beans packed with soluble dietary fibre) instead of with a drug whose possible side effects include kidney failure and liver damage?

Examining Diets with Absolutely, Positively Beneficial Medical Effects

Some foods and some diet plans are so obviously good for your body that no one questions their ability to keep you healthy or make you feel better when you're ill. For example, if you've ever had abdominal surgery, you know all about liquid diets — the water-gelatin–clear broth regimen your doctor prescribes right after the operation to enable you to take some nourishment by mouth without upsetting your gut.

Or if you have type 1 diabetes (an inherited inability to produce the insulin you need to process carbohydrates), you know that your ability to balance the carbohydrates, fats, and proteins in your daily diet is important to stabilizing your illness.

Other proven diet regimens include

✔ **The low-cholesterol, low-saturated-fat, and low-trans-fat diet:** The basic version, known as the Step 1 Diet, is used as a first step in lowering your cholesterol level. The diet limits cholesterol consumption to no more than 300 milligrams a day and total fat intake to no more than 30 percent of your total daily calories (see Chapter 16).

A nifty bonus to this diet is that it's a relatively painless way of losing weight.

✔ **The high-fibre diet:** A high-fibre diet quickens the passage of food through the digestive tract. This diet is used to prevent constipation. If you have *diverticula* (outpouchings) in the wall of your colon, a high-fibre diet may reduce the possibility of an infection. It can also alleviate the discomfort of irritable bowel syndrome (sometimes called a nervous stomach). Extra bonus: A diet high in soluble fibre also lowers cholesterol (see the section, "Defining Food as Medicine").

✔ **The sodium-restricted diet:** Sodium is hydrophilic (hydro = water; philic = loving). It increases the amount of water held in body tissues. A diet low in salt often lowers water retention, which can be useful in treating high blood pressure, congestive heart failure, and long-term liver disease.

By the way, not all the sodium in your diet comes from table salt. Check out Chapter 16 for a list of the sodium compounds used in food.

✔ **The extra-potassium diet:** People use this diet to counteract the loss of potassium caused by *diuretics* (drugs that make you urinate more frequently and more copiously, causing you to lose excess amounts of potassium in urine). Some evidence also suggests that the high-potassium diet may lower blood pressure a bit.

✔ **The low-protein diet:** This diet is prescribed for people with chronic liver or kidney disease or an inherited inability to metabolize amino acids, the building blocks of proteins. The low-protein regimen reduces the amount of protein waste products in body tissues, thus reducing the possibility of tissue damage.

Using Food to Prevent Disease

Using food as a general preventive is an intriguing subject. True, much anecdotal evidence ("I did this, and that happened") suggests that eating some foods and avoiding others can raise or lower your risk of some serious diseases. But anecdotes aren't science. The more important indicator is the evidence from scientific studies that track groups of people on different diets to see how things such as eating or avoiding fat, fibre, meat, dairy foods, salt, and other foods affect their risk of specific diseases.

Sometimes, the studies show a strange effect (meat fat increases the risk of colon cancer, high-fat dairy foods lower the risk). Sometimes studies show no effect at all. And sometimes — we like this category best — they turn up results nobody expected. For example, in 1996, there was a study designed to see whether a diet high in selenium would reduce the risk of skin cancer. After four years, the answer was, "Not so you'd notice." But then researchers noticed — by accident — that people who ate lots of high-selenium foods had a lower risk of lung, breast, and prostate cancers. Naturally, researchers immediately set up a second study, which happily confirmed the unexpected results of the first.

Foods that serve up a health benefit in addition to basic good nutrition have been christened "functional foods." Fruits and veggies rich in beta carotene are naturally functional foods that prevent night blindness (the inability to see clearly in low light) along with their low-calorie, low-fat goodness. A second kind of functional food is one created to produce a specific medical result, such as a food that can deliver a vaccine (which you can read more about later in this chapter).

Battling deficiency diseases

The simplest example of food as preventive medicine is its ability to ward off a *deficiency disease,* a condition that occurs when you don't get sufficient amounts of a specific nutrient. For example, people deprived of vitamin C develop scurvy, the vitamin C–deficiency disease. The identifying characteristic of a deficiency disease is that simply adding the missing nutrient to your diet can cure it; scurvy disappears when people eat foods such as citrus fruits that are high in vitamin C.

Fighting off cancer with food

Is there really an anticancer diet? Right now, the answer seems to be a definite maybe. The problem is that cancer isn't one disease; it's many. Some foods seem to protect against some specific cancers, but no single food seems to protect against all. For example:

- ✔ **Fruits and vegetables:** Plants contain some potential anticancer substances, such as antioxidants (chemicals that prevent molecular fragments called free radicals from hooking up to form cancer-causing compounds); hormone-like compounds that displace natural and synthetic estrogens; and sulphur compounds that interfere with biochemical reactions leading to the birth and growth of cancer cells. (For more about these protective substances in plant foods, see Chapter 12.)

- ✔ **Foods high in dietary fibre:** Human beings can't digest dietary fibre, but friendly bacteria living in your gut can. Chomping away on the fibre, the bacteria excrete fatty acids that appear to keep cells from turning cancerous. In addition, fibre helps speed food through your body, reducing the formation of carcinogenic compounds.

   For more than 30 years, doctors have assumed that eating lots of dietary fibre reduces the risk of colon cancer, but in 1999, data from the long-running Nurses' Health Study at Boston's Brigham and Women's Hospital and Harvard's School of Public Health threw this into question. By 2005, several very large studies — one with more than 350,000 people! — confirmed that dietary fibre has no protective effect against colon cancer. But even if dietary fibre doesn't fight cancer, it does prevent constipation. One out of two ain't bad.

Three degrees of vegetarianism

Vegetarianism isn't one diet; it's three, each one distinguished by what's allowed in addition to fruits, grains, and, yup, veggies.

✔ Variation #1 is a plant-based diet for people who don't eat meat but do eat fish and poultry or just fish. Those who just eat fish are called *pesco-vegetarians*. (Fairness dictates that we add that many strict vegetarians don't consider people who eat fish or poultry to be vegetarians.)

✔ Variation #2 is a plant-based diet for people who don't eat meat, fish, or poultry but do eat other animal products such as eggs and/or dairy products. Vegetarians who follow this regimen are called *ovo-lacto vegetarians* (ovo = egg; lacto = milk).

✔ Variation #3 is a diet for people who eat absolutely no foods of animal origin. Vegetarians who eat only plant foods are called *vegans*.

✔ **Low-fat foods:** Dietary fat appears to increase the proliferation of various types of body cells, a situation that may lead to the out-of-control reproduction of cells known as cancer. But all fats may not be equally guilty. In several studies, fat from meat seems linked to an increased risk of colon cancer, but fat from dairy foods comes up clean. In the end, the link between dietary fat and cancer remains up in the nutritional air . . . so to speak.

Because research shows that 30 to 35 percent of all cancers can be prevented by eating well, being active, and maintaining a healthy body weight, the Canadian Cancer Society recommends that you:

✔ **Base your eating habits on Canada's Food Guide.**

✔ **Choose most of the foods you eat from plant sources.** Plant foods are high in vitamins, minerals, and fibre and low in calories. Eat seven or more servings of fruits and vegetables every day. Eat other foods from plant sources, such as breads, cereals, grain products, rice, pasta (choose whole grain more often), or beans, several times a day. A diet that includes a variety of vegetables and fruit instead of higher-fat, higher-calorie foods can help you achieve and maintain a healthy weight.

✔ **Choose healthy fats.** Unsaturated fats are a healthier fat as compared to saturated and trans fats. Unsaturated fats seem to protect against cancer. They are found in avocados, nuts, seeds, and oils like olive, sunflower, and canola. A particularly healthy type of unsaturated fat is omega-3 fat, found in oily fish such as salmon, herring, and mackerel and also in plant foods such as canola, flaxseed, salba, and walnuts.

✔ **Limit your intake of high-fat foods, particularly from animal sources.** Choose foods low in fat; limit consumption of meats, especially high-fat meats. Choose leaner cuts more often.

✔ **Be physically active.** Achieve and maintain a healthy weight. Be at least moderately active for 30 minutes or more on most days of the week. Stay within your healthy weight range.

✔ **If you drink alcohol, drink in moderation.** Chapter 9 lays it out: Moderate consumption means no more than one drink a day for a woman, two for a man.

DASHing to healthy blood pressure

In Canada, roughly 22 percent of adults have high blood pressure (also referred to as hypertension), a major risk factor for heart disease, stroke, and heart or kidney failure. However, only about half of people with high blood pressure know that they have it, and blood pressure is controlled in just one out of every eight people who have high blood pressure.

As you can read in *High Blood Pressure For Dummies* (published by Wiley), the traditional treatment for hypertension has included drugs (some with unpleasant side effects), reduced sodium intake, weight reduction, alcohol only in moderation, and regular exercise. Recent data from a National Heart, Lung, and Blood Institute (NHLBI) study, "Dietary Approaches to Stop Hypertension" — DASH, for short — offer strong evidence that the diet that protects your heart and reduces your risk of some forms of cancer may also help control blood pressure.

The DASH diet is rich in fruits and vegetables, plus low-fat dairy products. No surprise there. But the diet is lower in fat than the ordinary low-fat diet. The Institute of Medicine's DRI recommendation is to get no more than 35 percent of your total calories from fat. DASH says to aim for no more than 27 percent.

The difference seems to make a difference. Your blood pressure is measured in two numbers that look something like this: 130/80. The first number is your *systolic pressure,* the force exerted against artery walls when your heart beats and pushes blood out into your blood vessels. The second, lower number is the *diastolic pressure,* the force exerted between beats.

When male and female volunteers with high blood pressure followed the DASH diet during clinical trials at medical centers in Boston, Massachusetts; Durham, North Carolina; Baltimore, Maryland; and Baton Rouge, Louisiana, their systolic blood pressures dropped an average 11.4 points and their diastolic pressures an average 5.5 points. And unlike medication, the diet produced no unpleasant side effects — except, of course, for that occasional dream of chocolate ice cream with real whipped cream, pound cake. . . . Oh well, nothing's perfect.

Food and sex: What do these foods have in common?

Oysters, celery, onions, asparagus, mushrooms, truffles, chocolate, honey, caviar, bird's nest soup, and alcohol beverages. No, that's not a menu for the very, very picky. It's a partial list of foods long reputed to be *aphrodisiacs,* substances that rev up the libido and improve sexual performance. Take a second look and you'll see why each is on the list.

Two (celery, asparagus) are shaped something like a male sex organ. Three (oysters, mushrooms, and truffles) are said to arouse emotion because they resemble parts of the female anatomy. (Oysters are also high in zinc, the mineral that keeps the prostate gland healthy and ensures a steady production of the male hormone testosterone. An 85-gram [3-ounce] serving of Pacific oysters gives you 9 milligrams of zinc, about 82 percent of the 11 milligrams a day recommended for adult men.)

Caviar (fish eggs) and bird's nest soup are symbols of fertility. Onions — and *Spanish fly* (cantharides) — contain chemicals that produce a mild burning sensation when eliminated in urine; some people, masochists to be sure, may confuse this with arousal. Honey is the quintessential sweetener: The Bible's Song of Solomon compares it to the lips of the beloved. Alcohol beverages relax the inhibitions (but overindulgence reduces sexual performance, especially in men). As for chocolate, well, it's a veritable lover's cocktail, with stimulants (caffeine, theobromine), a marijuana-like compound called anandamide, and phenylethylamine, a chemical produced in the bodies of people in love.

So do these foods actually make you feel sexy? Yes and no. An aphrodisiac isn't a food that sends you in search of a lover as soon as you eat it. No, it's one that makes you feel so good that you can follow through on your natural instincts. Which is as fine a description as you're likely to get of oysters, celery, onions, asparagus, mushrooms, truffles, chocolate, honey, caviar, bird's nest soup, and wine.

Conquering the common cold

This section is not about chicken soup. That issue has been settled, and Dr. Mom was right. In the 1980s, Dr. Marvin Sackler of Mount Sinai Medical Center in Miami, Florida, published the first serious study showing that cold sufferers who got hot chicken soup felt better faster than those who got plain hot water, and dozens of studies since have said, man, he's right. Nobody really knows why it works, but who cares? It works.

So let's move on to other foods that make you feel better when you have the sniffles — for example, sweet foods. Scientists do know why sweeteners — white sugar, brown sugar, honey, molasses — soothe a sore throat. All sugars are *demulcents,* substances that coat and soothe the irritated mucous membranes. Lemons aren't sweet, and they have less vitamin C than orange juice, but their popularity in the form of *hot lemonade* (tea with lemon and sugar) and sour lemon drops is unmatched. Why? Because a lemon's sharp flavour cuts through to your taste buds and makes the sugary stuff more palatable. In addition, the sour taste makes saliva flow, and that also soothes your throat.

Hot stuff — such as peppers, horseradish (freshly grated is definitely the most potent), and onions — contain mustard oils that irritate the membranes lining your nose and mouth and even make your eyes water. As a result, it's easier to blow your nose or cough up mucus.

Finally, there's coffee, a real boon to snifflers. When you're sick, your body piles up *cytokines,* chemicals that carry messages among immune system cells that fight infection. When cytokines pile up in brain tissue, you get sleepy, which may explain why you're so drowsy when you have a cold. True, rest can help boost your immune system and fight off the cold, but once in a while you have to get up. Like to go to work.

The caffeine in even a single cup of regular coffee (or one cup of decaf if, like us, you don't ordinarily drink regular coffee) can make you more alert. Caffeine is also a mood elevator (see Chapter 24) and a *vasoconstrictor* (a chemical that helps shrink swollen, throbbing blood vessels in your head). That's why it may help relieve a headache. But nothing's perfect: Drinking coffee may intensify the side effects of OTC (over-the-counter) cold remedies containing decongestants and/or caffeine that make some people feel jittery.

Check the label warnings and directions before using coffee with your cold medicine. Vasoconstrictors reduce the diameter of certain blood vessels and may restrict proper circulation. Couldn't hurt to check with your doctor, too, if you're taking meds for a chronic condition such as high blood pressure.

Eating for a Better Body (And Brain)

Citrus fruits are rich in vitamin C, an antioxidant vitamin that seems to slow the development of cataracts. Bran cereals provide fibre that can rev up your intestinal tract, countering the natural tendency of the contractions that move food through your gut to slow a bit as you grow older (which is why older people are more likely to be constipated). Getting enough calories to maintain a healthy weight helps protect against wrinkles. And although a diet with adequate amounts of fat doesn't totally prevent dry skin, it does give you a measure of protection. That's one reason virtually all sensible diet gurus, and *Eating Well with Canada's Food Guide,* recommend some fat or oil every day.

And now for a word about memory. Actually, two words: varied diet. A study of 250 healthy adults, ages 60 to 94, at the University of New Mexico School of Medicine, in 1983, showed that the people who ate a wide range of nutritious foods performed best on memory and thinking tests. According to researcher Philip J. Garry, Ph.D., professor of pathology at the New Mexico School of Medicine, overall good food habits seemed to be more important than any one food or vitamin. Maybe people with good memory are just more likely to remember that they need a good diet.

Or maybe it's really the food. In 1997, another survey, this time at Complutense University (Madrid, Spain), showed that men and women ages 60 to 90 who eat foods rich in vitamin E, vitamin C, folic acid, dietary fibre, and complex carbohydrates do better on cognitive tests. Is it the antioxidant vitamins? Does a low-fat diet protect the brain? No one knows for sure right now, but it may turn out that sticking with this same-old, same-old, low-saturated and trans fat, high-fibre diet as you grow older may help you remember to stick to the same-old low-saturated and trans fat, high-fibre diet — for years and years and years.

Delivering Meds with Dinner

If an adventurous band of plant biologists have their way, the world's children — and their needle-phobic parents — will someday get their vaccine inoculations with dinner rather than from a sharp stick in the arm.

Vaccines protect by introducing a substance called an antigen into your body. The *antigen* — a live or killed microbe particle — provokes an immune response in which you make antibodies to fight the antigen. This reaction inoculates you by teaching your body how to fight a specific infectious agent, such as the flu virus. If you're exposed later on, you're ready to beat the bug.

Most modern vaccines are injected. Some, like the polio vaccine, may be delivered on a sugar cube. Others can be inhaled. But for 15 years, Charles Arntzen, founder of Arizona State University's Biodesign Institute at Arizona State University, and his fellows across the country have been working toward creating "edible vaccines" — vaccines created via genetic engineering, by inserting the antigen, a viral gene, into food.

Not just any food, mind you. Heat destroys vaccines, so to get the benefits, you'd have to eat the food raw. To date, researchers have concentrated on potatoes, tomatoes, and bananas, with the emphasis on the latter two because — let's face it — raw potatoes are no treat.

The primary target for the vaccines is diarrheal diseases such as cholera and E. coli, which kill more than 2.5 million children under the age of 5 every year. Other possibilities include the Norwalk virus that's played havoc with cruise liner vacations, hepatitis B, and HIV, the virus that causes AIDS.

In trials with cows, mice, rabbits, and mink, antigen-containing tobacco leaves, alfalfa, tomatoes, and lettuce leaves have been able to trigger immune reactions to diseases as varied as anthrax and the common cold. In a handful of FDA-approved human studies at the National Vaccine Testing Center, the University of Maryland, and Roswell Park Cancer Centre in Buffalo, New York, human volunteers who ate about 100 grams (3.5 ounces) of raw potatoes containing anti-diarrheal or hepatitis vaccines showed an immune response similar to what you might expect from an injected vaccine.

Most researchers expect edible vaccines for animals to show up before edible vaccines for human beings. When the human versions do arrive, the plant scientists say they'll be cheap, administered without a needle and without a doctor.

Just don't expect to toss some seeds in the window box and grow your own. For one thing, fresh food has a relatively short shelf life. You can't stick your vaccine-laden banana in the fridge and use it sometime in the next six months. Second, unless the food is grown in controlled conditions, you can't be sure it has the correct amount of protective antigen. Finally, nobody wants these genetically modified foods to somehow slip into the general food supply.

In the end, the plant guys say, the banana, tomato, potato, or other vaccine-toting food will probably be sliced and diced, frozen, or ground to powder and pressed into chips, or tucked into a pill to make a stable med that can be produced with basic agricultural and food-processing technologies available virtually anywhere around the globe.

No needles, no doctors, no fuss. Now that's a med any mother could love.

The Last Word on Food versus Medicine

Sometimes, a person with a life-threatening illness is frightened by the side effects or the lack of certainty in standard medical treatment. In desperation, he or she may turn down medicine and turn to diet therapy. Alas, doing this may be hazardous to his or her already-compromised health.

No reputable doctor denies the benefits of a healthful diet for any patient at any stage of any illness. Food not only sustains the body but also can lift the spirit. But although food and diet may enhance the effects of many common drugs, no one has found them to be an adequate, effective substitute for (among other medicines)

- Antibiotics and other drugs used to fight infections
- Vaccines or immunizations used to prevent communicable diseases
- Anticancer drugs

If your doctor suggests altering your diet to make your treatment more effective, your brain will tell you, *Hey, that makes sense.* But if someone suggests chucking your doctor and tossing away your medicine in favour of food therapy alone, heed the natural warning in your head. You know there's no free lunch and — as yet — no truly magical food, either.

Part VI
The Part of Tens

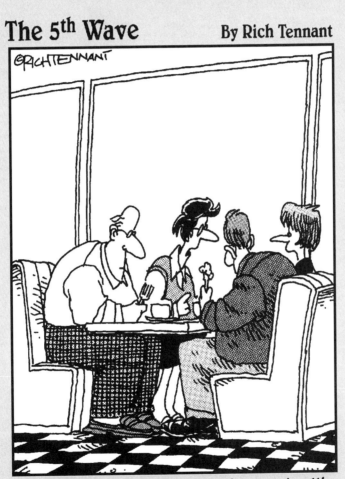

"Gordon's always had trouble controlling his appetite at restaurants. I had to explain to him that you're not supposed to pull your chair up to the salad bar."

In this part . . .

If you've ever read a *For Dummies* book, you know what to expect here — nifty lists of useful factoids that make great conversation starters and help you wind your way through the subject at hand.

In this book, that means ten great Web sites, ten (well, twelve) superstar foods, and ten easy ways to cut the calories without eliminating tasty food. What a bargain!

Chapter 27

Ten Nutrition Web Sites

In This Chapter

▶ Surfing the Web for accurate information about the food you eat

▶ Checking out the online home for Canada's dieticians

▶ Finding links between diet and disease

*T*he ten nutrition-oriented sites listed in this chapter give you reliable, accurate, balanced information: nutritional guidelines, medical news, interactive sites, directories, and more. And these sites are only a start. If Wiley Publishing had called this part of the book The Part of Hundreds rather than The Part of Tens, there would be many more super sources, but alas, there isn't room for them here.

Nevertheless, here's a sampling: the Canadian Nutrient File, the Canadian Diabetes Association, the Food Allergy and Anaphylaxis Network . . . well, you get the picture.

Click!

Canadian Nutrient File

```
www.hc-sc.gc.ca/fn-an/nutrition/fiche-nutri-data/index_
e.html
```

They say that necessity is the mother of invention, and this is certainly true for the Canadian Nutrient File (CNF). The CNF, a database of more than 5,000 foods, was created to fill in the gaps in Canada's Food Guide. It helps dietitians and other nutrition professionals assess and analyze what people eat. Unlike Canada's Food Guide, which simply categorizes food into one of four groups, the CNF offers information about foods that include multiple food categories. Assessing a piece of lasagna in terms of food groups isn't straightforward — meat lasagna has all four! The CNF reports nutrients found in commonly consumed foods, such as lasagna, in a variety of reasonable portion sizes, including the Food Guide serving, when possible.

To find a food item in the CNF, simply enter keywords related to the food you're looking for into the search engine. Keywords like "strawberry" and "milk" will return, for example, strawberry milkshake or milk mixed with strawberry-flavoured powder. Keep in mind that the search will return only food names that contain all the keywords you enter. Use the words "and" and "or" to refine your search. You can also use "not" to exclude a certain food from the search (for example, "beef not beef sauce").

The database also has nutritional analysis on various recipes, because recipes and therefore proportions of ingredients can vary for the same dish. The lasagna you make probably isn't the same as the one your grandmother makes, for example. For each recipe, the database gives the nutrient breakdown based on an estimate of the proportions and the ingredients used. Where possible, the proportions are provided.

Is your diet low in calcium? Do you need to boost your iron? You can also search for foods based on the nutrient content, to find the best sources for that nutrient.

The CNF site is great, but the variety of foods and recipes it offers is limited, although it is constantly being updated. For this reason you might want to check out the U.S. Department of Agriculture Nutrient Database (see the next section). Some may argue that food from the U.S. is not the same as the food here in Canada, and that would be a valid point — but remember, much of the food we eat, both fresh and packaged, is imported from the U.S. These sites are designed to give people best estimates of the nutrient profile of different foods. Don't worry about the accuracy of the nutrient values down to the decimal point.

U.S. Department of Agriculture Nutrient Database

`www.nal.usda.gov/fnic/foodcomp/search`

The USDA Nutrient Database is the U.S. equivalent to the Canadian Nutrient File (refer to the previous section). It contains nutrient data for more than 5,000 foods in several serving sizes and different preparations. Each entry is a snapshot of a specific food serving (for example, a raw apple with skin) that lists the amount of

✔ Water (by weight)

✔ Food energy (calories)

✔ Protein

✔ Fat

✔ Carbohydrates

✔ Dietary fibre

✔ Minerals: Calcium, iron, magnesium, phosphorus, potassium, sodium, and more

✔ Vitamins: Vitamin C, thiamin (vitamin B1), riboflavin (vitamin B2), niacin, vitamin B6, folate, vitamin B12, vitamin A, and more

✔ Lipids: Saturated, monounsaturated, and polyunsaturated fat, as well as cholesterol

✔ Amino acids

✔ Other substances, such as caffeine, alcohol, and beta carotene

When you visit this site, the first page that comes up is headlined "Search the USDA National Nutrient Database for Standard Reference." To find the food you're looking for, type its name — "apple," for example — into the empty box labelled "Keyword(s)." To refine the search, you can choose from another box labelled "Select Food Group." This list offers options such as "Fast Foods" and "Breakfast Cereals." If you're searching for information about a plain ol' apple, choosing "Fruits and Fruit Juices" would be the most appropriate selection. After you've made your selections, click Submit. Scroll down to something basic, such as "Apples, raw, with skin." Click on the circle next to that entry, then click Submit, and a new screen lists various forms of raw apple, such as "100 grams" or "1 cup, quartered or chopped" or "1 large (3¼" dia) (approx 2 per lb)." Choose the box in front of the serving you prefer, click the button marked Submit, and — bingo! There you are — calories and nutrients for one large apple. Neat!

To access a list of foods showing the content of a single nutrient such as protein or calories or vitamin C or calcium or beta-carotene, click the button marked Nutrient Lists on the main page. Then follow directions to get the list you want, with the foods arranged either in alphabetical order or by the amount of the nutrient in the food. The lists are displayed as PDF (portable document format) files; to read these files, you need Adobe Acrobat Reader, a program available free at `www.adobe.com/products/acrobat/reader main.html`.

Dietitians of Canada

www.dietitians.ca

Dietitians of Canada (DC) is the national professional organization for the more than 5,000 dietitians working in Canada. Their resource-rich site is for both professionals and the general public. Of particular interest are the following:

✔ "Healthy Bits and Bites," a continually updated list of three facts on nutrition or what's making news in the media, as well as a tip of the day. Follow the "Eat Well, Live Well" link on the home page to find this feature.

✔ "Let's make a meal," where you can build a one-day sample meal plan, then use the "Food Guide Calculator" to see how your meal plan compares to the Food Guide.

✔ "The Virtual Grocery Store," which helps you understand and use the Nutrition Facts table on packaged foods, so you can compare products to make healthier choices.

✔ "eatracker.ca," which allows you to enter the food you eat to determine if you're meeting your nutritional goals.

✔ "Find a dietitian," which is self-explanatory — just click on the magnifying glass on the home page.

Health Canada

www.hc-sc.gc.ca

The Web site for Health Canada, Canada's federal health department, is a great first stop to learn more about both basic nutrition and government policy around food and nutrition. On the Food and Nutrition page (which is accessible from the main page) you can explore a variety of topics:

✔ Advisories, warnings, and recalls: Here you can read about any warnings on food handling such as food-borne illness and how to prevent it, or an update on mercury in canned tuna, egg safety, or how to prepare fiddleheads and more!

✔ Nutrition and healthy eating: Issues discussed here include prenatal nutrition, healthy weights, nutrition policy reports, and more.

✔ Eating Well with Canada's Food Guide: Here you'll learn everything you need to kmow about Health Canada's latest version of the Food Guide. What's brand new is "Create my Food Guide," an interactive tool that allows you to get a suggested number of servings from the four food groups based on your own specifications such as age, sex, and activity level.

✔ Genetically Modified (GM) Foods and other Novel Foods: You can find out what GM foods have been approved in Canada. As well, there are fact sheets and an extensive list of questions on this controversial topic.

Heart and Stroke Foundation of Canada

ww2.heartandstroke.ca

This site tells you everything you ever wanted to know about diet and heart disease. On the home page, run your mouse down the left side to Healthy Living. Click on it and you'll find links to topics such as the following:

✔ Healthy eating: Here you'll find basic education on healthy eating, cooking, and topics such as fibre, salt, snacking, and vegetarian diets.

✔ Physical activity: This section gives you an overview of fitness basics, outlines the fitness needs of children, adults, and seniors, and includes tips on how to get started.

✔ Healthy weights: This section covers BMI, body shape, how waist circumference influences health, and how to achieve and maintain a healthy weight.

✔ Recipes: Need I say more? Appetizers, breakfasts, main courses — there's something for everyone.

✔ Heart and Stroke Position Statements: Read about the organization's stance on topics that affect heart health, such as trans fats, obesity, low-carb diets, and nutrition in schools.

The indisputable link between diet and heart disease risk, not to mention the Heart and Stroke Foundation site's user-friendly approach, makes this a must-stop on your nutritional tour of the Web.

The Canadian Cancer Society

www.cancer.ca

The Canadian Cancer Society Web site is dedicated to information about cancer: definitions, treatments, research, and support services. True, most of the nutrition news you find here is available elsewhere, but this site's defined focus provides easy access to other cancer-related topics.

Choose your province, then click on the word "Prevention" near the top of the screen. On the Prevention page, choose "Eat Well" from the topics list at the left side of the page. Choose from a menu of links to such topics as vegetables and fruit, high-fibre foods, healthy fats, and more.

Until now, the Canadian Cancer Society was barely a blip on the screen of nutrition sources. Today, a growing number of well-designed studies demonstrate that some foods and diet regimens may reduce your risk of certain types of cancer, while other foods put you in harm's way. The Canadian Cancer Society's Web site offers solid reporting on this area of nutritional research.

The Food Allergy and Anaphylaxis Network

www.foodallergy.org

The Food Allergy and Anaphylaxis Network (FAAN) is a nonprofit organization (membership fee: $30/year for individuals) whose participants include families, doctors, dietitians, nurses, support groups, and food manufacturers in the U.S., Canada, and Europe. The group provides education about food allergies, as well as support and coping strategies for people who are allergic to specific foods.

From FAAN's home page, you can link to updates, daily tips, newsletter excerpts, and all the usual service-oriented goodies. The site's best feature — an e-mail alert system — is free. Click the link under Special Allergy Alerts, fill out the form, and submit it to the site. You're now connected to an early warning system with allergy-linked news and information about recalls of troublesome products, such as small bags of cashews that may mistakenly contain peanuts.

This no-nonsense, easy-to-use site is required reading for people with food allergies. Families and friends can also benefit from its solid information and support services.

International Food Information Council (IFIC)

ific.org

The International Food Information Council (IFIC), created in 1985, is a nonprofit organization dedicated to improving the relationship between the nutrition community — scientists, food manufacturers, health professionals, government officials — and the news media. Although the council's membership includes corporations that make and sell food products, IFIC plays no role in marketing products or promoting its members. Its aim is to make sure that consumers get accurate information about diet and health.

The IFIC Web site allows you to access features in English and Spanish. You can bypass the professional stuff and head for links under "Nutrition and Food Safety Information," or click on "Food Insight Newsletter" or the terrific "Glossary of Food-Related Terms."

The site also offers articles on basic nutrition topics, such as functional foods, oral health, dietary fats and fat replacers, and additional resources. The writing is accessible, the information impeccable.

IFIC is a trade group, so purists may complain about some IFIC positions — for example, its endorsement of some food additives — but the site's intelligent approach to complex and emotional issues allows you to make up your own mind.

The Specialty Food Shop

`www.sickkids.on.ca/specialtyfoodshop/`

Located in the Hospital for Sick Children in downtown Toronto, The Specialty Food Shop is a retail outlet with an impressive inventory of various food products. It's also a resource centre for people with special nutritional and dietary needs. The Web site has valuable information on a variety of different conditions and diseases such as celiac disease, food allergies, and inborn metabolic disorders. Peruse their online catalogue (with 500 available items); you'll find gluten- and wheat-free, sodium-free, low-protein, and infant formula products. The Specialty Food Shop ships to anywhere in Canada.

Canadian Diabetes Association

`www.diabetes.ca`

The Canadian Diabetes Association site offers a wealth of information for people looking to understand diabetes. Click on the "About Diabetes" tab on the home page; it's your link to a range of subjects including medication, peer support, and nutrition — which is considered the cornerstone of diabetes management. The "Nutrition" link takes you to information on meal planning, carbohydrate counting, the "Top ten tips for tasty and healthy meals," sweeteners, the glycemic index, and much, much more.

Chapter 28

Twelve Superstar Foods

*E*ver since Eve pulled that apple (really a pomegranate) off the tree of knowledge in the Garden of Eden, people have been attributing special powers to one food or another.

This chapter is by no means the complete A+ list. For example, we haven't included chicken soup, because what more can anyone say about this universal panacea? Ditto for garlic and onions, both now honoured as probably heart healthy. Winnowing down the list was hard, but somebody had to do it! So here are our nominations for the Top Ten (actually, the Top Twelve, but who's counting?), plus a bonus list of baddies assembled by *Men's Health* magazine.

Eating Your Greens

No doubt you have memories of Popeye the sailor man squeezing open a can of spinach and gulping the contents down to gain superhuman strength. It may not make you a superhero, but spinach (and other green vegetables like it) is a remarkable food, packed with important nutrients. The nutrient most commonly associated with spinach is iron, but the iron in spinach isn't absorbed that well. However, spinach and other dark green leafy vegetables (such as kale, turnip greens, Swiss chard, collard greens, dandelion greens, green peas, and broccoli) contain another important nutrient: lutein.

Lutein is a *carotenoid*, and carotenoids are pigments responsible for giving plants their colour. In this case, lutein gives a distinctive yellow colour to plants. You're probably thinking: Why are these veggies green? Well, each also contains so much chlorophyll, which is green, that the yellow is masked.

Lutein is exciting on two fronts. First, higher consumption of lutein-rich foods is associated with lower rates of macular degeneration, which is the leading cause of vision loss and blindness in people older than 65. The *macula* is a small, sensitive part of the eye that's responsible for detailed central vision. Lutein acts as a powerful antioxidant and protects the macula from damage by sunlight. Because the macula has such a concentration of lutein, it's yellow. The body purposefully concentrates lutein into the macula because of its protective properties. The more lutein you get, the better protected your macula.

Second, lutein is a rising star when it comes to skin health. According to recent research, lutein is concentrated in the skin, more so than other carotenoids (like beta carotene). As it does in the macula, lutein acts as a powerful antioxidant; it seems to offer protection against the damaging effects of ultraviolet radiation. Lutein offers sun protection from the inside.

Enjoy your leafy greens, but don't stop being sun smart: Use sunscreen to prevent burns.

Finally, lutein will probably prove to be important for cardiovascular health. Research suggests that lutein has an important role in preventing plaque build-up in arteries, which can lead to heart disease. Keep your eye out for news on this topic in the next few years.

Loving Your Legumes

Modern science says that legumes such as chickpeas, kidney beans, fava beans, black beans, and lentils, for example, lower cholesterol levels with *gums* and *pectin,* soluble dietary fibres that mop up fats and prevent their being absorbed by your body. Oats, which also are rich in gums, particularly a gum called *beta glucan,* produce the same effect.

Legumes are also valuable for people with diabetes. Because legumes are digested very slowly, eating them produces only a gradual increase in the level of sugar circulating in your blood. As a result, metabolizing legumes requires less insulin than eating other types of high-carb foods such as potatoes. In one well-known study at the University of Kentucky, a diet rich in legumes made it possible for people with type 1 diabetes (their bodies produce virtually no insulin) to reduce their daily insulin intake by nearly 40 percent. Patients with type 2 diabetes (their bodies produce some insulin) were able to reduce their insulin intake by 98 percent.

Just about the only drawback to a diet rich in legumes is gas resulting from the natural human inability to digest some dietary fibre and complex sugars such as *raffinose* and *stachyose,* which sit in your gut as fodder for the resident friendly bacteria that digest the carbs and then release carbon dioxide and (ugh) methane, a smelly gas.

One way to reduce intestinal gas production is to reduce the complex sugar content of the legumes before you eat them. Here's how: Bring a pot of water to a boil. Turn off the heat. Add the legumes. Let them soak for several hours. The sugars leach out into the water, which means you can discard the sugars by draining the legumes and adding fresh water to cook in. If that doesn't do the job, try two heat-and-soak sessions before cooking. Canned legumes have the soaking part already done for you: All you have to do is drain the legumes and rinse them well under running water to remove most of the problematic gas-producing properties.

Picking Berries

Blueberries, raspberries, strawberries, blackberries, acai berries, goji berries, boysenberries, cranberries — the list goes on. Berries are hot right now. They're getting a lot of press because they're a source of powerful, health-promoting antioxidants called *anthocyanidins*. Researchers are discovering that the various pigments that give berries their distinctive colours of red, blue, and purple help prevent damage from *free radicals* (molecules that can wreak havoc on the cells and tissues of our bodies). These pigments help shore up the body's natural defenses. Berries are also a great source of vitamin C for the most part, and all are low in calories. A cup of strawberries has about 55 calories, and blueberries about 85.

Including berries into your everyday fare is easy. They go well with cereal, yogourt, in smoothies, topped on sherbet, or on their own as a light dessert or snack. Buy fresh when they're in season (they're cheap and plentiful). When they're not, buy frozen. It's equally healthy and the berries will keep as long as you need them: Just thaw and use!

Powering Up: Hemp

Hemp comes from the same plant species as marijuana (*Cannabis sativa l.*, a diverse plant with more than 500 varieties), but from a special variety that contains virtually no THC (tetrahydrocannabinol), the chemical responsible for marijuana's psychoactive properties. Hemp is truly a versatile product. In addition to being a food, it's used for nutraceuticals, body care products, and high-performance fibre products. As a food, hemp is available as whole and hulled seeds (often called hemp nut), hemp butter (ground hemp seeds), hemp oil, and hemp protein. Hemp food products include salad dressings, nutrition bars, bread, cookies, granola, nut butter, corn chips, pasta, ice cream, and cold-pressed oil supplements. The main nutritional advantage of hemp is the composition of its fat and protein.

Unlike other seeds such as sunflower or safflower, it contains both linolenic acid (LA), which is an omega-6 fat, and alpha-linolenic acid (ALA), which is from the omega-3 family (refer to Chapter 7 to read about fatty acids). People tend to over-consume omega-6 fats at the expense of omega-3 because sunflower and safflower oils are used widely in the food supply and because livestock is fed a lot of corn, which is another source of omega-6 fats. Hemp offers a better balance of both these essential fats.

Hemp is also a protein powerhouse. Most plant sources of protein are considered incomplete because, unlike animal proteins, they don't contain all the essential amino acids (those required for health; refer to Chapter 6 for more about protein). Hemp, however, contains all the essential amino acids in sufficient amounts to contribute to the body's protein requirement. Although hemp protein does have more fat than many other protein powders on the market, the majority of its fat is hearty-healthy essential fat, which you don't need to avoid.

Admittedly, hemp protein is an acquired taste. On its own it's very bitter, but try it in a smoothie with fresh fruit, yogourt, and a sweetener such as honey. You can also get your hemp protein in food products (such as hemp beverages, and energy bars), powders to add to smoothies, or naturally flavoured meal replacements (flavoured powders that are fortified with vitamins and minerals that are made into shakes with water or other beverages such as fruit juice).

Weighing in with Whey Protein

Little Miss Muffet, sat on her tuffet, eating her curds and whey, along came a spider . . . and, well, you know the rest. This nursery rhyme first appeared in print in 1805, so whey is really not new. Whey, or milk plasma, is the liquid that remains after milk has been curdled and strained in the cheese-making process. The whey is then dried and made into a powder. Whey is approximately 90 percent protein, with the remainder being a little carbohydrate and some fat. Whey is used to make ricotta and gjetost cheeses and is an additive in many processed foods, including bread, crackers, cereals, infant formula, and even animal feed.

More and more research is revealing just how nutritious this food product really is. What makes whey so nutritious? For one, whey has all the essential amino acids and is particularly rich in a group of amino acids referred to as *branched chain amino acids* (BCAAs): leucine, isoleucine, and valine. These amino acids collectively make up about one-third of muscle protein and are important in exercise because they're used by working muscles as fuel along with carbohydrate and fat. BCAAs are also used in the repair of muscle after exercise. (For more about amino acids, refer to Chapter 6.)

Whey has been shown to have a positive effect on muscle protein synthesis in those who have experienced muscle wasting, be it age related or part of a disease process such as cancer or HIV.

Whey protein is relatively inexpensive and very easy to use. It can be added to oatmeal or yogourt but is most popular as an ingredient in smoothies. For people looking to boost their protein intake or who have trouble meeting their protein requirements, adding whey is an easy way (pardon the pun) to get more protein.

Some medical conditions such as liver or kidney disease require a protein restriction. If you are under a doctor's care for any medical issue, be sure to check before adding protein or any natural health products to your diet.

Eating Your Seeds

Salba is actually a new twist on an old favourite. It's a variety of an ancient plant species belonging to the mint family, called Chia (yes, as in the Chia Pet). Chia was revered by the Aztecs, who used it as a staple in their diets. The Chia plant produces two different coloured seeds: black and white. Salba is the product of the white seeds, which are responsible for the nutritional profile of this newly discovered food. Move over flax, there's a new player in town.

So what makes salba the next big thing? Salba is a great source of omega-3 fat (alpha-linolenic acid), protein, potassium, magnesium, calcium, folate, niacin, copper, fibre, and antioxidants. A 15-millilitre (2-tablespoon) serving of salba has a whopping 127 milligrams of magnesium, 256 milligrams of calcium, 220 milligrams of potassium, and more omega-3 fat than an equal amount of ground flax seed. As well, unlike flax, salba has a better balance of omega-3 to omega-6 fats, making it a great source of essential fatty acids.

What's also remarkable about this ancient seed is that it can absorb much more water than flax. In this case, water retention is a good thing. By absorbing many times their weight in water, whole and ground salba seeds form a thick gel or bulking agent. This property makes salba a great additive to foods such as oatmeal, yogourt, applesauce, and smoothies. Foods that have added salba are digested more slowly, which helps keep you feeling full longer. Slow digestion can prevent swings in hunger, and may help reduce your total food intake by moderating your appetite. All this and a handful of vitamins and minerals. Why wouldn't you eat it?

Brewing Up: Coffee

For years, there was nothing but bad news about coffee. Pancreatic cancer. Cystic breasts. High cholesterol. High blood pressure. Heart disease. Stroke. Birth defects. Heartburn. Reflux. But the worm — okay, the coffee bean — has turned: Later studies show no link at all between drinking coffee and an increased risk of any of these conditions. Moderate intake, defined as three to four small cups per day, doesn't seem to cause any significant adverse health effects long term for the vast majority of people. True, coffee may upset your stomach and keep you up at night, but as *Heartburn & Reflux For Dummies* (published by Wiley) explains, for most people, these effects are almost always linked to intakes above the recommended amounts.

Coffee is also an excellent source of antioxidants. A new analysis of the Nurses Health Study II looked at the relationship between coffee intake and development of type 2 diabetes. Turns out that the rates of new cases of diabetes decreased as coffee consumption increased. The relationship held, regardless of the form of coffee — filtered, instant, caffeinated, or decaffeinated — and wasn't related to total caffeine intake. Coffee is a mixture of lots of different compounds, and it contains something — perhaps its antioxidants — that appears to protect against developing type 2 diabetes.

In the end, the simple fact is that taken in moderation, regular coffee definitely qualifies for anybody's list of super foods. Its most active ingredient, caffeine, elevates your mood and increases your ability to concentrate; may improve your athletic performance; can help shrink the swollen, throbbing blood vessels that make your head ache; and boosts the effects of painkillers, which is why caffeine is often included in over-the-counter analgesic (pain-relieving) products. Which is also why, time after time, the java really does the job.

Goin' Fishing

Did your great-grandmother call fish "brain food"? If so, it was because fish is rich in iodine, the mineral that allows your thyroid gland to churn out thyroid hormones vital to your ability to think and move. Once upon a time, back in great-granny's day, people living far from the ocean (our best natural source of iodine) were often sluggish, sometimes even mentally retarded, because they were lacking iodine.

But this condition became rare in Canada after the introduction of iodized salt in the 1920s. Fish's modern reputation for medical magic comes from its ability to reduce the risk of heart disease and stroke, in large part, because of its omega-3 fatty acids. These unsaturated fats make blood less sticky, thus reducing the incidence of clots. They also knock down levels of bad cholesterol.

You want proof? Here's proof: In 2002, data from the long-running Harvard Health Professionals Study indicated that people who eat 3 to 5 ounces of fish just once a month have a 40 percent lower risk of *ischemic stroke,* a stroke caused by a blood clot in a cranial artery. The Harvard study did not include women. But a report on women and stroke published in the *Journal of the American Medical Association* in 2000 says women who eat about 115 grams (4 ounces) of fish — think one small can of tuna — two to four times a week appear to cut their risk of stroke by a similar 40 percent. And in 2005, the *American Journal of Preventive Medicine* published several reports from the Harvard Center for Risk Analysis project concluding that "any fish consumption confers substantial relative risk reduction compared to no fish consumption, with the possibility that additional consumption confers incremental benefits," including a "17% reduction in death from heart attack, with each additional serving per week associated with a further reduction in this risk of 3.9%."

Of course, there are catches to this catch. First, some fish are high in mercury, a metal that can damage a developing fetus, but small amounts of fish, say two 85 gram (3-ounce) servings a week, seem to be safe for everyone else. Second, frequent servings of fish may increase the risk of a stroke caused by bleeding in the brain. This situation is common among Native Alaskans who eat lots of fish and have a higher than normal incidence of hemorrhagic, or bleeding, strokes. However, the amount of fish eaten by the Alaskans is very high — it's their main source of protein, and their consumption is higher than what would be found in a moderate, varied diet. The Harvard study found no significant link between fish consumption and bleeding strokes, but the researchers say more studies are needed to nail down the relationship, or lack thereof.

While we're waiting, pass the chips. Saturated fat– and trans fat–free, of course.

Going Nuts

Pass up the pretzels. Skip the chips. At snack time, reach for the almonds (or cashews, walnuts, pumpkin seeds, pistachios, macadamia, and so on). Although nuts are technically a high-fat food, a series of studies including several at California's Loma Linda University say that adding moderate amounts of nuts to a cholesterol-lowering diet or substituting nuts for other high-fat foods such as meats may cut normal to moderately high levels of total cholesterol and LDLs ("bad cholesterol") as much as 12 percent.

These guys should know. A while back, they made headlines with a walnut study in which volunteers were given one of two diets, both based on National Cholesterol Education Program (NCEP) recommendations. People on Diet #1 got 20 percent of their calories from fats in oils and fatty foods such as meat. Folks on Diet #2 got 20 percent of their calories from high-fat nuts instead of meat, but both controlled-fat diets appeared to lower cholesterol levels.

The take-home message here is that although nuts are high in fat, their fats are polyunsaturated and monounsaturated cholesterol busters (more about them in Chapter 7). And let us not forget that nuts also provide other heart-healthy nutrients such as arginine (an amino acid your body uses to make a clot-blocking compound called nitric oxide), folate (a B vitamin that lowers blood levels of homocysteine, a risk factor for heart disease), vitamin E, magnesium, and dietary fibre.

So feel free to go (sensibly) nuts for nuts. Crunch.

Brewing Up: Tea

Black and green? So 20th century. The hot new colour in tea is white. The leaves for all three teas come from one plant, *Camellia sinensis.* But those leaves meant for black and green teas are rolled and fermented before drying, while those destined for white teas — which actually brew up pale yellow-red — aren't. Nutritionwise, this small change makes a big difference.

Flavonoids are natural chemicals credited with tea's ability to lower cholesterol, reduce the risk of some kinds of cancer, and protect your teeth from cavity-causing bacteria. Fresh tea leaves are rich in flavonoids called catechins, but processing the leaves to make black and green teas releases enzymes that enable individual catechins to hook up with others, forming new flavouring and colouring agents called polyphenols (poly = many) that give flavour and colour to black and green teas. Because white tea leaves are neither rolled nor fermented, fewer of their catechins marry into polyphenols. According to researchers at the Linus Pauling Institute (LPI) at Oregon State University, the plain catechin content of white tea is three times that of green tea. Black tea comes in a distant third.

Why should you care about this? Because all those catechins seem to be good for living bodies. For example, when LPI researchers tested white tea's ability to inhibit cell mutations in bacteria and slow down cell changes leading to colon cancer in rats, white tea beat green tea, the former health champ. And when scientists at University Hospitals of Cleveland and Case Western Reserve University applied creams containing white-tea extract to human skin (on volunteers) and exposed the volunteers to artificial sunlight, the creamed skin developed fewer precancerous changes. To be fair, green tea preparations were also protective, but white tea has less caffeine than either green or black tea, which makes it the perfect brew for a recovering caffeine fiend. Sip.

Getting Your Grains

If you're a man who plans to live forever, a team of nutrition scientists at Harvard/Brigham and Women's Hospital in Boston have three words for you: whole-grain cereal. When the investigators took a look at the health stats for a one-year period in the lives of the 86,190 male doctors in the long-running Physicians' Health Study, they found 3,114 deaths among the study volunteers, including 1,381 deaths from heart attack and stroke. Then they looked a little closer and discovered that eating habits count. Men who ate at least one serving of whole-grain cereal a day were 27 percent less likely to die than were men who ate refined grain products. The whole-grain group was also as much as 28 percent less likely to succumb to a heart attack, regardless of how much they weighed, whether they smoked or drank alcohol or took vitamins pills, or had a history of high blood pressure or high cholesterol.

Nobody yet knows exactly why this should be so. But they do know that whole grains are a treasure trove of dietary fibre, vitamins, minerals, and other phytochemicals (plant compounds such as antioxidants) that protect by lowering blood pressure and cholesterol while improving the body's ability to process nutrients, particularly carbohydrates.

The question is, how much cereal must you eat to benefit? The studies say more is better, but one serving a day is better than none at all. To find the right cereal, haul out your magnifying glass or bifocals to check the Nutrition Facts label. If whole grain is the first ingredient and there's at least 2 grams of dietary fibre per serving, you've found breakfast. For those who absolutely, positively hate cereal, try whole-grain bread. And, yes, whole grains are an equal opportunity dish. Earlier studies suggest that women, too, may come out ahead by adding whole grain to their daily diets.

Eating Yogourt

Yogourt and kefir are milk with added friendly bacteria that digest milk sugar (lactose) to produce lactic acid, a natural preservative that gives the flavour of yogourt and kefir its pleasant bite. Yogourt and kefir are definitely magical for people who are *lactase deficient* (meaning they don't produce enough lactase to digest milk sugar, so they get gassy whenever they drink milk). Fermented dairy foods are a source of easily digested dairy nutrition: high quality protein, calcium, magnesium, and B vitamins.

Tracking the terrible ten

In 2003, while others whistled a happy tune about good foods, the worrywarts at *Men's Health* magazine compiled a list of the ten foods most likely to make you feel absolutely awful — mostly because of their tendency to harbour organisms that can seriously upset your intestinal tract. The top troublemakers are undercooked chicken, ground beef, ground turkey, oysters, and eggs, followed by unheated cold cuts, raw scallions, peaches, cantaloupe, and packaged salad greens. Luckily, thorough cooking (or reheating) can make the first seven safe to eat. As for peaches, the guys say, peel 'em to eliminate pesticides stuck in the fuzz. Scrub your bumpy cantaloupe before slicing to dislodge bacteria in the rind that may otherwise be transferred to the fruit. And rinse your packaged salad greens. Then rinse again. Even if the packaged says "washed." Splash.

But there's no evidence to show that these foods are a longevity tonic, a claim traced back to Ilya Ilyich Metchnikoff, a Russian Nobel Prize winner (1908; Physiology/Medicine) who believed that people die prematurely entirely because of the action of "putrefying bacteria" in the intestines. Searching for a way to disarm the putrefiers, Metchnikoff ended up in Bulgaria, a place where many people lived past 50 and a significant percentage made it into their late 80s.

Historians may argue that the only way to live that long in Bulgaria was to avoid Bulgarian politics, but Metchnikoff gave the credit to the organisms used to make Bulgarian cultured milk. He was wrong. The bugs, christened *L. bulgaricus,* make nice yogourt but don't take up residence in the human gut. This hardly mattered to Metchnikoff, who died in Paris in 1916, at the relatively young age of 71. His faith in yogourt, however, continues to cycle in and out of fashion.

Chapter 29

Ten Easy Ways to Cut Calories

....

In This Chapter

▶ Knowing the value of low-fat foods

▶ Cutting down, not cutting out

▶ Making substitutions that work

▶ Appreciating the real impact of proper portions

....

*L*osing weight isn't simple math. Because 0.5 kg (1 pound) of fat has an energy value of 3,500 calories, if you cut out 3,500 calories through increased activity and reduce the amount of calories you eat, you will lose 0.5 kg (1 pound) of fat — so goes the theory. But, as you cut calories with diet and activity, your body adapts and starts to use calories more efficiently, so this mathematical equation isn't entirely accurate. The rate of your weight loss will taper, which is often why people get frustrated when trying to lose weight. But here's the bottom line: By cutting calories and increasing activity, you will lose body fat over the long run. Keep your eye on that longer goal rather than obsessing over counting calories.

Yes, we know reading that last paragraph is easier than actually doing it, so we're ready to give you two tricks to make the job easier. First, cut your calories in small increments — 50 here, 100 there — rather than in one big lump. Second, instead of giving up foods you really love (and feeling deprived), switch to lower-fat versions of products where you really won't notice. This chapter tells you how to accomplish both.

Switching to Low-Fat Dairy Products

Milk and milk products are the best sources for the calcium that keeps bones strong. But these same products may also be high in cholesterol, saturated fat, and calories. You can reduce all three by choosing a lower-fat milk product.

Think twice before switching to fat-free altogether. This is because dairy foods are a source of a healthy fat called *conjugated linolenic acid* (CLA). It has been associated with lower rates of cancer and seems to help maintain a healthier ratio of muscle to body fat; in other words, CLA helps us achieve a better body composition. Unfortunately, in our effort to reduce saturated fat, we may have swung too far to the other side with the introduction of fat-free dairy products. You don't need to stick with full-fat dairy; there are still good amounts of CLA in 1 percent milk and yogourt, for example.

Here's how low-fat dairy can help reduce calories: A cup of whole milk has 150 calories, but a cup of 1 percent milk has only 100. If you have two 250-mL (8-ounce) glasses a day, you've saved 100 calories. One slice of regular processed cheese has 60 calories, but one slice of the low-fat version has only 30. A sandwich made with three slices of low-fat cheese is 90 calories lighter and still has all the minerals and protein in regular cheese slices.

Substituting Sugar Substitutes

Coffee has no calories, but every teaspoon of sugar you stir into your cup has 15 big ones. Multiply that by four (1 teaspoon each in four cups of coffee), and your naturally no-cal beverage can add 60 calories a day to your diet. Sixty calories a day times seven days a week, and yipes, that's 420 calories! That's about as much as you'd get from four or five medium slices of unbuttered toast or five medium apples. So is this a good time to mention that one packet of sugar substitute has absolutely zero calories? We thought so. The point is even more poignant with regular soft drinks. A 360-mL (12-ounce) can has on average about 136 calories and 33 grams (a little more than an ounce) of sugar, or the equivalent of 40 mL (8 teaspoons) worth.

Doing Away with Portion Distortion

One of the most confusing concepts around food is probably portions and serving sizes. In fact, we'd argue that it's probably one of the most important factors affecting weight gain. Gaining weight, at the end of the day, is still about getting more calories than the body needs. In the end, excess calories end up as extra body fat.

Serving sizes are getting larger. Bagels used to be about 56 g (2 ounces) twenty or so years ago and had about 150 calories; bagels today can be 113–140 grams (4–5 ounces) and clock in at around 330 calories. The story is pretty much the same for most prepackaged foods — and we haven't even mentioned meals at fast-food places.

Canada's Food Guide not only provides basic guidelines on the number of servings people should have, but it also provides examples of standardized serving sizes. The number of servings you'll need from each of the food groups will depend on factors such as age and activity level, but the Food Guide is still a good starting point. The key is to understand how a Food Guide serving compares to the portions that are provided by the food manufactures. Start with determining how many servings you need each day, and then, for the first few weeks, try measuring out and portioning most of your food, using the Food Guide to direct you. You'll probably be surprised as to how much you're actually eating. After a while you'll be able to eyeball portions and serve yourself appropriate amounts of food that are proportionate to your actual needs.

Cutting the Juice and Eating More Whole Fruit

Once upon a time, people used to drink juice in small glasses as part of breakfast. Growing up, we had juices glasses that were about 125 mL (half a cup) and typically had one of these with breakfast. This would provide, on average, about 50 or 60 calories. Juice is now sold in bottles that range from 384 mL (more than a cup and a half) to 500 mL (2 cups) and that contain 184 to 227 calories. You'd have to eat three pieces of medium-sized fruit to get the same calories, but because it would take time to chew and swallow the fruit, you'd be less likely to consume that many pieces in one sitting.

Fruit has fibre, which juice is missing. Fibre helps keep you full and is something that most people could get more of in their diets. We'd prefer it if people ate fruit instead of drinking juice — or at least limited their juice intake to about 125 mL (half a cup) per day, which is the suggested serving size in Canada's Food Guide for the average person who isn't very active. If you're active, then there is more room for juice and its concentrated calories. *Remember:* There's nothing magical or extra nutritious about fruit juice. If you eat fruit, then you don't need to drink juice.

Cooking with Little to No Added Fat

One of the easiest ways to cut or add calories is through the use of added fats and oils during cooking. A little goes a long way. If you're making a dish such as a stir-fry or need to sauté vegetables such as onions or garlic for a tomato sauce, then a little oil — 5 to 10 mL (1 to 2 teaspoons) — should be enough to prevent sticking. You can also prevent sticking by cooking on medium heat. Using a nonstick pan, try sautéing with 5 to 10mL (1 to 2 teaspoons) of oil and 15 to 30 mL (1 to 2 tablespoons) of water — the steam will help soften the vegetables. Bake with parchment paper instead of greasing the pan, and use muffin paper cups or vegetable spray instead of greasing the muffin tin. Every tablespoon of fat you don't use means approximately 100 fewer calories in the dish. Get your fat calories from nuts and seeds or from a healthy oil, such as virgin olive, when making a salad dressing.

Making One-Slice Sandwiches

Depending on the brand, one slice of bread in your daily luncheon sandwich may have anywhere from 65 to 120 calories. Eliminating one slice and serving your sandwich open-faced can cut up to 840 calories from your weekly total. The bread that's offered up by food manufacturers isn't the same as the standardized serving sizes in Canada's Food Guide. One slice of bread in the Food Guide is 35 grams, but many breads today contain 85 grams per slice, or the equivalent of two suggested serving sizes. And you know that making that one slice whole wheat adds dietary fibre to your menu, right? Just asking.

Using Low-Fat or Fat-Free Extras

A lot of fat-free and low-fat products aren't necessarily the best choice because when the fat is removed, other flavour enhancers are added, such as salt or sugar. This is especially true when it comes to fat-free and low-fat baked goods. Happily, lower-fat versions of sour cream, cream cheese, and mayonnaise are different. The fat is replaced with emulsifiers (ingredients that keep the product from separating) derived from plant fibres found in, for example, seaweed.

Avoiding Restaurant Pitfalls

If you've been to a restaurant lately, you've probably noticed that the portions are super sized. Most portions in restaurants are enough for two and sometimes three meals. Don't be fooled by what they put down in front of you. Stop when you're about halfway done (please don't feel like you have to clean your plate to get your money's worth). You can take the rest home for the next day's lunch or dinner.

Following the "Space on Your Plate" Model

Model your intake after the "Space on your plate" approach to portion control. The concept is simple: Fill

- Half your plate (about one and a half to two cups or two cupped handfuls) with low-starch vegetables (such as broccoli, cauliflower, asparagus, or bok choy)

- One quarter (113 grams, or 4 ounces, about the size of a computer mouse) with a lean protein (fish, pork, beef, or chicken will do)

- One quarter (about 250 mL, or one cup, or one cupped handful) with a starch (rice, pasta, potato, or barley)

These are estimates; how much food a person needs depends on age, sex, and activity level.

This approach helps keep calories in check because most of the plate is vegetables, which are bulky, lower in calories, and high in fibre, which helps keep you full and slows down the digestive process. Starch carbohydrates, although not inherently fattening, do pack a lot of concentrated calories. It's easy to overconsume them — who couldn't eat three cups of rice or pasta? That's about 665 to 725 calories right there. Because most of us don't get the recommended number of servings of vegetables and fruits every day, this model of eating will not only help keep calories in control but will help ensure you get enough good stuff.

Planning to Include Indulgences

You've heard the expression, "Extremes lead to extremes"? Many people who embark on the journey to eat healthfully or lose weight often go to the extreme of cutting out all junk food. They resort to eating lots of carrots or celery sticks, cutting out the very foods that make eating enjoyable. Eventually, these people snap, and go right back to their unhealthy habits.

No one food will make or break your health or weight-loss efforts; you need to focus on the big picture. As long as you make healthy choices, meet your nutritional requirements, and include some activity to help maintain a healthy weight, there's no reason to eliminate indulgences — and every reason to include them. Denying yourself can set you up for failure. Plan treats into your weekly healthy eating (how many you can afford to have depends on your personal situation and self-identified goals). You won't feel deprived and you'll be better able to control the amount you eat and the number of calories you consume.

Index

● *D* ●

Notes

Notes